The Supreme Court in the Federal Judicial System

THIRD EDITION

The Nelson-Hall Series in Political Science
Consulting Editor: Samuel C. Patterson
The Ohio State University

The Supreme Court in the Federal Judicial System

THIRD EDITION

Stephen L. Wasby

STATE UNIVERSITY OF NEW YORK AT ALBANY

NELSON-HALL PUBLISHERS/CHICAGO

Library of Congress Cataloging-in-Publication Data

Wasby, Stephen L., 1937-
  The Supreme Court in the federal judicial system.

  Includes index.
  1. United States.   Supreme Court.   2. Courts-United States.   I. Title.
KF8742.W38   1987   347,73'26   87-24712
ISBN 0-8304-1175-5 (pbk.)   347.30735

Manufactured in the United States of America

10   9   8   7   6   5   4   3   2

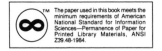

TM The paper used in this book meets the minimum requirements of American National Standard for Information Sciences—Permanence of Paper for Printed Library Materials, ANSI Z39.48-1984.

To the memory of my grandparents,
Frances and **Benjamin Bunshaft,**

and

Harold ("Hal") Chase,
> Constitutional law scholar, teacher,
> Marine, but more important: friend,
> and the one who made my first book possible.

The good people do is not interred with their bones,
> *but lives in the hearts*
>> *of those who cherish their memory.*

And

> for **Susan.**

Contents

Preface

THE UNITED STATES SUPREME Court receives much attention, adulation, and criticism. Yet the American public knows far less about it than about Congress or the president. Our national legislators and particularly the president, aided by media coverage, work at making themselves highly visible. The Court, however, has no public relations apparatus and remains generally secretive about its internal processes; its rulings are supposed to speak for themselves. Moreover, there has been little public education about the Court's functioning or its place in our government, a result of the "mystery of the law," lack of attention in the educational system and in the media, and lawyers' failure to inform the lay public.

In the last decade, the Supreme Court's work and the justices' activities have become more visible as a result of a journalistic exposé of strategic maneuvering in the Burger Court, a study of two famous justices' extrajudicial activities, and extended interviews with several justices. Further attention was produced by Chief Justice Burger's retirement, the elevation of Justice Rehnquist to the chief justiceship, and Justice Powell's retirement. Although the just-noted books and interviews add a significant dimension to our knowledge of the Supreme Court's workings, none provides the general reader with adequate information about the Court. This book is written in the hope of remedying such a deficiency in knowledge about the Supreme Court and of supplying a sufficient context in which to evaluate the Court's work. My intent is to provide not only understanding of what the Court has done thus far but also a basis for understanding its future actions. Justices, including chief justices, come and go, and the doctrine the Court announces may change, but the Court's basic method of deciding cases and the considerations that influence its decisions remain relatively stable.

Scholars who have devoted their attention to the Court provide much of the basis for what appears here. Their work is supplemented by data prepared specifically for this volume. I have also drawn on my own prior work while trying to avoid inflicting too much of it on the reader. As this book is basically a synthesis of others' studies, it reflects both emphases and gaps in the existing literature, and the reader should remember that it may take several years for detailed analyses of the Court's most recent terms to appear. This edition will appear after the new Chief Justice has served in that capacity for only slightly more than one term of Court, and when the "Rehnquist Court," about which we may be speaking for years, has only begun to develop. Basic information is presented through the end of the Court's 1985 Term (ending in July 1986), with salient information on personnel changes and the 1986 Term added where appropriate.

To understand the Supreme Court, one must know about its internal procedures, including how cases are accepted for review and how those cases are decided; the Court's role at the top of our nation's judiciary—how it fits into our dual court system of separate national and state courts; and its role in the overall political system. We must therefore look not only at the Supreme Court but also at the entire national court system, the relations between federal and state courts, the Court's relations with Congress and the executive branch, and the impact of the Court's decisions. An emphasis on the federal court system as a whole is imperative if we are to provide a full understanding of the Supreme Court, but we must also keep in mind that the federal courts are not fully representative of the nation's courts. For one thing, with the exception of judges on some specialized courts, federal judges are appointed to life terms, whereas most state judges are elected. For another, the number of cases in the federal courts is small enough—despite federal judges' complaints about caseload—to allow a more deliberate pace and greater emphasis on full-dress adversary proceedings than occurs in many high-volume state courts, particularly trial courts with their frenetic pace.

The primary emphasis throughout is on the Court's *operation* rather than on the doctrines the justices announce. However, in addition to the illustrative use of cases, particular attention is given to the Court's rulings on access to federal courts and on congressional and presidential actions. The book is divided into ten chapters. Chapter 1 presents a general discussion of the Court's role in the American governmental, legal, and political system, with some attention both to history and to contemporary political controversy concerning the Court. This is followed by discussion of the structure and administration of the federal court system (Chapter 2) and the selection of federal judges (Chapter 3). Chapter 4 deals with the role of lawyers and interest groups in pursuing litigation; Chapter 5, with rules for getting into courts and the relations between federal and state courts; and Chapter 6, with the Court's exercise of choice in determining what cases to decide. Chapters 7 and 8 provide an extended consideration of the way in which the Court handles cases accepted for review, judicial interaction in deciding cases, and major considerations that enter the writing of the Court's opinions. After an examination of the Court's review of congressional and executive branch actions in Chapter 9, the book concludes with a discussion in Chapter 10 of public opinion about the Court and of the communication of decisions to those affected and the impact of those rulings.

The structure of the book's second edition—based on a restructuring of the first edition to place discussion of basic institutional matters and judicial selection early in the volume—has been retained. The material of the second edition has been thoroughly updated, with newly available sources used where possible. No bibliography is included, but anyone wishing to read further can easily do so by following up items in the footnotes at the end of each chapter. A Table of Cases is provided where one can find citations to cases discussed or noted in the text.

Acknowledgments are many in a work of this sort, reflecting as it does study and exposure to others over a number of years. Over time, helpful and generous colleagues have provided many ideas and much information. All cannot be mentioned here, but I wish particularly to thank for their help with particular sections David Adamany, Wayne State University; George F. Cole, University of Connecticut; Jerry Goldman, Northwestern University; Maeva Marcus, Supreme Court of the United States; Karen O'Connor, Emory University; D. Marie Provine, Syracuse University; and Frank Way, University of California–Riverside. The fine editorial hand of sometime coauthor Joel Grossman, University of Wisconsin, Madison, is still evident from earlier endeavors on judicial selection. Special help was provided by Keith O. Boyum, California State University, Fullerton, and Elliot Slotnick, Ohio State University, who read the entire manuscript. I wish especially to express my gratitude to the late Harold Chase for his support and continuing interest in my work earlier in my career. It is to his memory that this book is in part dedicated.

Thanks also go to Denise Rathbun, formerly of Praeger Publishers, who first asked me to write this book; to Marie Schappert, my editor for the previous edition; and to Nelson-Hall, and particularly Stephen Ferrara, for his support during preparation of this edition. Suzanne Wickham, who effectively transformed my total lack of artistry into diagrams of the court system's structure, Addie Napolitano, who again did a superb job of manuscript preparation, and Mark Daly, who helped with proofreading, deserve special thanks. Most important have been the helpful suggestions and moral support of Susan Daly, who helped me get away from my work when I most needed to do so.

S.L.W.

1 The Supreme Court's Roles

THE SUPREME COURT OF the United States is seen in many different ways by the American public. To some the Court is lawgiver, the nation's high tribunal and protector of the Constitution—and perhaps upholder of our liberties. Not only do some see the Court as performing these functions, but they expect it to do so; they would assign it these roles, as something the Court *should* do. To others the Court is not the finder of the law but a policymaker perhaps usurping the legislative prerogative or acting as an obstacle to change—that is, as doing things it *should not* do. Whether they evaluate the Supreme Court positively or negatively, many people see it as different both from other courts in the United States and from the highest courts of other nations.

After World War II, courts in an increasing number of nations were granted a power previously possessed by few courts outside the United States—the power of *judicial review*, the power to invalidate acts of other branches of the government as violating the Constitution. The U.S. Supreme Court remains unusual among highest courts of the world in being not solely a *constitutional court*, one created to hear only questions of the validity of legislative and executive actions and questions of the Constitution's meaning. Instead it has both the power of judicial review *and* the authority to handle all types of litigation, including cases involving interpretation of statutes and application of already-developed policy to particular fact situations (norm enforcement), such as determinations in employee injury cases under federal law. The Supreme Court also differs from most other courts—which *must* accept and decide most cases brought to them—in being able to choose the cases it hears.

If this were not enough to make the Supreme Court exceptional, it is the

1

highest court in the national judicial system, not only the highest among the federal courts but also the court of last resort for cases from the judicial systems of all the states. Such a position leads to the Court's performing certain functions (see pages 31-36). As the highest court, the Supreme Court thus has the final judicial word in any case involving the U.S. Constitution, which is binding on state courts as well as on federal judges. The Court's ability to choose its cases, coupled with its paramount position, gives its rulings the widest possible influence. Although Alexander Hamilton wrote in *The Federalist* that because it did not possess "either the sword or the purse" the Supreme Court would be the "least dangerous" branch, the Court has become very important—and powerful— indeed.

Although the Supreme Court may have the final judicial word, its statements are final only after Congress, the executive, state officials, and even the public have been able to respond; in short, the law is what the judges say it is, after everyone else has had their say. To the extent that the Court's interpretation of a statute or a constitutional provision is accepted as appropriate, it is perhaps only because the Court is the *highest* court. As Justice Jackson admonished, "We are not final because we are infallible, we are infallible only because we are final."[1]

People expect the Supreme Court to act like a court—or like what they think a court is. Indeed, like any other court, the Supreme Court acts within a particular legal system. In the United States, the legal system is supposedly adversary in nature, and judges are expected to rely on *precedent*, that is, decisions in past cases, just as they are also expected to decide on the basis of *principle*—some use the term *neutral principles*—rather than personal likes or whim. Both of these elements, along with the further expectation that the justices will respect the position of the states in our federal system, are part of the expectation that they will exercise *judicial restraint* rather than engage in *activism*. All these matters are elements that some feel should enter the opinions the justices write (see Chapter 8).

People do, however, react to the Court not only in terms of its procedures but in terms of its results as well. They treat it not only as a legal institution deciding specific cases but also as another agency of government, making policy by its decisions just as legislatures make policy by enacting statutes and executive agencies do by promulgating regulations; as it makes policy, the Court interacts with these other branches of government (see Chapter 9).

All courts—even trial courts sentencing defendants after accepting guilty pleas—are policymakers. However, the Supreme Court's policy-making is far more visible than the actions of most lower courts, such as state supreme courts' decisions in the business cases that constitute a larger proportion of their caseload. Because Supreme Court rulings potentially apply to the entire nation, they have far greater significance than those of most other courts. Public reaction to the Court's decisions (its policy statements) forces the Court to become an actor in the political system: if the Court's actions are to have an effect and if, in the long run, the Court is to survive, the justices must take the Court's environment into account.

This chapter provides some context for our subsequent, more detailed examination of the Supreme Court in the federal judicial system. We begin with a discussion of the current controversy about the courts and the reach of their decisions. This is followed by a description of changes in the Court's importance in our political system over the course of our nation's history. Then we turn to an examination of the Warren Court (1953–69) and the just-concluded Burger Court (1969–86). We end the chapter by returning to the theme of this introduction—the roles of the Supreme Court.

The Courts and Current Controversy[2]

Judicial Imperialism

Courts, we have been told repeatedly since the late 1970s, are "activist" rather than "self-restrained." Judges have changed "the very nature of judicial review," so that "what was once a distinctively judicial power, essentially different from legislative power, has become merely another variant of legislative power," with the judge's function no longer limited to "ascertaining and applying the will of the law." After Earl Warren became Chief Justice, the Supreme Court "assumed a role in policy-making unknown in previous American history."[3] Judges, we are told by others, are an "imperial judiciary" making decisions on "social policy" issues that judges should not decide. Moreover, we are told of "judicial incapacity"—that courts lack the skill, competence, or capacity to resolve such social policy issues.[4] Complaints of this sort have come even from within the judiciary, with Chief Justice Rehnquist commenting several years ago that it was "unhealthy" to have "so much authority" given to a small number of life-tenured justices.

In the late 1950s and early 1960s, the Court's internal security rulings produced cries of "Impeach Earl Warren!" and efforts to limit the Court's jurisdiction. Attacks on the courts, particularly the federal courts and most specifically the Supreme Court, in the 1980s have been more serious and carried out on a broader front than at that time or than in 1937, when President Franklin Roosevelt tried to pack the Supreme Court. Decisions on abortion, school prayer, and school desegregation ("forced busing") have particularly provoked intense reaction and efforts to remove the Court's appellate jurisdiction or the jurisdiction of all federal courts (see pages 308-9) over the subjects of those cases. Rulings by lower federal courts on conditions in state prisons and mental hospitals—in which some judges have specified in considerable detail how the institutions should be restructured and administered—have also produced considerable hostility. Judges in such cases are seen as particularly intrusive, displacing state and local officials and becoming administrators of school systems or state institutions.

The fact that federal judges are appointed for life increases the frustration of the critics of their actions: judges are seen as not only intrusive but also unaccountable. Such a view is reinforced by the Supreme Court's 1978 ruling in *Stump v. Sparkman** that judges were immune from lawsuits for damages resulting from actions they had undertaken as judges. A judge who had ordered the sterilization of a 15-year-old female at the request of the girl's mother was sued for his part in the sterilization when the daughter and her husband learned years later why she could not have children. The Supreme Court refused to say the judge's act—normally one not performed by judges—was not "judicial." However, dissenting Justice Stewart argued that "the conduct of a judge surely does not become a judicial act merely on his own say-so. A judge is not free, like a loose cannon, to inflict indiscriminate damage whenever he announces that he is acting in his judicial capacity." (The Court did rule later in *Pulliam v. Allen* (1984) that judges violating people's civil rights may be enjoined from such action and made to pay attorney's fees to a successful plaintiff.)

Criticism of the courts is deeply felt; it is intellectually appealing in a political system in which the elected branches of government are expected to be dominant; and it carries considerable political weight, particularly when the criticized rulings are seen as liberal while the nation's political tone has become more conservative. In evaluating the criticism, one must keep several matters in mind. One is that, like previous attacks on the courts, current criticism is largely prompted by critics' dislike of the courts' *results*. The attack on "government by judiciary," in the 1930s, resulted from a preference for the program of economic regulation the Court had struck down, just as the earlier attack on "government by injunction" stemmed from a preference for laws benefiting labor unions. The liberals who criticized the Court's "activism" then did not also criticize it in the 1950s and 1960s when the Court supported civil liberties. Another point is that "social policy" issues, such as labor-management relations, taxation, and economic regulation of business, have long been brought to the courts for disposition. However, the users of the courts—those raising current social policy questions—have changed: those representing racial minorities, women, and the poor or disadvantaged have joined the advantaged elements of society, such as major commercial interests, in using courts to seek redress of grievances, leading to the filing of many more civil rights cases with which the judges must deal. Here it must be kept in mind that litigation on school desegregation and institutional conditions is particularly complex and drawn out. Because considerable time is needed to prove a constitutional violation and then, once the violation is proved,

---

*Citations to cases mentioned in the text may be found in the Table of Cases, page 391.

to develop a remedy, a court tends to remain involved in overseeing the implementation of its decree for an extended period, perhaps many years.

The "imperial judiciary" and "judicial incapacity" arguments also tend to focus on the courts to the exclusion of other political actors, although the *general* growth of government and additional action by legislatures and executives is a major reason for the expansion of litigation aimed at the government action; indeed, growth in judicial authority is necessary to provide continued "checks and balances" when legislative and executive authority have grown. Much recent litigation concerning rights of the disadvantaged is based on congressional statutes, not on the Constitution, and such litigation results from the need to have judges interpret and enforce vague and ambiguous statutory provisions and the regulations developed to implement the statutes. (The same is true of efforts to clean up the environment.) Judges did not enact the statutes and regulations on which people base their cases nor are they to blame for the lack of clarity. Yet it is the courts, not Congress or executive agencies, that are blamed.

Similarly it is judges, not the officials whose actions (or inaction) have led to litigation, who are criticized. Critics attacked a judge's involvement in administering the Boston school system to produce desegregation, but not the Boston School Committee's adamant refusal to obey *state* laws on school desegregation. Long-standing prison and mental hospital conditions, often so appalling that even conservative federal judges have found the conditions in violation of the Constitution, are given less attention than judges' orders to remedy the violation. Critics of the "imperial judiciary" also seem to forget that, although judges have been willing to provide officials with considerable leeway in remedying conditions on their own, more severe remedial orders often result from officials' resistance to the initial judicial rulings.

Even if judges do not shirk their duty when cases are brought before them, they may remain *reluctant* to become deeply involved in such litigation. Moreover, they cannot impose their views concerning schools or prisons until someone brings a case to court, often as a last resort after complaints to unresponsive legislators and executives. This use of courts as a "last resort" is evidence of courts' connections to, rather than isolation from, the political process. As this indicates, it is litigants, not judges, who initiate cases and thus establish courts' agendas.

Critics of judges' lack of capacity to handle complex social policy issues claim that courts carve up problems that are in reality intertwined, and that the problems with which judges deal in any one case may provide an unrepresentative slice of a larger problem that is better addressed as a whole. Preoccupied with individual cases, judges are said not to think about whether the cases represent typical situations from which precedents for later cases might be properly derived. The resultant judicial policy-making is thus piecemeal, with correction of problems only intermittent rather than continuous. Perhaps this is an accurate description of judicial policy-making, but it is an accurate description of policy-making in the other branches of government as well.[5]

Legislators, administrators, *and* judges generally begin developing policy with a problem presented by particular instances. Most legislative action, for example, occurs only after a series of complaints by constituents or interest groups, not unlike litigants' filing of cases. To some degree, however, officials in all three branches contemplate other situations to which the policy they announce is intended to apply. Judges, who are expected to be subject-matter generalists, may have difficulty dealing with new areas of the law, but so do legislators, who are also generalists not always adequately informed who also lack an adequate basis for choosing experts to assist them. Time and preparation can, however, overcome these difficulties for both judges and legislators. Judges' supervision of institutions can also be facilitated by required periodic reports, reliance on complainants' attorneys to return to court if something is amiss, and appointment of judicial masters who can "compensate for judges' lack of familiarity with organizational routines and procedures in defendant institutions."[6]

Judicial Accountability[7]

The intensity of contemporary criticism of "imperial" judges insufficiently responsive to current political sentiment should not make us forget the strongly and widely held view that judges *should* be independent. Although independence can result in judges' exercising discretion in ways we dislike, we do not wish judges' decisions to be purchased nor to have their decisions reflect partisan political considerations. Similarly, there is a strong argument that because of the substantial pressures against the rights of the disadvantaged, the courts, particularly the Supreme Court, need to serve as a beacon light for such rights.

The wish by many people that judges be independent does not eliminate influences that help to keep them at least somewhat accountable, if we define accountability to mean "keeping an institution's decisions in line with community political and social values and otherwise imposing constraints on the exercise of discretion."[8] Indeed, Shapiro argues that the "universal pattern" is that judging is "an integral part of the mainstream of political authority rather than . . . a separate entity,"[9] thus suggesting clear connections with—and accountability to—the political system.

Judges are accountable *within* the legal system (legal accountability) and *to* the broader political system (political accountability), similar to the "legal subculture" and "democratic subculture" in which all judges operate.[10] Legal accountability includes judges' socialization, their exposure to and learning of norms; legal precedents and the public nature of judicial action; reversal of judges' decisions by higher courts; and constraints imposed by courts' organizational needs. Political accountability derives from the role of public opinion—including resistance—in the judicial process, in addition to the selection and removal of judges. Within the legal system, judges are accountable primarily to lawyers or other judges, while political accountability propels judges toward the broader public or at least its more attentive members. Overlap and convergence between the types of accountability occur both because lawyers participate in judicial selection and because they are part of the political elite.

In the United States, judges receive no formal judicial training before they become judges and only limited formal judicial training after they reach the bench. Before they become judges their most extensive relevant socialization is to their roles as lawyers. As judges, they learn most from contact with other judges, not from nonjudges and even less from nonlawyers. Legal education and training produce thorough exposure to the norm of judicial independence; to the expectation that decisions should be derived from precedent; to the idea that, when applicable precedent is lacking, they should look to "the law" as the source of decisions; and to the norm that decisions should be explained in written opinions. Precedent (see pages 264-70) affects the process by which judges arrive at the reasoned decisions expected of them; the requirement of written (or at least public) opinions, in addition to making the judicial process more open, assists in producing accountability because others can examine the justifications that judges have offered for their actions.

Cutting against accountability is the increasing proportion of unpublished opinions in the lower courts, the fact that the Supreme Court does not provide—and does not have to provide—reasons for denying review of cases, and courts' secrecy about their own internal operations. Although there is considerable freedom of action for lower courts, the potential sanction of reversal by higher courts helps produce accountability, at least to the higher courts, in those cases litigants choose to appeal; litigants thus become an important part of the process of producing judicial accountability. Within any court, trial or appellate, as part of the dynamics that within any organization have a strong effect on everyone's everyday actions, there is accountability (lateral or horizontal accountability) to other judges of the court, to other court officials, and to the lawyers who regularly practice there.

We are more likely to think of the effect of judicial decisions on public opinion (see pages 342-53) than of the reverse. Nonetheless, political account ability may take place through the effect of public opinion on judges, many of whom became accustomed to responding to it while holding elective public office before their judicial appointment, and we can see the continuing pull of constituency particularly in controversial cases such as those involving race relations.[11] Certain aspects of public opinion are also increasingly pressed upon judges by single-issue interest groups. Even in the absence of such activity, judges are not unaware of the political environment relevant to their decisions; the comment has been made that the judges "follow the election returns." Judges certainly are aware of public opinion in the form of resistance to their decisions. Because such resistance certainly lessens the effects of "judicial imperialism"— when disliked decisions are not fully implemented or when they are ignored, resisted, attacked, and overturned in other arenas (see Chapters 9 and 10)—such action may be an important way of holding courts accountable to the views held by significant segments of the public.

A key principal means by which judges might be held accountable, one directly at the intersection of legal and political accountability, is the process by which they are selected. A particular method of judicial selection can affect which political actors play a dominant role and can help to establish the values to which judges may be accountable: partisan election is likely to magnify the importance of political party leaders, but appointive methods—such as that used in the federal judiciary (see pages 97-107)—and "merit systems" increase the relative importance played by the organized bar. Accountability may be built in before a judge takes the bench through the choice of appropriate nominees and through participation by lawyers' groups and other interested individuals and groups in the selection process, thus potentially reducing the need for continuing mechanisms of accountability. On the other hand, there has been increased development of means for disciplining judges and even removing them (see pages 91-96).

The Present Court and the Historical Pattern: The Court's Relative Importance

Historical perspective is important when one examines the Supreme Court's place in our political system. In order to evaluate competing claims that, from a critic's perspective, the Court is too "conservative" (or too "liberal") or too "activist" (or too "restrained"), one must first be able to penetrate such rhetorical terms as "strict construction," "self-restraint," and "activism"—terms that refer to adherence to precedent, injection of personal values, and willingness to intervene in controversial matters (see chapter 8). Second, one must also understand how the Court's performance at any one time compares with its performance in other periods.

Statements that the Burger Court was conservative on civil liberties issues, for example, are based on a comparison with the Warren Court, which decided a substantial majority (upward of 80 percent) of civil liberties cases in favor of the civil liberties claim; the Burger Court, by contrast, ruled against the claim over half the time, although it often faced less clear-cut questions than its predecessor. A different picture of the Burger Court would be produced by comparing it with the Vinson Court (1946–53), generally conservative and not supportive of civil liberties claims. In this section, based on a brief historical recapitulation of the Court's history, we focus on the variation over time on the Court's importance as a major political actor. Particular attention is paid to the Warren and Burger Courts, and to the latter's decisional output.

The Court has not always been as central or important as it now appears. It may come as somewhat of a shock, for example, to realize that when, early in the Court's history, partisan conflict between Congress and the Court led to cancellation of a term of Court (something quite unlikely to happen now), the nation's business went on without interruption. The Supreme Court did not even have its own building until the 1930s: the Court met in the basement of the Capitol, and the justices did much of their work in their Washington, D.C., homes. Although the Supreme Court edifice across from the Capitol (brought in under cost, a miracle not likely to recur) is properly impressive, one of the first justices to work in it said that he and his colleagues felt like "Nine Black Beetles in the Temple of Karnak."

The significance of the Supreme Court's role in the American system has varied across time and between issues. At times, the Court has seemed central to the nation's development; at other times, it has been more in the background. One of the periods of the Court's greatest centrality came in the early nineteenth century under Chief Justice John Marshall, who helped the Court achieve its earliest prominence. Through Marshall, the Court established its power to invalidate acts of Congress. Through decisions such as *Gibbons v. Ogden*, establishing Congress' power over interstate commerce broadly defined, and *McCulloch v. Maryland*, striking down a state tax on the National Bank, the Court played a major role in establishing the national government's place in our scheme of federalism. Under Chief Justice Roger Taney, the Supreme Court was perhaps less obtrusive. In that period, the Court allowed the states more authority over commerce, ruling in *Cooley v. Board of Port Wardens* that where diversity was needed, states could act where the federal government had not done so. Unfortunately for Taney's reputation, in the *Dred Scott* case—the Court's second exercise of judicial review at the national level and one of its "self-inflicted wounds"[12]—the Court seriously exacerbated the tensions that led to the Civil War by upsetting Congress's regulation of slavery in the territories and ruling that a slave was not a person who could sue in the courts. Prior to the Civil War, there was a much closer link between the Court's rulings and party policy than would be found later. This link reduced the Court's independence and thus the centrality of its role. During and after the Civil War, the Court also played a subordinate role—its usual posture with respect to war efforts—generally sustaining Lincoln's actions and his theory of the relation between Union and Confederacy.

The Court's general prestige in the late nineteenth century was great, but the Court did not play a positive leadership role. The Court undercut post-Civil War civil rights legislation, for example, in the *Civil Rights Cases*, and then, in *Plessy v. Ferguson*, sustained state legislation requiring Negroes to ride in separate railroad cars. At the same time, the justices were saying that the Fourteenth Amendment's Due Process Clause did not include the Bill of Rights' procedural protections for criminal defendants.[13] Later the Court's conservatism led it to uphold convictions of "subversives" in cases brought in the atmosphere of World War I.[14] The Court's importance in the late nineteenth and early twentieth centuries also resulted from its striking down most state attempts to regulate the economy even when Congress had not acted. This was the period when "substantive due process" was at its height—with the judges reading into the Constitution their views of what was "reasonable" for the states to legislate. The Court also undid Congress's attempts to regulate the economy, defining the commerce and taxing powers narrowly[15] and even saying that powers not expressly delegated to the federal government were reserved to the states—language like that of the Articles of Confederation.

During the New Deal period, the Court became a principal political actor as a result of its actions striking down much early New Deal legislation.[16] These decisions ran contrary to the political realignment reflected in President Roosevelt's election. (It was during this time that in calling a Supreme Court session to order, the court crier is alleged to have said, "May God save the United States from this Honorable Court.") Whether or not as a result of President Roosevelt's attack on the Court and his proposal to add justices (see pages 314-15), the Court changed position, sustaining a wide variety of economic regulatory measures.[17] This change was reinforced by the departure of its four most conservative members and their replacement by justices chosen for their support of New Deal programs. After 1937, the Court regularly accepted Congress' determinations about the reach of the Commerce Clause as a vehicle for regulation of the economy—and other types of regulation, such as race relations. Although in 1976, the Court moved toward restricting Congress' regulatory authority over state and local governments, it undid this ruling several years later and upheld Congress' authority to extend the minimum wage to state employees.[18]

The Court's post-1937 restraint concerning economic regulation was not immediately accompanied by consistent judicial protection for civil liberties. In cases stemming from World War II, the Court again showed its unwillingness to protect civil liberties in war-related matters (see pages 319-20). Most important, the Court showed its deference to the president in sustaining the relocation of Japanese-Americans in the *Korematsu* case. After World War II, blacks began to win some support for their rights in housing and graduate education,[19] but the Vinson Court, as noted previously, had an otherwise conservative record on civil liberties.

The Warren Court

Although it is now almost 20 years since Chief Justice Earl Warren stepped down from the Court, the Warren Court commands our attention because, in the areas of civil liberties and civil rights, it remains the benchmark against which subsequent periods of the Supreme Court will be measured. Certainly it served as such a benchmark for the Burger Court and it is likely to remain one for the Rehnquist Court as well. The Warren Court period was the first one in which the Court gave substantial attention to civil liberties and civil rights claims. In the long view of the Court's history, that attention, coupled with the Warren Court's *support* of civil liberties claims, made it something of an aberration. Aberration or not, its position on civil liberties and civil rights and the controversy surrounding its decisions made it a central force in the American political system. Even if it was not as important as the president and Congress, it was highly involved in key policy issues, and the public became accustomed to the Court's being in that position.

Only with the Warren Court were minorities able to win victories they had not been able to obtain from reluctant legislatures and executives. Through its civil liberties "activism," most of it evident in decisions striking down state restrictions on individual rights, the Court again became extremely prominent and central in the nation's life. The Court was also pretty much "the only game in town" for civil liberties and civil rights policy until Congress enacted the Civil Rights Act of 1964 and the Voting Rights Act of 1965 and the executive branch developed implementing regulations for those statutes, leading to a sharing of civil rights policy-making among the three branches but only slightly diminishing the Court's centrality.

The Warren Court's first major step was the invalidation of racial segregation ("separate but equal") in education in *Brown v. Board of Education* (1954). Whether, in making this landmark ruling, the Court was leading the nation or was following public opinion—at least elite public opinion—is unclear; arguments have been made on both sides. The ruling is thought to have led the nation, but it can be argued that it came only because the time was ripe, a position that does not suggest leadership as much as consonance with the nation's tone.

The Court followed up its schools ruling with a series of decisions in 1956 and 1957 protecting political dissidents caught up in government internal security investigations aimed at suspected Communists and other radicals. The Warren Court also required that both houses of each state legislature be apportioned on the basis of population; expanded free speech in the areas of obscenity and libel; invalidated prayers in public schools; and overturned convictions of those protesting against racial discrimination in transportation and places of public accommodations, also regularly sustaining Congress' actions to protect civil rights with respect to public accommodations, voting, and housing.[20] The justices also turned their attention to the poor, invalidating the poll tax and durational residence requirements for receiving welfare benefits.[21]

In what produced probably the greatest controversy, the Court adopted a series of broad rules protecting criminal defendants and suspects. Of these the most notable were *Mapp v. Ohio* (improperly seized evidence inadmissible at trial—the "exclusionary rule"), *Gideon v. Wainwright* (right to counsel for indigents at trials for felonies and major misdemeanors), and *Miranda v. Arizona* (no confession admissible without suspect being warned of rights). That the Court also approved "stop and frisk" practices, lifted restrictions on material that could be taken in a search, approved the use of informants, and supplied the basis for electronic surveillance with a warrant received far less attention.[22] Also receiving less attention was the Court's avoidance of some problems, such as implementation of school desegregation for over a decade after the *Brown* decision and the basic constitutional question of the right of a private proprietor to refuse service on the basis of race—never reached despite all the sit-in convictions the Court reversed. Furthermore, the Court was criticized for having subordinated the interests of racial minorities to the concerns of whites and having too closely followed public opinion. The Court, it was said, had "struck down only the symbols of racism," leaving racist practices intact, and "had waltzed in time to the music of the white majority—one step forward, one step backward and sidestep, sidestep."[23]

The Warren Court's civil liberties record, reinforced by its easing of access to the courts for those wishing to challenge government action, led groups increasingly to turn first to the federal courts for redress of their grievances, particularly against state and local officials, instead of using the courts as a last resort. This development gave some pause even to supporters of the Court's decisions, who wondered whether reliance on the courts might lead to atrophy of the legislative process, central to a democratic political system.

When we talk of the "Warren Court," we must keep in mind that its level of support for civil liberties was not uniform throughout the entire 1953–69 period, but was highest at the end of Chief Justice Warren's tenure. Just as there was more than one Roosevelt Court, several Warren Court periods can be identified. Although the transition from the Vinson Court to the Warren Court was immediately visible in the 1954 *Brown v. Board of Education* school desegregation ruling, several terms passed before the Court "succeeded impressively in freeing itself from the self-doubts that deterred constitutional development during the 1940–1953 period."[24] It took Chief Justice Warren more than one term to locate himself firmly among the liberals; not until the 1956 Term did one see, in the Court's internal security rulings, a distinctly liberal posture, and this may have resulted at least as much from Justice Brennan, said to be the Warren Court's intellectual leader, as from the Chief Justice. In part because of congressional reaction to those rulings, the next four terms were "characterized by an abatement of the liberal trend that had occurred during the first four terms of the Warren era,"[25] and the Court supported civil liberties claims less than half the time in 1958–60. The Court's support of such claims at rates of close to 80 percent came only when Justice Felix Frankfurter retired in 1962 and was replaced by Justice Arthur Goldberg. Goldberg and Abe Fortas, who replaced him, provided the Court's fifth reliable civil liberties vote, and they were reinforced by Thurgood Marshall, the Court's first black member, who replaced the more conservative Tom Clark.[26] Their presence allowed the Warren Court to "finish strong" in support of civil liberties claims. (For a list of members of the Warren and Burger Courts, see Figure 1.1.)

Because the Warren Court's strongest support for civil liberties came in its last terms, the transition to the Burger Court did not begin before Earl Warren's departure, unlike the transition from the Marshall Court (1801–35) to the Taney Court (1836–63), which is said to have begun before the end of one chief justice's tenure. Instead, another aspect of the Marshall to Taney transition—considerable continuity accompanying change or transformation—can be said to have characterized the Warren Court to Burger Court transition, and some have said the two are not easily marked off.

Perhaps all courts pass through transitional periods. As they change personnel, their policy direction changes, and so does the relationship of the Court to public sentiment—at times moving closer to public opinion, at times appearing to lead that opinion. Such changes also involve shifts in the predominant role the courts assume, whether as restrained discoverers of the law or more actively as developers or makers of policy. During a transitional period, several years may elapse before a pattern is clear. Moreover, different patterns may characterize different policy areas. The "new" Court may extend earlier rulings; maintain, consolidate, or clarify those rulings; or curtail or erode the precedents of previous years—often with substantial cumulative effect. Direct reversal of precedent may occur, but usually only after several years have elapsed. As one observer put it: "After the Marshall era, a period of great constitutional creativity, the Court experienced a period characterized by limitation and modification but not by major departure from established precedent."[27] In some ways that was the Burger Court's position vis-à-vis the Warren Court.

The transition to the Roosevelt Court, which began prior to a change in personnel and then was reinforced by new justices such as Hugo Black and William O. Douglas, did not take place until FDR's second term, when his first opportunities to nominate justices occurred. However, it has been suggested that the "Constitutional Revolution of 1937" took place before the personnel changes, indicating that they are only one part of shifts in Supreme Court direction. Even with replacements of justices or a change in the person in the "center chair," there may be relatively little change, at least at first, as in the change from Chief Justice Edward White to Chief Justice William Howard Taft. In that situation, the change did not occur until several years later.[28]

The Burger Court

If the transition to the Burger Court did not begin before the end of Earl Warren's term, it began shortly thereafter, as President Nixon was able to name not only a Chief Justice but three associate justices as well within the first three years of taking office. The departures of Warren and of Abe Fortas in 1969 were followed by those of Hugo Black and John Marshall Harlan in 1971. Warren Burger became Chief Justice and was joined first by Harry Blackmun, and then by Lewis Powell and William Rehnquist. After William O. Douglas, who had joined the Court in 1939 and served on it longer than anyone else, departed in 1975, President Ford named John Paul Stevens to replace him. President Nixon,

Figure 1.1   Membership of the Supreme Court (1953 - present)

WARREN COURT

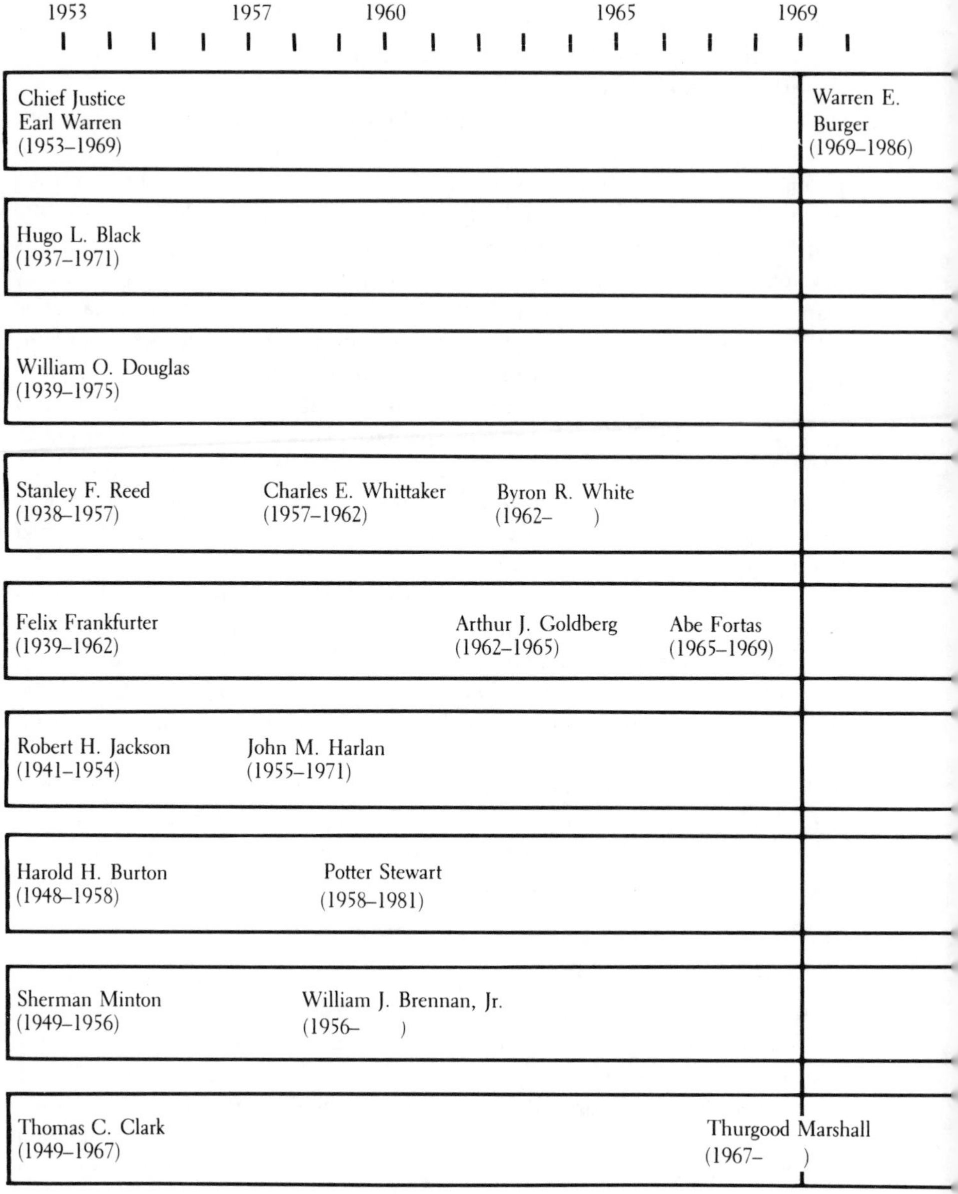

1953	1957	1960	1965	1969

Chief Justice Earl Warren (1953–1969)	Warren E. Burger (1969–1986)

Hugo L. Black (1937–1971)

William O. Douglas (1939–1975)

Stanley F. Reed (1938–1957)   Charles E. Whittaker (1957–1962)   Byron R. White (1962–   )

Felix Frankfurter (1939–1962)   Arthur J. Goldberg (1962–1965)   Abe Fortas (1965–1969)

Robert H. Jackson (1941–1954)   John M. Harlan (1955–1971)

Harold H. Burton (1948–1958)   Potter Stewart (1958–1981)

Sherman Minton (1949–1956)   William J. Brennan, Jr. (1956–   )

Thomas C. Clark (1949–1967)   Thurgood Marshall (1967–   )

14

1975	1981	1986

William H. Rehnquist (1986 –   )

Lewis F. Powell, Jr. (1972–1987)

John Paul Stevens (1975–   )

Harry A. Blackmun (1970–   )

William H. Rehnquist (1972–1986, then to Chief Justice)

Antonin Scalia (1986–   )

Sandra Day O'Connor (1981–   )

having made the Supreme Court, and particularly its criminal procedure rulings, a subject of campaign controversy—thereby increasing expectations that the new Court would indeed change Warren Court policy—gave particular attention to his nominees' ideology. Thus it should be no surprise that the changes in personnel brought changes in doctrine (discussed below) and in the Court's relationship to public opinion; what is perhaps surprising is that the changes were not greater than they now appear.

Without doubt, the Burger Court—like most other periods in the Court's history—will look different to us in 10 or 20 years from the way it looks now, shortly after Warren Burger stepped down as Chief Justice. Yet even some years down the road, our picture of it may remain unclear because the Burger Court did not establish the clear direction of the Warren Court, perhaps because it lacked firm leadership, and because Justice Brennan's intellectual leadership remained although he was more frequently in the minority. On balance, the Burger Court was most certainly more conservative than the Warren Court; it would have been unlikely for the Court to move in any other direction. In certain areas of the law, particularly criminal procedure and most particularly search and seizure and confessions, the Court adopted a proprosecution stance, but lacked direction. Moreover, its overall record across the wide range of the civil liberties/civil rights spectrum is also studded with liberal outcomes: support, although with unclear doctrine, for affirmative action programs; development of a woman's right to an abortion; the opening of criminal trials to the public and the press; and the development of protection for "commercial speech."

Initially, Chief Justice Burger produced no great across-the-board policy change, although some areas saw more change than others. Although the Burger Court did reinforce or even advance some Warren Court doctrine and developed rights in some previously unexplored areas, on the whole the Court's decisions demonstrated considerable withdrawal from and undercutting of Warren Court policies affecting the entire range of civil liberties problems; this was particularly noticeable in criminal procedure cases. The Court limited expansion of Warren Court doctrine, but the basic picture for several years was one of marginal change and a generally unsettled pattern. The Burger Court did not at first directly overrule precedent; instead it whittled away at prior rulings. Thus the 1974 Term left a picture of a "reluctant Court" that tried to make potentially important cases stand for as little as possible; a Court whose theme song was the refrain "we *only* decide"; a Court that loved to decide issues "in these particular circumstances," that performed contortions to avoid announcing new principles even when new principles were inescapably needed, and that pretended not to be announcing them even while it was announcing them.[29] However, in the 1975 Term the Court consolidated its position and overruled 1968 Warren Court precedents that had allowed picketing of a store in a shopping center.[30]

The Court's mid-1970's consolidation, which had led some liberals to say,

"If the president gets one more appointment, watch out!", was not, however, to mean that the Court would become unremittingly conservative, and observers are still making the same comments. In 1980, the Court was best characterized by the headline, "Pragmatism, Compromise Marks Court: Tricky Track Record Harder to Categorize Than Pundits Predicted." That characterization continued to be true even once the Court moved in a more conservative direction when Justice Sandra Day O'Connor replaced Justice Potter Stewart for the 1981 Term and even after the 1983 Term, when the Court was thought by the media to have shifted considerably to the right. The Court limited suits for discrimination in government programs and employment, and followed an "accommodationist" church-state position. The majority, which had earlier overturned two Warren Court rulings on the use of informants' tips as the basis for obtaining a warrant, also created a "public safety" exception to *Miranda* and the "good faith" exception to the exclusionary rule, placed limits on prisoners' rights, and approved preventive detention for juveniles.[31]

Increased tenure by the Chief Justice and his Nixon-appointed colleagues did not result in increased stability of position, leading to "drift and division" and a "lack of consistent vision" in what was called "one of the most fragmented Courts" in our history,[32] with the Court acting pragmatically rather than as the result of an agenda—except perhaps in the area of criminal procedure, where the justices were most (and most consistently) conservative. Thus in its final term, despite the upholding of antisodomy laws as applied to homosexuals and action taken against a high school student for an off-color speech,[33] there were rulings supporting affirmative action, facilitating challenges to "vote dilution" of minorities' votes, and preventing prosecutors' use of peremptory challenges to eliminate minorities from juries.[34]

For all the rhetoric accompanying the appointment of its members, the Burger Court was not noticeably less "restrained" than its predecessor had been. Restraint might be inferred from the Court's increased deference to the legislative and executive branches, and by its subjecting state laws and actions to less strict tests than the Warren Court had used. This was done, however, in aid of conservative rulings, reinforced by the Court's decreased willingness to have the federal courts serve as a forum for resolving complaints against the government. For example, when a policeman complained that he had been improperly discharged without a hearing, the Court said, "The federal court is not the appropriate forum in which to review the multitude of personnel decisions that are made daily by public agencies. . . . The United States Constitution cannot feasibly be construed to require federal judicial review for every such error."[35]

Although such a ruling indicates judicial self-restraint, the Court's overall record of invalidating federal and state legislative acts provides evidence to the contrary. Decisions on both types of legislation produced sharp breaks from a pattern of more than 30 years. As noted in 1979,

In no decision did the Warren Court—nor, for that matter, did any Supreme Court since the mid-1930's—hold that an act of Congress was invalid on the ground that the lawmaking branch had exceeded its delegated powers and invaded ground reserved to the States by the tenth amendment. The Burger Court has done so twice. . . . In no decision did the Warren Court—nor, for that matter, did the Supreme Court for a period of over thirty-five years—hold any state law in violation of the contract clause of the Constitution. In the last two years, the Burger Court has done so twice. . . . In no decision did the Warren Court—nor, for that matter, did any Supreme Court in nearly twenty-five years—invalidate an act of Congress or an act of the President on the ground that it usurped the other branch's constitutional powers.[36]

Yet the Burger Court had done so, and later, in its ruling invalidating the legislative veto, struck down portions of 200 federal statutes at one swell foop.

As the legistlative veto ruling indicates, the Burger Court handed down important rulings on the separation of powers. Most notable was the crisis-resolving Watergate Tapes case (see pages 324-25) and its recent invalidation of a key section of the Gramm-Rudman-Hollings Budget Act (*Bowsher v. Synar*, 1986). These and further historic decisions like those in *Roe v. Wade* (1973), providing protection for the right to an abortion, and the Court's follow-up decisions reaffirming that ruling, have served to keep the Court almost continuously in the limelight as *a*—not *the*, but *a*—central government institution.

Civil Liberties. The Burger Court's rulings on civil liberties and civil rights received the most attention, because that was where retrenchment from the Warren Court's doctrine was thought most likely. In Burger's first term, support for civil liberties claims fell to 55 percent. By the 1972 Term, it was down to 43.5 percent, the lowest since 1957. Indicative of the change is that, in the 1974 Term, when the Court was divided, the justices rejected civil liberties claims 29 of 46 times. Its support for civil liberties claims decreased into the 30 percent range starting with the 1980 Term. (See Figure 1.2.) One specific indication of trends in the Burger Court is the progressive decline, from the 1969 through 1979 Terms, in the rate at which interests of poor people prevailed—from 65 percent at the beginning of the period to only 30 percent in the post-1975 period.[37] And, as Figure 1.2 indicates, support for civil liberties claims in the criminal procedure area have, with but one exception, been lower—at times as much as 15 points lower—than for all civil liberties claims.

Of particular importance is that state officials who challenged assertions of rights replaced civil liberties claimants as the principal victors in civil liberties cases. This can be seen in the Court's treatment of cases brought directly from state court where one party was a state official and the other a private rights claimant. Roughly *one-fourth* of all state-initiated petitions were successful in some way, with challenged lower court rulings being reversed, vacated, or granted full review; the same was true of *less than 10 percent* of petitions from civil liberties claimants.[38] Closely related was the Court's willingness to upset state court decisions interpreting rights expansively. Furthermore, although during

Figure 1.2 Supreme Court Support for Civil Liberties Claims, 1976–85 Terms

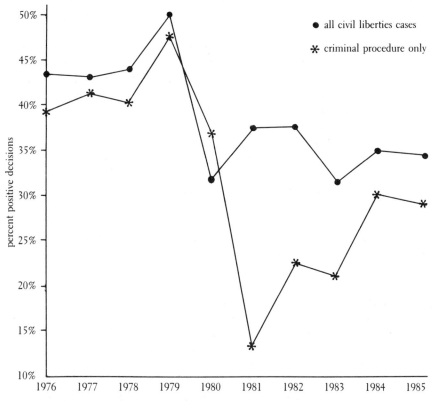

Source: Data gathered by author; graphics by Thomas Church, Jr.

the heyday of the Warren Court *no* state civil liberties ruling was overturned for exceeding the Supreme Court's civil liberties standards, the Burger Court did so both directly and, more frequently, by sending cases back to state courts for clarification of the constitutional basis of prorights rulings. It has, however, been suggested that the Burger Court's "bias against liberal state court decisions extends only to search-and-seizure and *Miranda* warning cases, and not to criminal procedure or civil rights and liberties generally," with the Court having overturned a large proportion of cases "which the state courts decided *antithetically* to civil liberties and civil rights claimants."[39] Such a view, from the 1969–83 Terms, indicates the importance of not focusing on one or two terms of Court such as the 1982 and 1983 Terms, but of examining longer trends.

The Burger Court's civil liberties decisions, particularly those on criminal procedure, moved the Court closer to public opinion than was the Warren Court at the height of its support for civil liberties claims. Congress also reflects public opinion, for example, in its opposition to "forced busing," in some important civil liberties areas, but it has been more sympathetic to some civil rights claims, for example, on pregnancy-based discrimination and voting discrimination.

The Court's change in position—both its real changes and the considerable change perceived by those who had become accustomed to the Warren Court's liberalism—coupled with this somewhat more conducive congressional atmosphere, led some to turn away from the Supreme Court for resolution of their grievances. In addition to Congress, civil liberties activity was mounted on other fronts; this included the extended if unsuccessful effort to obtain ratification of the Equal Rights Amendment (ERA). It also included turning to state courts in states where such courts were liberal; suggestions to take such action even came from liberal members of the Court such as Justice Brennan. That some state high courts were willing to overturn property-tax financing of public education (when the Supreme Court was not), to invalidate zoning laws that excluded moderate- and low-income housing (after the Supreme Court refused to grant standing to those challenging such laws), and to enforce the "wall of separation" between church and state more strictly gave some substance to the hope that assistance in enforcing civil liberties could be found there.

These developments, coupled with the events surrounding Watergate, which further deflected attention from the Court toward the president and Congress, moved the balance of influence between the courts and the elected branches of government toward the situation predating the Warren Court, making the Court not as predominant or central a political actor as it had been during the 1950s and 1960s. Yet it remained more central than the Court of the 1940s, in part because of the high "surprise level" in its actions and in part because of political activity, provoked by its own rulings, to overturn those rulings (on "forced busing" and abortion). The Court certainly had not left the political arena, and the importance of its civil liberties rulings—both those retaining strength from the Warren Court era and the Burger Court's own decisions— continue to give the Court greater prominence than it had before Earl Warren became Chief Justice, with people continuing to turn to it for whatever assistance they can obtain. "After all," said one lawyer, "it's the only Supreme Court we have."

The Burger Court did not cut back on Warren Court rulings as much as had been expected, in part because of the strength of those rulings as precedent and the civil liberties education they had provided the public. The Burger Court actually moved forward with Warren Court doctrines in some areas and broke new ground in other areas not considered by the Warren Court. In the *Swann* case, the justices upheld lower court judges' authority to order broad remedies for school segregation, including busing; they invalidated schemes for evading desegregation; and they told private schools they could not discriminate on the basis of race.[40] The Court took a strong stand against discrimination in employment. It reinforced Congress' action in passing Title VII of the 1964 Civil Rights Act, by ruling in the *Griggs* case that, even though no discrimination was intended, employment tests not related to the job could not be used if they had a discriminatory effect; the justices also supported back pay and seniority remedies for job discrimination.

However, the Court then moved in a more conservative direction by imposing tests for proving employment discrimination—tests it imported into cases on housing discrimination and voting rights—that were far more difficult to satisfy and by sustaining seniority provisions despite the claim that they locked in past discrimination.[41] The Court also handed down three major cases on affirmative action, the most troublesome topic in the employment discrimination area—indeed, in the whole race relations field. The first, and perhaps best known, is the *Bakke* case (1978), where one five-justice majority narrowly invalidated a medical school's action in setting aside a specific number of seats for minorities, but another five-justice majority said that race *could* be taken into account in remedying past discrimination. In the *Weber* and *Fullilove* cases, the Court then upheld programs established by private industry and by Congress that provided positions for minorities in training programs and construction employment. Although the Court seemed to have come to the end of the road in its support for affirmative action programs when, in the *Stotts* case, it overturned agreements to protect minorities in the event of layoffs, the justices ended the 1985 Term with strong affirmation of affirmative action programs involving preferences in hiring.[42]

Where schools instead of jobs were at issue, the Court's pattern was mixed. In *Milliken v. Bradley*, a 1974 ruling in a Detroit case—seen by some as the end of the road for desegregation—the Court struck down busing across school district lines because districts outside the center city had not been shown to have discriminated. The Court also limited lower court judges' discretion to order desegregation, requiring that remedies for school segregation be tailored more narrowly than in the past. Showing its lack of predictability, the Court ruled that northern cities like Dayton and Columbus, Ohio, were subject to the full range of desegregation remedies for having maintained segregated school systems since before the Court's 1954 *Brown* ruling.[43]

The Warren Court had not decided cases on sex discrimination, so this was an area in which the Burger Court could set its own tone; while women were not given as complete protection as was given racial minorities, the tone was moderate-to-liberal, not conservative. In its initial cases, the Court invalidated an automatic preference for men as executors of estates, statutes making it easier for men than women to obtain dependents' benefits, automatic exemptions of women from jury duty, and forced maternity leave requirements for school teachers.[44] Perhaps most significant as well as most controversial was the Court's invalidation, in *Roe v. Wade* and *Doe v. Bolton* (1973), of laws interfering with the right to obtain an abortion, particularly during the first trimester of pregnancy.

In the continuing controversy over abortion, the Court struck down a variety of requirements that interfered with a woman's right to obtain an abortion, although by only a 5-4 vote in 1986.[45] However, efforts by federal, state, and local governments to impose severe restrictions on funding of abortions were upheld.[46] Although the Court expanded the basis for complaints of sex discrimination in employment and pay, the justices declined to adopt the controversial "comparable worth" theory in doing so, and also severely limited the reach of federal antidiscrimination provisions that had assisted women (and minorities); in addition, the Court upheld Congress' adoption of male-only draft registration.[47]

With respect to the First Amendment, at first the Court continued—and advanced—a strong position on separation of church and state, outlawing virtually most other forms of aid to elementary and secondary parochial schools. However, the Court then showed willingness to approve more forms of aid to parochial schools, although it was unwilling to have public school teachers teach in religious school facilities under "shared time" programs.[48] Toward the close of the Burger Court, the justices handed down a number of rulings said to represent not a separationist but an "accommodationist" posture, most notable among which was Lynch v. Donnelly, which upheld a city's providing a creche at Christmastime, and a decision sustaining a state law allowing parents tax credits for tuition for parochial schools.[49] However, the Court reinforced a major Warren Court ruling by invalidating a statute providing for a moment of silence in the classroom.[50]

The Court's free speech posture was mixed. In New York Times v. United States (1971) the justices refused to allow the government an injunction against publication of the "Pentagon Papers" and struck down "gag orders" on the press in criminal trials. However, grand juries were allowed to question reporters about their confidential sources, and free speech by military officers and on military bases was restricted.[51] The Court distinctly moved away from the Warren Court's position on obscenity in Miller v. California (1973), rewriting the definition of the concept to give greater scope to local community values. Its most important advance concerning free speech involved "commercial speech," to which the justices gave protection, for example, by striking down restrictions on advertising by pharmacists and lawyers.[52] The Court also tried to deal with the relation between freedom of the press and defendants' rights. After first saying, in a case involving pretrial proceedings, that judges could close the courtroom in trials, the Court did find a First Amendment right to open trials, and it reinforced the openness of criminal proceedings in its subsequent rulings on the subject, even providing for open preliminary hearings in some situations.[53] The Court— which refused to allow radio or television coverage of its own open proceedings (oral argument)—also ruled in Chandler v. Florida (1982) that states could allow live electronic media coverage of trials even if defendants objected.

Criminal Procedure.   The Burger Court's greatest retrenchment from Warren Court doctrine occurred with respect to criminal procedure, particularly searches and confessions, with the majority adopting a "crime control" model rather than the "due process" model that for the most part the Warren Court preferred. This continued to be the area in which the Court most strongly supported government officials—police, prosecutors, and prison administrators. The *legal* guilt of a factually guilty defendant meant less to the Burger Court majority, which tended to rule on a case-by-case basis instead of establishing broad (or "bright-line") rules, despite claims that law enforcement officers needed the latter. And when the Court encountered constitutional errors in criminal trials, it often said they constituted "harmless error" so that the conviction did not have to be reversed.

Continuing to confound observers' expectations, the Court left standing both the *Miranda* requirements and the exclusionary rule, despite a campaign by Chief Justice Burger and Justice Rehnquist against the latter. However, both rules were restricted, and the "good faith" exception carved out of the latter is a major victory for law enforcement officers. The Court held the exclusionary rule inapplicable to grand jury proceedings, and made it more difficult to challenge improper searches by limiting *who* could bring such challenges and *where* they could bring them: federal court review of claims about improper searches were prohibited where the state courts had been able to pass on the claims *(Stone v. Powell*, 1976). (The Court generally made it more difficult to use the writ of habeas corpus in federal courts to challenge alleged constitutional violations in state trials; see pages 186-87.)

The Court did extend Fourth Amendment protections in ruling that arrest warrants were necessary before police could make felony arrests in the suspect's home and that search warrants were required where the person was in someone else's home.[54] However, searches of people and of cars were generally made easier. Following up on the Warren Court's "stop-and-frisk" ruling, the Burger Court permitted detentions of alleged drug smugglers in airports and of other individuals at crime scenes. They also ruled that when police properly stop an automobile, they may search not only the passenger compartment of the car but also items found within the car *(United States v. Ross*, 1982). Catching up with technology, the Court also approved following cars on the basis of beepers placed by government agents in items transported in those cars; aerial surveillance of the area near homes and of industrial complexes was also upheld.[55] The justices also supported law enforcement efforts by allowing searches of newspaper offices for evidence relating to a crime and warrantless covert entry of property to install a "bug," and by permitting school officials to search students' lockers.[56] (The Court had earlier upheld wiretapping and other electronic surveillance carried out under the 1968 Safe Streets Act.)

Miranda was not overturned, but was weakened, first by a ruling that confessions obtained without warnings could be used to impeach a witness's testimony at trial.[57] Then the majority said that questioning of a suspect could be resumed several hours after it had initially been terminated, and that grand jury investigations and tax investigations could be carried out without persons being warned of their *Miranda* rights.[58] Rulings that someone asking to see a lawyer—which would terminate interrogation—had to do so "clearly and unequivocally" (*Edwards v. Arizona*, 1981) or that police did not have to tell a defendant that an attorney had called (*Moran v. Burbine*, 1986) were in a way only refusals to extend *Miranda*, not reductions in its "core holding." However, in *New York v. Quarles*, where the Court created a "crime scene" exception to *Miranda*—that, at the scene of a crime, where weapons needed to be retrieved quickly for public safety, the warnings need not be given before questions were asked—the Court was limiting even the core of *Miranda* and its "bright-line" rule.

Perhaps the two most important "*Miranda*" cases of the Burger Court involved confessions obtained by subtle techniques, in which the police officers, through their statements (not explicit interrogations) played on a suspect's mental state and religious concerns to learn the whereabouts of a murder victim's body or of a murder weapon. In *Brewer v. Williams* (1977), which state prosecutors tried to use as a vehicle to seek to have *Miranda* overturned, the Court avoided doing so by ruling that the officers had interfered with the defendant's post-indictment right to counsel. (After the defendant was reconvicted, the Supreme Court, ruling that the little girl's body would have been found even without his statement, upheld admission of the evidence under the "inevitable discovery" rule.[59]) Three years later, in *Rhode Island v. Innis* (1980), the Court defined "interrogation" broadly, to extend beyond direct questions to statements likely to elicit an answer, but said that, on the facts of the case, the defendant had *not* been interrogated in violation of *Miranda*.

In another important criminal procedure area, the Court did extend the right to counsel at trial to all cases where a person was in fact to be jailed (*Argersinger v. Hamlin*, 1972). However, the right to counsel at police lineups and on appeal was limited, and neither the standard the Court established for "ineffective assistance of counsel" claims nor its application was particularly helpful to defendants. The justices also refused to make counsel automatically available for those whose probation or parole was being revoked or to provide counsel in prison proceedings for rule violations. However, in all those situations procedural protection was provided for the first time.[60] Yet the Court seemed to be returning to the old "hands off" posture concerning prison matters when it turned aside attacks on conditions for pretrial detainees (those not yet convicted), double-celling and other deficiencies in prison conditions, and searches of prison cells, and rejected prisoners' suits against prison officials for contributing to their injuries.[61] The Court also legitimized and encouraged plea bargaining, and strictly limited challenges to a conviction once a defendant, with assistance of counsel, had entered a guilty plea.[62]

With an increasing number of executions of those convicted of murder, capital punishment is a topic of continuing controversy; the Court's rulings are at the heart of that controversy. The Court at first struck down the death penalty *as then applied (Furman v. Georgia*, 1972), but then, directly confronting its constitutionality, held that the death penalty did *not* violate the Eighth Amendment's prohibition against cruel and unusual punishment, at least if the penalty were not mandatory and if aggravating *and* mitigating circumstances were considered in sentencing (*Gregg v. Georgia*, 1976). The Court went on to rule that the death penalty for rape was excessive and grossly disproportionate to the crime (*Coker v. Georgia*, 1977), required some procedural protections for imposition of the death sentence, and refused to allow execution of those insane at the time of execution.[63] The justices reinforced the position that a defendant had to be allowed to introduce mitigating evidence so that his case would receive individualized consideration.[64] However, the Court's majority did not hold state courts tightly to these standards and became increasingly impatient with death penalty appeals and increasingly abrupt in its treatment of them. Thus the majority complained about repeated petitions for habeas corpus, and even denied stays of execution when the issues raised by the Death Row inmate were before Court in other as-yet-undecided cases.[65]

The majority's deference to state prosecutorial and judicial officials produced an increasingly harsh tone in exchanges among the justices in criminal procedure rulings, with Justice Brennan accusing the majority of showing "an unseemly eagerness to act as 'the adjunct of the State and its prosecutors in facilitating efficient and expedient conviction,'" and of exhibiting "willingness to take special judicial action to assist the prosecutor."[66] The Court's proprosecution tilt was also often noted by Justice Stevens, who said, "It is particularly striking to compare the Court's apparent willingness to forgive constitutional errors that redound to the prosecutor's benefit with the Court's determination to give conclusive effect to trivial errors that obstruct a defendant's ability to raise meritorious constitutional arguments."[67]

Burger's Legacy.   What legacy has Chief Justice Burger left? With respect to doctrine, the headline "Burger Court Leaves an Unclear Legacy" is accurate, and it may be that the Burger Court, without a strong Chief Justice, will be remembered as the period between the Warren Court and the Rehnquist Court. The Burger Court's conservatism in criminal procedure is obvious, but the picture otherwise is less clear. Thus one can agree that "the continuity and stamp of identity on the Court that Chief Justice Burger wants to personify . . . proved increasingly elusive in his Court's performance" and, as Justice Powell told the American Bar Association after Burger's last Term, "there has been no conservative counter-revolution by the Burger Court."[68] One reason is that Burger appears neither to have led the Court as a whole or even his own "bloc," nor was he able to prevent his "Minnesota Twin," Justice Blackmun, from moving far away from their early joint voting, suggesting ineffective leadership.

Burger's contributions were primarily *outside* the Court rather than inside it. He was the first Chief Justice since William Howard Taft (1921–29) to devote considerable effort to judicial administration, particularly but not exclusively in the federal judiciary, as he took seriously his official title of Chief Justice of *the United States*. The range of his activities was greater than Taft's. In addition to creating institutions like the Institute for Court Management, which has provided training for court administrators, and the National Center for State Courts, which provides technical assistance to state courts and conducts research on topics of concern to them, Burger was the first Chief Justice to appoint an administrative assistant to help with his administrative tasks for both the Court and the judicial system as a whole; and his efforts at legislative-executive-judicial contact led to annual meetings among leaders of the three branches to discuss administration of justice issues.[69]

Burger did not hesitate to comment on a wide range of issues and made many speeches, most notably annual State of the Judiciary addresses to the American Bar Association, in which he called attention to problems like training of lawyers or excessive litigation; his comments on the latter led federal judicial districts to impose special requirements for admission to practice before the federal courts. He also called for restructuring of the circuits; elimination of three-judge district courts (now accomplished: see pages 47-48) and diversity of citizenship jurisdiction (not accomplished: see pages 182-83); and for limitations on federal judicial power over state criminal cases, a position consonant with his votes in the Court's decisions.[70] In this, Burger is like most other recent Chief Justices, whose "administrative and legal philosophies . . . have complemented one another." Indeed, he may have found it "advantageous to rephrase as a judicial administration issue a question having far-reaching substantive public policy implications."[71] He certainly managed to place on the national agenda some matters that probably would not otherwise have been placed there—most specifically, the proposal for a National Court of Appeals, or Intercircuit Tribunal, to handle cases on national interpretation of the law that the Supreme Court, because of its workload, cannot handle (see pages 62-63). Burger's retirement may well reduce much of the thrust behind that proposal.

Burger's willingness to speak out was not matched by a willingness to engage in debate. His many formal appearances were held under strict conditions of his choosing, and he would not otherwise meet with the press, justifying this in terms of a First Amendment "right to be left alone." The American Bar Association, after at first acceding to Burger's wishes that his State of the Judiciary addresses to them not be televised, later decided he would not be allowed to control media coverage of *their* activities, and the Chief Justice adjusted his position. These matters raise, and leave unresolved, the question of how "public" a figure the Chief Justice is expected to be. Perhaps a Chief Justice who is going to venture into the "outer world" beyond the Court has to accept more graciously the "costs" of having to deal with the media and others in part on their terms.

Burger's retirement also leaves unresolved the larger issue of how much time we wish a Chief Justice to devote to judicial administration—a question of importance but not of burning political significance. The chief justice of a lower court, where not all judges sit on all cases, can shed some caseload to provide time for administrative duties, but the Chief Justice, sitting on a court where all justices are expected to sit on all cases, cannot do so. The result is thus a trade-off between attention to internal court leadership and to supervision of judicial administration. Do we want to continue a situation in which the Chief's judicial administration efforts lessen the effectiveness of a within-Court leader, producing more division in its rulings? (By going outside the Court to press policies that complement his jurisprudence but that his colleagues have not approved, the Chief Justice may actually increase within-Court friction.[72]) Or, if we want a Chief Justice to focus on the Court and to be less interested in judicial administration, how is supervision of judicial administration to occur? Warren Burger's tenure as Chief Justice raises these questions, but they are a long way from being answered.

Some First Thoughts on the Rehnquist Court

At the end of only one term with William Rehnquist, the sixteenth Chief Justice, in the center chair and Justice Scalia on the Court, it is far too early to tell what the Rehnquist Court is going to be like. Its first term saw expected conservatism in the criminal procedure area, as the Court upheld searches in a variety of situations; upheld the death penalty in most cases it considered, most significantly against a challenge based on its racially discriminatory application; and upheld preventive detention. The Court supported property rights by ruling that land-use regulations constitute "takings" requiring compensation, and upheld state laws making takeovers of corporations more difficult. Important rulings on federalism upheld a law requiring withholding of federal transportation funds if a state did not adopt 21 as the minimum drinking age, and allowed federal courts to order governors to comply with valid extradition requests. At the same time, the Court was liberal on many important civil liberties and civil rights matters, most notably in upholding affirmative action programs involving hiring and promotion. In addition, it upheld a state law providing for pregnancy leaves; allowed Arabs and Jews to sue under a civil rights statute protecting against racial discrimination; ruled that communicable diseases are "handicaps" within the protection of the Rehabilitation Act; and said Rotary Clubs could be required to admit women. The Court also struck down a state requirement that "creation science" be taught along with evolution.

Justice Powell, important as a "swing vote," retired at the end of the first term of the Rehnquist Court, and the ages of some of its other members, Brennan, Blackmun, and Marshall, all around 80, means the likelihood of changes in its membership through death. President Reagan's opportunity to name a replacement for Justice Powell means the strong possibility the Court's tone would become increasingly conservative. However, the intransigence of the Reagan administration's conservatism on social policy matters increased the resolve of Justice Blackmun to remain on the Court and decreased President Reagan's chances of naming another justice. Until changes in personnel occur, and the new justices have been on the Court for a while, the "Rehnquist Court" is likely to remain unpredictable; a "Court," under anyone's chief justiceship, does not immediately establish itself. That was true of the Warren Court, which we remember primarily from its middle and later years, and is not any less likely to be true with the Rehnquist Court.

Expectations about the Rehnquist Court derived initially from perceptions of Rehnquist and Scalia. In Rehnquist's case, those perceptions are based on over 14 years of Supreme Court rulings, and stem from his "willingness to stake out a position in the strongest of terms" and his "well-formed jurisprudence," particularly his attention to the Framers' "original intent," as well as his "genuine warmth" and the "regard among both his colleagues and others who work at the Court"—interpersonal skills, not possessed by his predecessor, that could assist him in bringing his colleagues together during the Court's decision making.[73] We must be careful not to give too much weight to the frequency of Rehnquist's dissents as an associate justice (see page 239), as being Chief Justice might exert a moderating influence on him. However, the frequent dissents of his first term as Chief Justice limited his ability to exercise leadership, often leaving assignment of opinions in the hands of Justice Brennan. Indeed, it can be said that Brennan controlled the Court in important cases, with Justice Powell in the position of "swing" justice, and with Justice Scalia not joining Chief Justice Rehnquist as often as had been expected. ("Scalia Making Conservatives Nervous," read one headline.)

Justice Scalia clearly brought more "intellectual firepower" to the conservative position on the Court, which might lead to a clearer doctrinal line even if results are not significantly more conservative than those decided to date. Comparisons of Scalia and Burger, in which Scalia is said to be more conservative, are out of place because if Burger had been associate justice, his record would likely have been more conservative than he was as Chief Justice. Likewise, Scalia as an associate justice can be less moderate than someone in the "Chief's" chair.

Over the longer run, one might expect continuing retrenchment in the protection of civil liberties and civil rights both by the Supreme Court and by the federal courts, although the latter may come at least as much from President Reagan's appointees to those courts as from the Supreme Court's direction. If this leads to continuation of the period of increased state lawmaking begun during the Burger Court as people recognized that rights might receive greater protection there, the Supreme Court, while continuing to be an important actor in the American scheme, will be less central, perhaps by far, than it has been over the last three decades.

The Longer Term

Before leaving the subject of the Court's centrality in our political scheme, we should stand back from our detailed attention to the Warren and Burger Courts to get a broader perspective. In doing so, it is helpful to look at the debate over whether the Supreme Court has interfered with the work of the other, elected branches of government, and has followed them; certainly it would be less central if the latter were the case. In the 1950s, Robert Dahl asserted that the Court does not block the legislature and executive but, as a part of the dominant national alliance, actually legitimizes their work. In making his argument, Dahl relied on the 78 cases through 1957 in which the Supreme Court had exercised judicial review to invalidate 86 provisions of federal law. He also considered the timing of that review. Only half of the Court's actions came within four years of the legislation's enactment, with more than one-third of the "prompt" overrulings occurring during the Court's emasculation of the New Deal. In most instances when recent legislation was overturned, Congress reversed the Court or the Court itself did so somewhat later.

Seldom is the Court outside the dominant alliance for long, according to Dahl; moreover, the Court generally can do little without support from president and Congress. The Court might win small battles, but the justices are not likely to be successful "on matters of *major* policy, particularly if successive presidents and Congresses continue to support the policy the Court has called unconstitutional." When other political actors are unable to decide important questions, the Court can take action, but even then it does so at great risk and can succeed only if its actions are in tune with the norms of the political leadership.[74]

This position has been met directly. One argument is that Dahl overestimated the Court's ability to legitimize; another, that Dahl *under*estimated the Supreme Court's effectiveness. In arguing the first of these two positions, David Adamany says the Court cannot legitimize unless it strikes down the acts of other branches at least occasionally. If all statutes and administrative actions were sustained, the Court's ability to legitimize would be meaningless. During constitutional crises, the Court cannot grant legitimacy because at such times justices, having been appointed earlier, are of the party opposite to that controlling the elected branches; the Court's actions invalidating legislation, more likely when one political party has dominated Congress and nominees of the other party controlled the Court, certainly do not grant legitimacy to the new coalition. Instead, conflict between the Court and the elected branches after realigning elections—those in which party control of the presidency changes and there is substantial shift in the voters' partisan identification—has "somewhat discredited and sometimes checked the lawmaking majority." In each such situation, however, the result has been "a clash that left doubtful the Court's capacity ultimately to legitimize the new regime and its policies." One hardly has legitimization when as a result of changes in personnel or its own strategic movement the Court finally adopts the dominant coalition's position. Instead there is "more the appearance of surrender to superior force."[75]

The public also does not seem to know about the Court's legitimizing role; what little the public does know is principally about cases in which majorities have been checked, not legitimized (see pages 348-49). The Court's decisions also do not eliminate substantial opposition to policies the Court has enunciated or prevent legislative attacks on the Court and efforts to reverse its rulings. It is important to note, however, that the Court's opinions do provide ammunition for those defending the Court's position. Moreover, the views of political elites, who know more than does the general public about the Court and its decisions (see page 349), are largely conditioned by the elites' political attitudes, not the Court's actions. Thus the Court does not legitimize policy for the nation through the elites; elites confer legitimacy on the courts. The Court does not itself help create respect for the political system, but commands respect because it is part of the political system. This ultimately saves the Court when a new political coalition considers limiting the justices.

In a response to Dahl from another direction, Jonathan Casper noted that the Court has intervened decisively in the policymaking process, holding 32 provisions of federal law unconstitutional in 28 cases from 1957 through 1974— roughly one-fourth of the instances in which national legislation had been invalidated up to that time. Even when ultimately overturned, Court decisions delay implementation of policies for some years after they are enacted, further indication of the Court's effectiveness. (Prompt overrulings of legislation—within four years of enactment—occurred in only a few of the cases. In only one, on the 18-year-old-vote, and in no case involving older legislation, was the Court reversed.) Also important in evaluating the Court's effects are the Court's statutory interpretation rulings, which have produced important policy on a wide range of subjects. When one assesses the Court's effectiveness, its initiatives not involving invalidation of national legislation, such as Marshall's *McCulloch v. Maryland* and *Gibbons v. Ogden* rulings, must also be taken into account, as should the Court's introduction of new issues and new participants into the political process, which may assist actors' ability "to attract adherents, mobilize resources, and build institutions."[76]

The Supreme Court's Roles

Out of this look at the controversy in which courts are often embroiled, at the Supreme Court's changing place in the American political system, and at the Court's recent pattern of decisions, we can begin to get some sense of the roles the Court has played, does play, and is expected to play, from its "unique position as the only institution in our society capable of an authoritative, final judicial resolution of a controversy governed by federal law."[77]

Article III of the Constitution mentions "judicial power" and indicates the reach of that power. "Judicial power" is not otherwise explained nor is the

Supreme Court's work otherwise indicated. There are, however, functions, or tasks, generally associated with the highest appellate court in a nation's legal system. These functions include:

- marking boundaries between national power and state power;
- maintaining boundaries between decision-making units at any level of government;
- interpreting and clarifying statutory law and common (judge-made) law;
- delineating limits of governmental authority against claims of individual liberty;
- insuring its place as final interpreter of the Constitution and laws; and
- overseeing lower courts' interpretation and application of legal rules.[78]

The judicial power shall extend to all cases, in law and equity, arising under this Constitution, the laws of the United States, and treaties made, or which shall be made, under their authority; to all cases affecting ambassadors, other public ministers and consuls; to all cases of admiralty and maritime jurisdiction; to controversies to which the United States shall be party; to controversies between two or more states; between a state and citizens of another state; between citizens of different states; between citizens of the same state claiming lands under grants of different states; and between a state, or the citizens thereof, and foreign states, citizens or subjects. (Art. III, Sec. 2)

These multiple tasks do not necessarily fit together well and may in fact conflict with each other. Thus the Supreme Court, "a court of law operating within a malleable but recognizable set of rules," is both "a tribunal dispensing justice between litigants" and "a coequal branch of the federal government with a responsibility for formulating national policy while deciding specific cases."[79] While it is generally agreed that the Court "can no longer act to ensure that justice is done in each individual case," there is "an unwillingness or inability to resolve conflicting visions of the Court's responsibilities." Yet the functions the Court is supposed to perform or might perform are not important simply in the abstract but affect how the Court conducts its business.[80]

When the Supreme Court performs the functions or tasks identified above for a highest appellate court, the Court becomes a principal national policymaker. Some expect the Court to be such an actor; they assign it such a role. Many other actors in the American governmental system have not, however, fully or easily accepted that broad role. For many years the principal belief about the Supreme Court—still believed by many (see pages 351-52)—was that the Court did not make, but only found, the law. The idea that there was an external, immutable truth that could be found through "right reason" (an idea that is part of the philosophical view known as *natural law*) took the form that judges found preestablished law in statutes, regulations, and particularly the Constitution, applying in specific cases the intentions of the authors of those documents. Reverence for the Supreme Court, which was thought to be "above politics," reinforced this view: the Constitution became our Bible and the Supreme Court justices our high priests, and the public transferred "our sense of the definitive and timeless character of the Constitution to the judges who expound it."[81]

The belief that courts found rather than made the law has had considerable force and has been enunciated by the justices themselves. It was stated perhaps most starkly by Justice Owen Roberts just one year before President Franklin Roosevelt attempted to "pack" the Court because of its obstruction of the New Deal:

> When an Act of Congress is appropriately challenged in the courts as not conforming to the constitutional mandate the judicial branch of the Government has only one duty—to lay the article of the Constitution which is invoked beside the statute which is challenged and to decide whether the latter squares with the former. All the court does, or can do, is to announce its considered judgment upon the question. The only power it has, if such it may be called, is the power of judgment. This court neither approves nor condemns any legislative policy. Its delicate and difficult office is to ascertain and declare whether the legislation is in accordance with, or in contravention of, the provisions of the Constitution; and, having done that, its duty ends.[82]

This disingenuous statement—by a justice who was soon to shift his vote on the validity of economic regulation in the famous "Switch in Time That Saved Nine" (by blunting FDR's 1937 attack on the Court)—has been called the *slot machine theory of judicial intepretation*: if you get two apples and a lemon, you lose; if three oranges appear, you win. Despite its amazingly simplistic character, this myth of what judges do has been perpetuated even by some who realize it to be a myth because they believe that the myth makes the Court's decisions legitimate in the eyes of those affected by them. Perhaps this explains Justice Potter Stewart's recent remark, "For me there is only one possible way to judge cases and that is to judge each case on its own facts of record, under the law and the United States Constitution, conscientiously, independently, and with complete personal detachment."[83]

Myth or no myth, the Supreme Court is without doubt a policymaker, "not an impartial arbiter but a participant in social conflict [seeking] to serve twin goals of system stability and responsible government through conflict management."[84] The Court may do this in part by giving legitimacy to existing policy (but see pages 29-30). It also helps manage conflict by providing an arena in which major national issues can be debated, even when the Court itself does not resolve the issues that are raised, "by clarifying and sharpening political conflicts," by making choices in disputes "intelligible and explainable."[85] As deTocqueville noted long ago, most political, economic, and social issues in the United States are transformed into legal questions that end up in court. When legislative and executive arenas are not open to debate on major issues, such as racial equality before the 1960s, those issues are particularly likely to be moved to the courts for resolution. Even when elected officials do consider important issues, they may prefer to allow ultimate resolution of those issues to be made by the justices rather than assuming responsibility themselves. However, the Court's actions may raise the level of conflict or provoke dispute rather than resolving it, a major result of the 1973 abortion decision. And we must remember that, for all its importance, the Supreme Court is "in vital respects a dependent body"— dependent on others for its jurisdiction, for its funding, for the nomination and confirmation of its members, and, perhaps most important, for the carrying out of its mandates.[86]

The Supreme Court's policy-making role was made clear by the Judiciary Act of 1925 (the "Judges Bill," because justices strongly urged its adoption), which gave the Court its present power to select the cases it would hear. A court required to decide all cases brought to it, like the U.S. courts of appeals, could be more easily seen as a regular "court of law," or what might be called a "court of errors and appeals," engaging primarily in "error-correction" (review of trial court decisions for error) rather than "law-making" (or "institutional review," in which the court would "announce, clarify and harmonize" the law).[87] Yet it is hard to say that a court is not making policy when it can choose cases affecting broad classes of people and use them to announce rules intended to have general application. Indeed, the justices themselves have made clear that the Court is expected to decide "cases of broad significance" and not "to correct every perceived error coming from the lower. . . . courts,"[88] although the Court does take some cases because of "human concerns" and dissenters have argued that it engages in too much "error-correction" instead of attending to its "broader responsibilities."

Because cases of broad significance more often than not produce division in the Court, indicating that the law can hardly be clear or obvious, it is quite difficult to maintain the view that the justices are only finding the law. If a trial judge decides a case one way, only to be reversed by an appellate court by a vote of, say, 8-7, and the Supreme Court reverses in turn by a 5-4 vote, can one claim the law is being "found"? (One is reminded of the joke, "There stands the Supreme Court like a rock, 5-4.") The law-finding myth may not have been difficult to believe when the Court's rulings conformed closely to the nation's predominant ideology, as in the probusiness era of the late nineteenth century before the Court obtained the authority to choose its cases. However, the conflict between President Franklin Roosevelt and the Court over New Deal programs helped considerably both to alter the view that the Court found law and to produce a realization that "judicial decisions are not babies brought by judicial storks, but are born out of the travail of economic circumstances."[89] Chief Justice Charles Evans Hughes' statement that the law is what the judges say it is, a recognition that judges exercise discretion in interpreting ambiguous language in statutes and the Constitution, further confirmed the realization. Although debate continued about what the Supreme Court *should* do, doubt about its policymaking role and the political effects of its decisions was further extinguished by resistance to and attacks on rulings of the Warren Court on such subjects as internal security, reapportionment, school prayer, and criminal procedure. The hold of the myth of the Court as lawfinder may be further reduced by the portrayal in *The Brethren* of the very human traits of the Burger Court's justices and of their bargaining and negotiating over the Court's opinions, and from revelations about continuing involvement in extrajudicial political activities by Justices Louis Brandeis and Felix Frankfurter (see pages 289-90).[90]

Virtually all who follow the Court's work now admit that the Court does make policy and cannot avoid doing so. Some of the judges have even openly acknowledged that this is the case. Justice Byron White, dissenting in *Miranda v. Arizona*, argued that the majority's ruling, while not exceeding the Court's powers, served to "underscore the obvious—that the Court has not discovered or found the law in making today's decision, nor has it derived it from irrefutable sources." Instead it had made new law "in much the same way that it has done in the course of interpreting other great clauses of the Constitution. This is what the Court historically has done. Indeed, *it is what it must do* and will continue to do until and unless there is some fundamental change in the constitutional distribution of governmental powers."[91]

Yet from time to time judges try to say that they do not engage in policy-making based on their personal values—that they act differently as judges from the way they would act in other situations. As Justice Frankfurter put it in 1943 while dissenting when the Court invalidated the compulsory flag salute for school children:

> As judges we are neither Jew nor Gentile, neither Catholic nor agnostic. As a member of this Court I am not justified in writing my private notions of policy into the Constitution. . . . The duty of a judge who must decide which of two claims before the Court shall prevail . . . is not that of the ordinary person.[92]

Justice Blackmun, dissenting in 1972 when the majority invalidated the death penalty as then applied, said the punishment "violates childhood's training and life's experience" and that as a legislator he would sponsor legislation to repeal the penalty and as a governor he would use executive clemency to prevent people from being executed. But, he said, "There—on the Legislative Branch of the State or Federal Government, and secondarily, on the Executive Branch—is where the authority and responsibility for this kind of action lies."[93]

Such statements may continue to provide support for those who continue to believe that the Court finds the law and that it should act in special, nonpolitical ways. These beliefs are part of the context within which the Court, like any other policymaker, must act and which serve to constrain its actions. Indeed, the Supreme Court must continue to act like a court if it is to be effective. However, such statements, even if deeply felt by the person making them, may not only distract us from seeing the political values supported by the justices' votes but may well be irrelevant for those most directly affected by the Court's decisions.

Whatever a judge's anguish and however moving the statement of that anguish, the ultimate consumer is interested in the judge's votes, in the specific outcome of the case, not in the judge's rhetoric, no matter how much that rhetoric interests other judges and lawyers. Thus someone on Death Row would be more interested in Justice Blackmun's vote to uphold capital punishment than in the justice's personal unhappiness about the death penalty.

Judges cannot put past experience and personal values, particularly their policy views, fully to one side, particularly if they are members of a high appellate court that decides controversial cases. It has been argued that judges are readily interchangeable one for another (fungible). Were that true, however, senators and interest groups would not display such concern about the values of the potential members of the High Court, as Right-to-Life advocates did about Sandra Day O'Connor's votes in the Arizona Senate on abortion issues; as women's groups did about Antonin Scalia's lack of sympathy with feminist concerns; and as civil rights groups did about William Rehnquist—first, at the time of his initial appointment to the Court, about his opposition to a public accommodations ordinance in Phoenix, and, then, at the time of his nomination to be Chief Justice, about his harassment of minority voters and the racial and religious restrictive covenants attached to deeds on property he owned.

Personal values do not, however, always dominate judges' decisions (see pages 246-56). Judges vary in the degree to which they can put their personal views of policy to one side rather than making themselves as highly predictable as was William O. Douglas at the liberal end of the political spectrum and as William H. Rehnquist has been at the conservative end. *Judicial role conceptions*—expectations, based on others' views, of what a judge should do—can affect judges' actions, as can other factors, including the Court's internal institutional norms. This is true even in a court like the U.S. Supreme Court, which can choose the cases it hears, although the presence of a high proportion of the most controversial cases will result in judges' policy positions being more evident. Because the justices' policy positions do play a major part in the Supreme Court's decisions, the Court is thus quite clearly a policymaker, although the political *effects* of its decisions would make it one even if judges kept personal views fully under wraps.

As a policymaker, the Supreme Court does not play a single uniform policymaking role. There are differences from one policy area to the next in the degree to which the Court makes policy. At times policy-making is evident in major single decisions; at other times policy develops cumulatively through several decisions in a policy area. In some areas, the Court may be a "policy leader"; in others, it may avoid such leadership. It may accept Congress' statement of the need for a statute or an administrative agency's rationale for a regulation, or it may make its own determination of the need and evaluation of the rationale. Such variation "might seem rather strange in an isolated and insulated court administering The Law by processes of rigorous legal logic" but is not unusual "in a political agency faced with a wide range of problems, each entailing a different constellation of political forces."[94] However, although the Court is a policy-maker, it is not just any old political actor. It wears special garb, proceeds by means of special forms, and uses specialized language. It is *both* a political institution and, because of its format, procedures, and language, a legal one.

Notes

1. *Brown v. Allen*, 344 U.S. 443 at 540 (1953).

2. This section is drawn from Stephen L. Wasby, "Arrogation of Power or Accountability: 'Judicial Imperialism' Revisited," *Judicature* 65 (October 1981): 209–19.

3. Christopher Wolfe, *The Rise of Modern Judicial Review: From Constitutional Interpretation to Judge-made Law* (New York: Basic Books, 1986), pp. ix, 3, 60, 204, 259.

4. See Donald Horowitz, *The Courts and Social Policy* (Washington, D.C.: The Brookings Institution, 1977); Nathan Glazer, "Toward an Imperial Judiciary," *The Public Interest* 40 (Fall 1975): 104–23; Raoul Berger, *Government by the Judiciary: The Transformation of the Fourteenth Amendment* (Cambridge, Mass.: Harvard University Press, 1977).

5. For a well-developed set of criteria for examining the relative capacity of policymaking institutions, see Lief Carter, "When Courts Should Make Policy: An Institutional Approach," *Public Law and Public Policy*, ed. John Gardiner (New York: Praeger, 1977), pp. 141–57.

6. Ralph Cavanagh and Austin Sarat, "Thinking About Courts: Toward and Beyond a Jurisprudence of Judicial Competence," *Law & Society Review* 14 (Winter 1980): 406.

7. For a more complete discussion, see Stephen L. Wasby, "Accountability of the Courts," *Accountability in Urban Society*, ed. Scott Greer et al. (Beverly Hills, Calif.: Sage, 1978), pp. 143–68.

8. Ibid., p. 145.

9. Martin Shapiro, *Courts: A Comparative and Political Analysis* (Chicago: University of Chicago Press, 1981), p. 20.

10. Richard J. Richardson and Kenneth N. Vines, *The Politics of Federal Courts: Lower Courts in the United States* (Boston: Little, Brown, 1970), pp. 8–11.

11. See Jack Peltason, *Fifty-Eight Lonely Men* (New York: Harcourt, Brace and World, 1961); Charles Hamilton, *The Bench and the Ballot: Southern Federal Judges and Black Voters* (New York: Oxford University Press, 1973); Micheal Giles and Thomas Walker, "Judicial Policy-Making and Southern School Segregation," *Journal of Politics* 37 (November 1975): 917–36.

12. Others were said by Chief Justice Hughes to have been *Hepburn v. Griswold*, 75 U.S. 603 (1870), the first Legal Tender Case, in which the Court invalidated use of paper money to pay debts, and *Pollock v. Farmers' Loan and Trust Co.*, 157 U.S. 429 (1895), holding the income tax unconstitutional. Some have referred to more contemporary cases, like *Miranda v. Arizona*, 384 U.S. 436 (1966), or the 1973 abortion rulings (*Roe v. Wade*, 410 U.S. 113, and *Doe v. Bolton*, 410 U.S. 179), in such terms.

13. For example, *Hurtado v. California*, 110 U.S. 516 (1884) (grand jury indictment), and *Twining v. New Jersey*, 211 U.S. 78 (1908) (Fifth Amendment).

14. *Abrams v. United States*, 250 U.S. 616 (1919), and *Schenck v. United States*, 249 U.S. 47 (1919). See also *Gitlow v. New York*, 268 U.S. 652 (1925).

15. On child labor legislation, see *Hammer v. Dagenhart*, 247 U.S. 251 (1918) (commerce), and *Bailey v. Drexel Furniture*, 259 U.S. 20 (1922) (taxation).

16. For example, *Schechter Poultry Corp. v. United States*, 295 U.S. 495 (1935); *United States v. Butler*, 297 U.S. 1 (1936); *Carter v. Carter Coal Co.*, 298 U.S. 238 (1936).

17. *National Labor Relations Board v. Jones & Laughlin Steel Corp.*, 301 U.S. 1 (1937); *United States v. Darby*, 312 U.S. 100 (1941).

18. *National League of Cities v. Usery*, 426 U.S. 833 (1976); *Garcia v. San Antonio Metropolitan Transit Authority*, 105 S.Ct. 1005 (1985).

19. *Shelley v. Kraemer*, 334 U.S. 1 (1948) (restrictive covenants); *Sweatt v. Painter*, 339 U.S. 629 (1950) and *McLaurin v. Board of Regents*, 339 U.S. 637 (1950) (law school and graduate education). Whites-only primary elections had been invalidated during the war: *Smith v. Allwright*, 321 U.S. 649 (1944).

20. Reapportionment: *Reynolds v. Sims*, 377 U.S. 533 (1964); obscenity: *Roth v. United States/Alberts v. California*, 354 U.S. 476 (1957); libel: *New York Times v. Sullivan*, 376 U.S. 254 (1964); school prayer: *Engel v. Vitale*, 370 U.S. 421 (1962) and *Abington School District v. Schempp*, 374 U.S. 203 (1963); public accommodations: *Heart of Atlanta Motel v. United States*, 371 U.S. 241 (1964) and *Katzenbach v. McClung*, 379 U.S. 294 (1964); voting: *South Carolina v. Katzenbach*, 383 U.S. 301 (1966); housing: *Jones v. Mayer*, 392 U.S. 409 (1968). See generally Stephen L. Wasby, *Continuity and Change: From the Warren Court to the Burger Court* (Pacific Palisades, Calif.: Goodyear, 1976), pp. 71–77.

21. *Harper v. Virginia Board of Elections*, 383 U.S. 663 (1963); *Shapiro v. Thompson*, 394 U.S. 618 (1960).

22. *Terry v. Ohio*, 392 U.S. 1 (1968); *Warden v. Hayden*, 387 U.S. 294 (1967); *Lewis v. United States*, 385 U.S. 206 (1966) and *Hoffa v. United States*, 385 U.S. 293 (1966); *Berger v. New York*, 388 U.S. 41 (1967).

23. Lewis M. Steel, "Nine Men in Black Who Think White," *New York Times Magazine*, October 13, 1968, pp. 56, 117.

24. Robert G. McCloskey, "Reflections on the Warren Court," *Virginia Law Review* 51 (November 1965): 1234.

25. Russell W. Galloway, Jr., "The Second Period of the Warren Court: The Liberal Trend Abates (1957–1961)," *Santa Clara Law Review* 19 (1979): 947.

26. See Galloway, "The Third Period of the Warren Court: Liberal Dominance (1962–1969)," *Santa Clara Law Review* 20 (1980): 773–829.

27. Richard Funston, "Foreword: The Burger Court: New Directions in Judicial Policymaking," *Emory Law Journal* 23 (Summer 1974): 656.

28. Russell W. Galloway, Jr., "The Taft Court (1921–1929)," *Santa Clara Law Review* 25 (1985): 5, 11.

29. Paul Bender, "The Reluctant Court," *Civil Liberties Review* 2 (Fall 1975): 101.

30. *Hudgens v. National Labor Relations Board*, 424 U.S. 507 (1976), overruling *Food Employees v. Logan Valley Plaza*, 391 U.S. 308 (1968).

31. *Grove City College v. Bell*, 465 U.S. 555 (1984) and *Firefighters v. Stotts*, 467 U.S. 561 (1984) (discrimination and affirmative action); *Illinois v. Gates*, 462 U.S. 213 (1983) (informants); *New York v. Quarles*, 467 U.S. 649 (1986) (*Miranda*); *United States v. Leon*, 468 U.S. 897 (1984) and *Massachusetts v. Sheppard*, 468 U.S. 981 (1984) ("good faith" exception); *Hudson v. Palmer*, 467 U.S. 517 (1984) (prisoners' rights); *Schall v. Martin*, 467 U.S. 253 (1984) (detention of juveniles).

32. See Benno C. Schmidt, Jr., "As Burger Continues, His Court Becomes Unstable," *New York Times*, September 30, 1984.

33. *Bowers v. Hardwick*, 106 S.Ct. 2841 (1986); *Bethel School District v. Fraser*, 106 S.Ct. 3159 (1986).

34. *Local 28 v. E.E.O.C.*, 106 S.Ct. 3019 (1986) and *Local 39 v. City of Cleveland*, 106 S.Ct. 3063 (1986) (affirmative action); *Thornburgh v. Gingles*, 106 S.Ct. 2752 (1986) (vote dilution); and *Batson v. Kentucky*, 106 S.Ct. 1712 (1986) (jury selection).

35. *Bishop v. Wood*, 426 U.S. 341 (1976).

36. Jesse Choper, "The Burger Court: Misconceptions Regarding Judicial Restraint and Insensitivity to Individual Rights," *Syracuse Law Review* 30 (Spring 1979): 771–72. The first two cases are

Oregon v. Mitchell, 400 U.S. 112 (1970) (18-year-olds' right to vote) and *National League of Cities v. Usery*, 426 U.S. 83 (1976) (application of the minimum wage to state and local employees); the last case is *Buckley v. Valeo*, 424 U.S. 1 (1976) (method of selecting the Federal Election Commission).

37.   Gayle Binion, "The Disadvantaged Before the Burger Court: The New Unequal Protection," *Law & Policy Quarterly* 4 (January 1982): 39–41.

38.   Robert C. Welsh, "Whose Federalism? The Burger Court's Treatment of State Civil Liberties Judgments," *Hastings Constitutional Law Quarterly* 10 (Summer 1983): 846. The data is based on "paid" cases only.

39.   Harold J. Spaeth, "Burger Court Review of State Court Civil Liberties Decisions," *Judicature* 68 (February–March 1985): 285.

40.   *Runyon v. McCrary*, 427 U.S. 160 (1976) (admission to racially discriminatory private schools). See also *Bob Jones University v. United States*, 461 U.S. 574 (1983).

41.   *Washington v. Davis*, 426 U.S. 229 (1976) ("intent" rather than effect required to show a constitutional violation) (employment); *Village of Arlington Heights v. Metropolitan Housing Development Corp.*, 429 U.S. 252 (1977) (housing); *City of Mobile v. Bolden*, 447 U.S. 55 (1980) (voting); *Teamsters v. United States*, 431 U.S. 324 (1977) and *American Tobacco Co. v. Patterson*, 456 U.S. 63 (1982) (seniority).

42.   *Local 28 v. E.E.O.C.*, 106 S.Ct. 3019 (1986); *Local 93 v. City of Cleveland*, 106 S.Ct. 3063 (1986).

43.   *Dayton Board of Education v. Brinkman*, 443 U.S. 527 (1979) and *Columbus Board of Education v. Penick*, 443 U.S. 449 (1979).

44.   *Reed v. Reed*, 404 U.S. 71 (1971); *Frontiero v. Richardson*, 411 U.S. 676 (1973); *Taylor v. Louisiana*, 419 U.S. 522 (1975); *Cleveland Board of Education v. LaFleur*, 414 U.S. 632 (1974).

45.   *City of Akron v. Akron Center for Reproductive Health*, 462 U.S. 416 (1983); *Thornburg v. American College of Obstetricians*, 106 S.Ct. 2169 (1986).

46.   *Harris v. McRae*, 448 U.S. 297 (1980).

47.   *North Haven Board of Education v. Bell*, 456 U.S. 512 (1982) (employment); *County of Washington v. Gunther*, 452 U.S. 161 (1981) (pay); *Rostker v. Goldberg*, 453 U.S. 57 (1981) (draft); *Grove City College v. Bell*, 465 U.S. 555 (1984) (sex discrimination in education aid).

48.   See *Wolman v. Walter*, 433 U.S. 229 (1977) (allowed: books, standardized testing and scoring, diagnostic services, therapeutic and remedial services; not allowed: instructional materials, equipment, field trips). *Grand Rapids School District v. Ball*, 105 S.Ct. 3216 (1985), and *Aguilar v. Felton*, 105 S.Ct. 3232 (1985) (shared time programs).

49.   *Mueller v. Allen*, 463 U.S. 388 (1983).

50.   *Wallace v. Jaffree*, 105 S.Ct. 2479 (1985).

51.   *Nebraska Press Association v. Stuart*, 427 U.S. 539 (1976) (gag order); *Branzburg v. Hayes*, 408 U.S. 665 (1972) (journalists' testimony about sources); *Parker v. Levy*, 417 U.S. 733 (1974) (military officers' free speech); *Greer v. Spock*, 424 U.S. 828 (1971) (military bases).

52.   *Virginia State Board of Phamacy v. Virginia Citizens Consumers Council*, 425 U.S. 748 (1976) (pharmacists); *Bates v. State Bar of Arizona*, 433 U.S. 350 (1977) and *Zauderer v. Office of Disciplinary Counsel*, 105 S. Ct. 2265 (1985) (lawyers); *Consolidated Edison Co. of New York v. Public Service Commission*, 447 U.S. 530 (1980) (bill inserts on controversial topics); *Central Hudson Gas & Electric Corp. v. Public Service Commission*, 447 U.S. 557 (1980) (promotional advertising). The most recent ruling is *Posadas de Puerto Rico Associates v. Tourism Company of Puerto Rico*, 106 S.Ct. 2968 (1986) (upholding ban on advertising of lawful casinos to residents of Puerto Rico although advertising to tourists allowed).

53.   *Gannett v. DePasquale*, 443 U.S. 368 (1979); *Richmond Newspapers v. Virginia*, 448 U.S. 55 (1980); *Press-Enterprise Co. v. Superior Court*, 106 S.Ct. 2735 (1986).

54.   *Payton v. New York*, 445 U.S. 573 (1980); *Steagald v. United States*, 451 U.S. 204 (1981).

55.   *United States v. Knotts*, 460 U.S. 276 (1983) (beeper); *California v. Ciraolo*, 106 S.Ct. 1809 (1986) and *Dow Chemical Co. v. United States*, 106 S.Ct. 1819 (1986) (aerial surveillance).

56.   *Zurcher v. Stanford Daily*, 436 U.S. 547 (1978); *Dalia v. United States*, 441 U.S. 236 (1979); *New Jersey v. T.L.O*, 105 S.Ct. 733 (1984).

57. *Harris v. New York*, 401 U.S. 222 (1971), reinforced by *Oregon v. Hass*, 420 U.S. 714 (1975).

58. *Dunaway v. New York*, 442 U.S. 200 (1979) (illegal stop); *Michigan v. Mosley*, 423 U.S. 96 (1975) (resumption of questioning); *United States v. Mandujano*, 425 U.S. 564 (1976) (grand jury); *Beckwith v. United States*, 425 U.S. 341 (1976) (tax investigation).

59. *Nix v. Williams*, 467 U.S. 431 (1984).

60. *Kirby v. Illinois*, 406 U.S. 682 (1972) (line-up); *Ross v. Moffitt*, 417 U.S. 600 (1974) (discretionary appeals); *Morrissey v. Brewer*, 408 U.S. 471 (1972) (parole); *Gagnon v. Scarpelli*, 411 U.S. 778 (1973) (probation); *Wolff v. McDonnell*, 418 U.S. 539 (1974) (prison discipline).

61. *Bell v. Wolfish*, 441 U.S. 520 (1979) (pretrial detainees); *Rhodes v. Chapman*, 452 U.S. 337 (1981) (double-celling); *Hudson v. Palmer*, 468 U.S. 517 (1984) and *Block v. Rutherford*, 468 U.S. 568 (1984) (searches of cells); *Daniels v. Williams*, 106 S.Ct. 662 (1986) and *Davidson v. Cannon*, 106 S.Ct. 668 (1986) (suits for injuries).

62. *North Carolina v. Alford*, 400 U.S. 25 (1970) and *Santobello v. New York*, 404 U.S. 527 (1971); *Brady v. United States*, 397 U.S. 542 (1970).

63. See *Gardner v. Florida*, 430 U.S. 349 (1977) (sentencing procedure); *Estelle v. Smith*, 451 U.S. 454 (1981) (limiting psychiatrist's testimony); *Bullington v. Missouri*, 451 U.S. 430 (1981) (application of double jeopardy); *Ford v. Wainwright*, 106 S.Ct. 2595 (1986) (mentally ill Death Row inmates).

64. *Lockett v. Ohio*, 438 U.S. 586 (1978); *Eddings v. Oklahoma*, 455 U.S. 104 (1982).

65. For basic procedures for handling stays, see *Barefoot v. Estelle*, 463 U.S. 880 (1983).

66. *Colorado v. Connelly*, 106 S.Ct. 785 (1986).

67. *Rose v. Clark*, 106 S.Ct. 3101 at 3112 (1986).

68. Benno C. Schmidt, Jr., "As Burger Continues, His Court Becomes Unstable," *New York Times*, September 30, 1984; "Court Under Burger Foiled Conservative Hopes, Powell Says," *Los Angeles Times*, August 13, 1986, p. 20.

69. See Edward A. Tamm and Paul C. Reardon, "Warren E. Burger and the Administration of Justice," *Brigham Young University Law Review* 1981: 447–521, particularly 452; and William F. Swindler, "The Chief Justice and Law Reform, 1921–1971," in *The Supreme Court Review*, ed. Philip Kurland (Chicago: University of Chicago Press, 1971), pp. 241–64.

70. See, for example, Warren E. Burger, "Annual Report to the American Bar Association by the Chief Justice of the United States," *American Bar Association Journal* 67 (March 1981): 290–93, and "Isn't There a Better Way?" *American Bar Association Journal* 68 (March 1982): 274–77. See also Arthur B. Landever, "Chief Justice Burger and Extra-Case Activism," *Journal of Public Law* 20 (1971): 523–41.

71. Peter G. Fish, "The Office of Chief Justice of the United States: Into the Federal Judiciary's Bicentennial Decade," *The Office of Chief Justice* (Charlottesville, Va.: University of Virginia, 1984), pp. 77, 115.

72. Ibid., p. 137.

73. A. E. Dick Howard, "A Key Fighter in Major Battles," *ABA Journal* 72 (June 15, 1986): 47–48.

74. Robert Dahl, *Democracy in the United States* (Chicago: Rand McNally, 1972), pp. 201–02. The original statement was Dahl, "Decision-Making in a Democracy: The Supreme Court as a National Policy-Maker," *Journal of Public Law* 7 (Fall 1957): 279–95.

75. David Adamany, "Legitimacy, Realigning Elections, and the Supreme Court," *Wisconsin Law Review* 1973: 825, 822.

76. Jonathan D. Casper, "The Supreme Court and National Policy Making," *American Political Science Review* 70 (March 1976): 3.

77. Samuel Estreicher and John E. Sexton, "A Managerial Theory of the Supreme Court's Responsibilities: An Empirical Study," *New York University Law Review* 59 (October 1984): 717.

78. Arthur D. Hellman, "The Business of the Supreme Court Under the Judiciary Act of 1925: The Plenary Docket in the 1970's," *Harvard Law Review* 91 (June 1978): 1716; D. Marie Provine, *Case Selection in the Supreme Court* (Chicago: University of Chicago Press, 1980), p. 101.

79. Walter F. Murphy, *Elements of Judicial Strategy* (Chicago: University of Chicago Press, 1964), pp. 208–09.

80. Estreicher and Sexton, "A Managerial Theory," 717, 710.

81. Max Lerner, "Constitution and Court as Symbols," *Yale Law Journal* 46 (1939): 1294–95.

82. *United States v. Butler*, 297 U.S. 1 at 62–63 (1936).

83. Potter Stewart, "Reflections on the Supreme Court," *Litigation* 8 (#3, Spring 1982): 8.

84. S. Sidney Ulmer, "Researching the Supreme Court in a Democratic Pluralist System: Some Thoughts on New Directions," *Law & Policy Quarterly* 1 (January 1979): 55.

85. Vincent Blasi, "The Rootless Activism of the Burger Court," in *The Burger Court: The Counter-Revolution That Wasn't*, ed. Blasi (New Haven, Conn.: Yale University Press, 1983), p. 209.

86. Robert H. Jackson, *The Supreme Court in the American System of Government* (Cambridge, Mass.: Harvard University Press, 1955), p. 10.

87. Paul D. Carrington, Daniel J. Meador, and Maurice Rosenberg, *Justice on Appeal* (St. Paul, Minn.: West Publishing Co., 1976), pp. 2–3.

88. *Boag v. MacDougall*, 454 U.S. 364 at 366 (1982) (Justice O'Connor, concurring).

89. Max Lerner, *Ideas for the Ice Age* (New York: Viking, 1941), p. 259.

90. Robert Woodward and Scott Armstrong, *The Brethren: Inside the Supreme Court* (New York: Simon and Schuster, 1979); Bruce Allen Murphy, *The Brandeis/Frankfurter Connection: The Secret Political Activities of Two Supreme Court Justices* (New York: Oxford University Press, 1982).

91. 384 U.S. 436 at 531–532 (1966); emphasis supplied.

92. *West Virginia State Board of Education v. Barnette*, 319 U.S 624 at 647 (1943).

93. *Furman v. Georgia*, 408 U.S. 238 at 405–6, 410–11 (1972).

94. Martin Shapiro, *Law and Politics in the Supreme Court* (New York: Free Press, 1964), p. 328.

2   Elements of the Federal
Judicial System

THIS CHAPTER IS INTENDED to provide a picture of the federal court system's overall structure. We look at the basic levels of the national court system and at associated specialized courts, starting with the district courts and moving to the courts of appeals, followed by a discussion of judicial administration. An examination of the Supreme Court and its position in the federal judicial system concludes the chapter.

The United States has a dual court system of separate national and state courts, a result of our system of federalism. There is a set of national courts including territorial courts, and each state has its own courts, giving us 52 separate court systems (the federal system, 50 states, and the District of Columbia). Each state has trial courts of general jurisdiction, that is, courts with legal authority to hear all civil and criminal cases; they are usually called district, superior, or circuit courts. All states also have specialized courts of one or more types, for example, for probate (wills and estates) or juvenile and family proceedings. Most states have an intermediate appellate court, to which all or most appeals are taken first, and a supreme court (in some states, called the court of appeals). Many states retain a fourth level of limited jurisdiction courts—the "inferior" (meaning lower) or "petty" courts—including justice-of-the-peace courts, mayors' courts, police courts, and some municipal courts established to assist with the higher volume of litigation in large urban areas. Appeals from these courts, instead of going directly to an appellate court, are often directed to the general jurisdiction trial court, sometimes for a new trial (trial *de novo*).

Although the Supreme Court of the United States, the only court specifically designated in the Constitution, is our principal interest as the apex of the federal judicial system, we must also pay attention to the lower federal courts. The national judicial structure—the Supreme Court, courts of appeals, district courts, and magistrates (connected to and generally subordinate to the district courts), as well as some specialized courts such as the bankruptcy courts—is similar to most states' court systems. The Supreme Court cannot initiate cases but must rely on the lower federal courts (and the state courts) as the source of its business, the place where cases are initiated and where they take the shape in which they arrive at the Supreme Court and with which the justices must then work. The lower federal courts are also where most federal litigation terminates so that they make much law in areas of litigation not reviewed or seldom reviewed by the Supreme Court. The basic relations among federal courts, discussed in this chapter, are portrayed in Figure 2.1. (For relations between state courts and federal courts, see Figure 5.1 in Chapter 5.)

Development of the Federal Court System

The federal court system as we now know it assumed its present basic form only late in the nineteenth century. The system of federal courts established by Congress in the Judiciary Act of 1789 was relatively elementary. In addition to the Supreme Court, specified by the Constitution itself (see Art. III, Sec. 1), the Congress created district courts and circuit courts. The district courts' jurisdic-

> The judicial power of the United States shall be vested in one Supreme Court, and in such inferior Courts as the Congress may from time to time ordain and establish. (Art. III, Sec. 1)

tion was not broad, and they dealt mainly with admiralty cases. The circuit courts, although they had some appellate jurisdiction over the district courts, were primarily trial courts for diversity of citizenship cases (suits between citizens of different states). These courts, created under the Judiciary Act of 1789, had final authority on most matters within their jurisdiction, with appeals limited by various technical provisions. This made the Supreme Court largely a court of review for *state* court rulings.

In the circuit courts, which did not have their own judges, a district judge and two Supreme Court justices were to sit twice a year in each district of the circuit. Almost immediately (in 1793), Congress reduced the burden on Supreme Court justices of attending court in the districts so that each year only one justice would have to sit once in each district. In 1801, the Federalists created 16 circuit court judgeships for six circuits, but in 1802 the Jeffersonian Democrats promptly repealed this action. The Act of 1801 also granted the circuit courts what we now call "federal question" jurisdiction, but the courts' opportunity to develop it was eliminated by the repealer, which the Supreme Court upheld.[1]

District judges were used increasingly in the circuit courts until after the Civil War, and the Supreme Court justice assigned to the circuit (the *circuit*

Figure 2.1. The Federal Court System

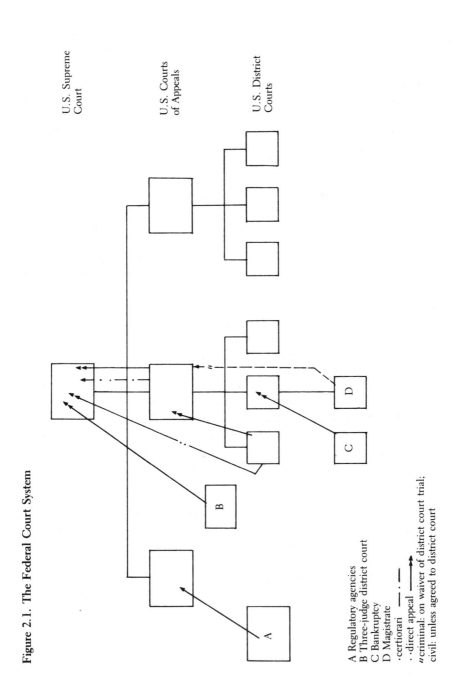

U.S. Supreme Court

U.S. Courts of Appeals

U.S. District Courts

A Regulatory agencies
B Three-judge district court
C Bankruptcy
D Magistrate
·certiorari   —·—
··direct appeal ——▶
"criminal: on waiver of district court trial;
civil: unless agreed to district court

justice) often did not visit certain parts of large western circuits. Because of the extreme distance from the East Coast to California, a separate circuit court—with its own circuit judges—was established for California. In 1869, nine judgeships were created specially for the circuit courts: these circuit judges had the same authority as the Supreme Court justices assigned to the circuit, who were now required to attend only one term of circuit court in each district of the circuit every two years. A circuit justice, circuit judge, or district judge could hold circuit court, or any two could sit as a panel. Nonetheless, district judges held circuit court most of the time, creating a dual role in which they sat in review over their own district court decisions. Supreme Court justices also had this dual role when they sat on circuit and later had to review their rulings appealed to the Supreme Court, a matter that concerned them. The justices handed down some very important rulings on circuit. Included were one of the first rulings on judicial review (*Hayburn's Case*, 1792), John Marshall's ruling on executive privilege in the Aaron Burr treason trial (*United States v. Burr*, 1807), Justice Bushrod Washington's opinion in *Corfield v. Coryell* (1823) on "privileges and immunities," and, later, Chief Justice Roger Taney's ruling—ignored by President Lincoln—on the detention of civilians by the military (*Ex parte Merryman*, 1861).

Supreme Court justices are no longer subject to the rigors of riding circuit. In the early days, they had to put up with "the dangers and miseries of overturned vehicles, runaway horses, rivers in full flood, or icebound and scruffy taverns."[2] There were even more serious dangers: the life of Justice Stephen Field, on circuit in California, was threatened by a disgruntled litigant who was shot and killed by the U.S. marshal assigned to guard the justice. After the state indicted the marshal for murder, he was transferred to the federal court's jurisdiction and was exonerated, the Supreme Court ruling that his action was part of properly enforcing the nation's laws (*In re Neagle*, 1890). Circuit duty was continued for many years because the lower courts needed help with their caseload and because the Supreme Court's caseload was not overwhelming; in addition, Congress felt that if the justices stayed in Washington, they might be dominated by the capital's lawyers, with whom they often shared rooming houses. If anything, the risk now is that the justices will not have sufficient contact with the hinterlands. However, they usually attend their circuit's judicial conference and in 1984 Justice Rehnquist, who had no experience as a trial judge, "rode out to Richmond" to preside over one trial. (His ruling in that case was reversed by the court of appeals.)

In the Judiciary Act of 1875, the district courts for the first time received general federal question jurisdiction, allowing them to hear civil suits involving at least $500 if the case arose "under the Constitution, laws, or treaties of the United States." (At the same time, the jurisdictional minimum for cases coming to the Supreme Court from the circuit courts was $5,000.) Congress did not provide for review of capital (death sentence) cases until 1889 and for all cases involving "infamous crimes"—those where a sentence of imprisonment was possible—until 1891.

The failure to create any lower federal courts in the Constitution, and the limited jurisdiction given them in the early years resulted from arguments that the state courts, bound by the Supremacy Clause (Art. VI), could be expected to enforce the Constitution. Whatever the force of such arguments in connection with the Constitution's ratification, competing considerations later came to the fore. Particularly important were the feelings of those wanting a strong national government that because the state courts were not enforcing federal law adequately, a federal judicial mechanism was necessary for that purpose.

In 1891, the U.S. Courts of Appeals (as they are now called) were established, to be staffed by two circuit judges and a Supreme Court justice, for whom a district judge could substitute. The old circuit courts, which thus became courts without full-time judges, were finally abolished in 1911, at last making district courts the dominant federal court of original jurisdiction. The presence of a regular set of intermediate appellate courts meant that the Supreme Court no longer had to accept all the cases in which its decision was sought, and the movement toward giving the Court control over what cases it would hear then began. This process of providing the Supreme Court with discretionary jurisdiction began in 1914, continued in 1916, and was fully consummated in the Judges Bill of 1925, which provided authority to hear large categories of cases on petition for a writ of certiorari (see page 73).

The District Courts

District courts are the federal judicial system's basic trial court, with which litigants having federal cases come in contact, and where both jury trials and nonjury (bench) trials take place. They can hear all civil and criminal cases for which Congress has provided, and their cases cover both a wide range of criminal offenses and diverse types of civil cases, including antitrust, commerce, patent and copyright, contract, and tort suits. Most district court civil cases involve private individuals or businesses raising federal questions or bringing suit under diversity of citizenship jurisdiction, but the United States government is a party in roughly one-fourth of the civil cases.

Each of the nation's 94 district courts, which sit at locations designated by statute, is located in a single state or territory, except for the District of Wyoming, which includes the Montana and Idaho portions of Yellowstone National Park. Twenty-six states, the District of Columbia, and the nation's four territories each constitute one district; the remaining states have two to four districts each. There are now 577 district court judgeships—more than double the number in 1960—with each judge appointed by the president with the advice and consent of the Senate (see pages 96-107). A district judge generally is appointed to a single district, although in some "floater" positions a judgeship is assigned to more than one district (for example, Eastern and Western Districts of Oklahoma), only eventually being assigned to a single district. District courts vary considerably in the number of judgeships. There are no more single-judge districts, but some have as few as two judges while the largest districts—like the Southern District of New York, which includes Manhattan—have more than 20. Other large districts include the Northern and Central Districts of California, centered at San Francisco and Los Angeles, respectively; the Northern District of Illinois (Chicago); and the Eastern District of Pennsylvania (Philadelphia).

District court caseloads have increased substantially in recent years in absolute numbers, up 178+ percent from 1969 to 1985, greatly exceeding the increase in district judgeships (69%). (Filings may increase when judgeships are added because potential litigants believe the judges will be able to decide cases more promptly.) Case filings per year—over 200,000 civil cases and 30,000 criminal cases—have not necessarily paralleled increases in population or economic growth,[3] but may reflect social trends, shifts in the nation's political agenda, and Supreme Court decisions, such as those in the 1960s protecting defendants' rights and facilitating state prisoners' access to federal courts. Growth in criminal cases has resulted both from increases in crime, for example, drug offenses, and from increased public pressure to "do something" about it, and from new federal criminal statutes. The Speedy Trial Act, by imposing a strict calendar on the stages of federal criminal cases from arrest and indictment through trial and providing for dismissal of a case for failure to meet designated deadlines, means that district courts must attend to criminal cases ahead of civil cases.

On the civil side, there have been increases in cases on environmental protection, job discrimination, education of the handicapped, and prison conditions, but Burger Court rulings restricting state prisoners' use of federal court and use of new prison grievance mechanisms have deflected some of the latter from the courts. The increase in the number of priority civil cases, a growing proportion of which involve challenges to actions of national, state, and local government agencies, coupled with the Speedy Trial Act's requirements, has strained the busier district courts' capacity to keep up with routine civil cases, leading to delay in processing them. Although the Supreme Court ruled in 1976 that district judges may *not* use workload as a reason for refusing to accept cases that are within their jurisdiction,[4] Chief Justice Burger and some of his colleagues, as well as many other lawyers, have advocated having Congress eliminate diversity of citizenship cases as one way of reducing caseload. District courts by no means have identical dockets, which vary depending on business or industry and other activities (such as major prisons) located in the district. Thus the Southern District of New York (S.D.N.Y.) has a large number of admiralty cases, as does the Eastern District of Louisiana (E.D.La.), which also has many Jones Act (personal injury to those working on the high seas) cases because of the Gulf of Mexico oil rigs.

Most district court decisions are final.[5] They are either not appealed, if appealed are settled prior to an appellate ruling, or, in the vast proportion of cases reviewed by the courts of appeals, are sustained—often in brief affirmances without opinion. In 1965–67, for example, roughly one-third of completed district court cases were taken to the appellate courts, but because of terminations before final submission, the proportion finally reviewed was only about one-fifth. When we add the fact that by no means all court of appeals rulings are carried to the Supreme Court, which grants review to only a very small percentage of those cases in which review is sought, "the great majority of district court decisions are neither reviewed nor reversed."[6] Thus district court decisions are *the* rulings in all but a very small percentage of cases decided there.

Moreover, appellate court review of district court output is not uniform across the districts within each circuit or across subject matters; indeed courts of appeals provide "sustained supervision" of district court decisions "in only a few areas of public policy."[7] In part because district court rulings on various subjects are not appealed in the same proportions, appellate review is not necessarily focused to produce uniformity in federal law or protection of important national interests. For example, where district judges resisted appellate rulings in civil rights cases, so that appellate supervision was most needed, appeal rates were among the lowest. The low rate of review and of appellate court reversal means that district courts follow appropriate legal doctrine less as a result of the explicit sanction of reversal by superiors than through informal controls, which include precedent, professional socialization including service with the court of appeals, anticipation of appellate judicial action, and ideological unity provided by shared regional and political backgrounds.[8]

District court cases are ordinarily heard by one judge. However, in special situations, three-judge district courts, composed of two district judges and a court of appeals judge, have been convened. Three-judge district courts were first established in 1903 to deal with requests for injunctions against Interstate Commerce Commission (ICC) orders. Because it was felt that allowing single district judges to invalidate state laws, particularly those regulating the economy, was giving them too much power, the jurisdiction of three-judge district courts was extended in 1910 to injunctions against state laws, in 1913 to those against state administrative actions, and in 1937 to those against federal statutes. Appeals from such panels do go directly to the Supreme Court—because of the importance of the cases and because an appeals court judge has already participated in hearing them—and are among those the Supreme Court must hear, although it disposes of most of them summarily.

Increased use of three-judge courts came from the mid-1960s through the early 1970s, as litigants sought injunctions against state laws said to interfere with civil rights. As a result, more cases came directly to the Supreme Court without benefit of prior treatment by the courts of appeals. Because the justices felt that these mandatory appeals, which accounted for a significant portion of the Court's decisions, hindered their ability to use their certiorari (discretionary) jurisdiction to choose the cases they would consider fully, they developed doctrines to limit use of three-judge district courts and called upon Congress to eliminate them.

Direct appeals were first eliminated with respect to ICC orders and government civil antitrust cases, and then, in 1976, Congress eliminated three-judge district courts except in legislative reapportionment cases or when Congress specifically provided for them, as in the Civil Rights Act of 1964 and the Voting Rights Act. A single judge now handles preliminary matters in such cases, and requests for injunctions against state laws now reach the Supreme Court only after the court of appeals has heard the case. When a district judge invalidates a federal statute, the case still goes directly to the Supreme Court.

District of Columbia and the Territories. In addition to the usual national courts—a district court and a court of appeals—the District of Columbia has a set of courts, established under Congress' authority to make laws for the nation's capital (Art. I, Sec. 8, cl. 17), that is closer in function to state courts. These courts, whose judges serve fixed terms, apply laws passed by Congress specifically for the District and those passed by the D.C. City Council. Prior to 1971, cases from the District of Columbia Court of Appeals went to the U.S. Court of Appeals for the District of Columbia, not directly to the U.S. Supreme Court, as they would from the highest state courts. In 1970 a new District of Columbia Superior Court assumed most local jurisdiction, including some cases formerly in the federal district court. Most cases from the District of Columbia Court of Appeals now go directly to the U.S. Supreme Court, but those involving a law "not applicable exclusively to the District of Columbia" still go to the U.S. Court of Appeals.

The district courts in Guam, the Virgin Islands, and the Northern Marianas (the newest federal judicial district) were established under Congress' power to regulate the territories (Art. IV, Sec. 3). (The District Court for the Canal Zone, created under the same authority, went out of existence in 1982 when authority over the Zone was transferred to the government of Panama.) The territorial courts hear cases under local as well as federal laws. Decisions concerning the district court's authority to hear appeals from local courts—for example, whether that authority should be transferred to local supreme courts—must be made by Congress because such review at times turns on questions of federal law. In earlier years, the territorial courts were treated much like regular district courts; although the judges sometimes had legislative as well as judicial duties, they had tenure "during good behavior," that is, for life, under Article III of the Constitution. By the mid-nineteenth century, however, Congress shifted the basis for creating their positions to Article IV concerning governing of the territories, so the territorial judges lost their lifetime positions, and presidents even treated the judges as removable summarily. Judges of the territorial courts now have terms of from four to eight years. When a territory becomes a state, the territorial court is abolished and is replaced by a regular Article III court with lifetime judgeships.

Since 1966, district judges in Puerto Rico have had lifetime appointments. The Supreme Court has treated Puerto Rico, which has commonwealth status, much like a state, for example, extending the protections of the Fourth Amendment to it and giving great weight to its courts' interpretations of Puerto Rico law.

Native Americans. Relations of native Americans with the federal judicial system have given rise to special problems as a result of treating Indian tribes as separate, although dependent, nations, and as a result of the many treaties signed with them (and often dishonored by the government). The tribes have traditional courts, consisting of a tribal chief and council of elders. In addition, as part of Bureau of Indian Affairs activities on the reservations, Indian agents have appointed Courts of Indian Offenses, known as CFR courts because they operate under guidelines in the Code of Federal Regulations. Modern tribal courts, operating under modern tribal legal codes, were established under the Indian Reorganization Act of 1934. Even though the tribes are not states, decisions of these courts are given deference under the idea of comity and the Full Faith and Credit Clause (Art. IV, Sec. 1). The 1968 Indian Civil Rights Act made available habeas corpus petitions to federal district court to test their orders, and the Major Crimes Act (18 U.S.C. §§1154, 3242), under which designated offenses by an Indian against an Indian or non-Indian are to be tried in federal court, serves as a restriction on tribal courts' ability to try criminal cases. The Supreme Court has had to deal with jurisdictional conflicts from time to time when states have sought to assert jurisdiction over certain matters Indians claim to be within tribal court jurisdiction or have tried to limit Indians' access to state courts unless the Indians allow themselves to be sued there.

Magistrates[9]

The position of U.S. magistrates resulted from the reorganization of the U.S. commissioner system. The authority of the commissioners, about one-third of whom were not lawyers, was limited; they were paid by a fee system with a $10,500 limit. Under the Federal Magistrates Act, fully effective in 1971, full-time magistrates must be lawyers and serve for eight years, and part-time magistrates serve for four years. As of 1986, there were 266 full-time and 183 part-time magistrates as a result of a trend toward full-time positions. Roughly a quarter of the districts have only one full-time magistrate, with only a few having only a part-time magistrate. More than two-thirds of the full-time ones serve in the 25 largest district courts. Subject to congressional funding, the Judicial Conference allocates magistrate positions to districts on the basis of recommendations from district courts, circuit councils, its own Magistrates Committee, and the Administrative Office, but the magistrates are selected by the district judges in the district in which they serve. A provision in the 1979 Magistrates Act requires the district judges to appoint merit panels (with some nonlawyers) to advertise magistrate positions, evaluate the applicants, and submit a list of five nominees. The result has been the appointment of more women and minorities, but an earlier pattern of appointing people with close connections to the court (and thus known to the judges) continues.

Magistrates started with all the commissioners' former duties and were given additional duties by statute or by assignment, to relieve the district judges of their increasing caseload. Such additional duties have accounted for an increasing proportion of the magistrates' work each year. Although most magistrates are assigned most tasks the district judges can designate, with handling of Social Security cases and prisoner petitions most likely to be assigned, more magistrates are *designated* to perform certain duties than are actually *assigned* them. Depending on the tasks assigned, they may serve as subject-matter specialists (on Social Security and prisoner matters); as "team players," taking cases through the early stages before district judges take them; and as additional judges, handling their own caseload.

Although magistrates previously could hear only those criminal cases involving minor offenses (those with a maximum fine of $1,000, a year's prison sentence, or both) and could not hear jury trials, under the Federal Magistrates Act of 1979 they may now hear, and impose sentence in, all jury and nonjury misdemeanor criminal cases if the defendant waives the right to trial by a district judge; in such situations, appeals go directly to the courts of appeals. Their juvenile jurisdiction, which depends on the juvenile's consent, is still limited to petty cases and they may not impose a term of imprisonment on juveniles.

Magistrates also conduct pretrial criminal proceedings and preliminary review of applications for posttrial relief, and evidentiary hearings on federal habeas corpus petitions. The Supreme Court has said authority may be delegated to a magistrate to hear testimony concerning suppression of evidence as long as the district judge is the ultimate decisionmaker.[10]

Magistrates' civil jurisdiction has also been expanded. Prior to the 1979 Act, they could conduct civil pretrial and discovery proceedings, act as special masters in civil cases, and review administrative records in Social Security cases. The Supreme Court upheld district judges' referrals to magistrates of Social Security benefit entitlement cases as "substantially assist[ing] the district judge in the performance of his judicial function, and benefit[ing] both him and the parties"; the district judge had the opportunity to review—and object to—the magistrate's findings and could hear the matter *de novo*.[11] The 1979 statute confirmed existing practice of referring civil cases, with the parties' consent, to a magistrate for trial: any full-time and some part-time magistrates the district court designated could hear and confer judgment in any jury or nonjury civil cases with the parties' consent.

Prior to the 1979 Act, appeal of a magistrate's order to the district court for trial *de novo* was thought to protect the right to be tried by an Article III judge, even though the district judge usually based a ruling on the magistrate's report. Under the new statute, civil cases tried to a magistrate were to be appealed to the court of appeals, unless when the case was referred the parties agreed the appeal would go to the district judge. (When an appeal is taken from a magistrate's decision to the district court, further appeal—to the courts of appeals—is not a matter of right but is by petition for leave to appeal.) The U.S. Court of Appeals for the Ninth Circuit has ruled that the parties' consent cures any constitutional problem about the right to be tried by an Article III judge, but also said that district judges have extensive control over management of the magistrate system and can resume control over individual cases in the magistrates' hands.[12]

Bankruptcy Court

Bankruptcy judges were called referees in bankruptcy until 1973; prior to 1946, they were paid by fees they collected, but now are salaried, with their salaries subject to adjustment by Congress. Until the Bankruptcy Reform Act of 1978, they were appointed by district judges for six-year terms, and served on a full-time or part-time basis, with an increasing proportion full-time. The then 222 bankruptcy judges dealt with over 350,000 bankruptcy petitions a year, over three-fourths of which involved little or no assets. The 1978 statute changed bankruptcy judges' status in important ways. Starting in 1984, they were to be appointed by the president for 14-year terms; before then, merit screening committees could recommend termination of those whose terms expired and chief judges could terminate them and appoint replacements. In another important change, most supervision of bankrupts' assets was to be placed in the hands of bankruptcy trustees appointed by the attorney general rather than in the hands of individuals appointed by the judges for particular cases. That gave rise to judicial-executive conflict concerning the preferred method of administering such a program. When Congress considered making the trustee program—started as a pilot program in 18 districts—permanent, the Judicial Conference objected. Its position was that there would be potential confusion and overlap as judges handled bankruptcy cases and U.S. trustees separately administered the underlying estates, and that it would be more efficient and cheaper to house such a program in the judiciary, to be run by bankruptcy administrators appointed by the courts of appeals.

Bankruptcy courts' jurisdiction was also expanded under the new statute, to encompass *all* civil proceedings related to bankruptcy cases, including state law as well as federal law questions. The scope of bankruptcy judges' new authority led to legal challenges. In 1982, in a bankruptcy case involving a matter otherwise typically within state court jurisdiction (a contract by a company in the bankruptcy court's jurisdiction), a badly divided Supreme Court ruled that Congress had unconstitutionally granted too much authority to these judges who did not have lifetime tenure. Justice Brennan said judges with most attributes of "judicial power"—including authority over matters normally handled through the common law—had to be Article III judges with the necessary independence provided by lifetime appointments and protection against salary reduction so that they would not slant decisions to increase the chances of reappointment.[13] (He did, however, find constitutional justification for having judges of limited terms—Article I judges—serve on territorial and District of Columbia courts, courts-martial, and courts and administrative agencies established to adjudicate cases involving "public rights," those granted by the government against itself such as pensions.)

To avoid invalidating prior decisions of bankruptcy judges appointed under the old procedures but exercising authority under the new statute, the Court did not make its ruling retroactive. In a move unusual because it usually makes rights effective upon its declaration of those rights,[14] the justices also stayed implementing the ruling to give Congress several months either to curtail bankruptcy judges' jurisdiction or to give them Article III status. However, after extending this stay for several months when Congress was unable to agree on a new statute, at the end of 1982 the Court refused any further extension. Congressional inaction continued until mid-1984, well past the 1978 statute's March 31, 1984, deadline for authority of the former bankruptcy judges and presidential appointment of new ones. During this period, matters were made more complicated by challenges to bankruptcy judges' jurisdiction to hear cases, although the Judicial Conference provided guidelines for dividing jurisdiction between the bankruptcy and district courts and all federal judicial districts adopted emergency interim rules based on the guidelines.

These unfolding events, and what followed, created a fascinating case study in the politics of the courts. Congressional stalemate stemmed from disagreement about (1) bankruptcy judges' proper status—whether, as the House wished, they should be Article III judges, or, as the Judicial Conference and the Senate preferred, they should have a lesser status, with district judges handling complex matters relating to bankruptcy; (2) whether, if lifetime appointments were involved, one president should be able to appoint a large number of bankruptcy judges; and (3) whether the bankruptcy law's substantive provisions, which had facilitated bankruptcies by individuals, should be changed, with business wanting to make bankruptcy more difficult and labor wishing to eliminate the Supreme Court's ruling in *N.L.R.B. v. Bildisco*, which allowed firms going into bankruptcy to abrogate their collective bargaining agreements with labor.

Congress finally reached a compromise in midyear 1984, which included creation of 85 new district and appellate judgeships. There were to be 232 bankruptcy judges; since then, Congress has authorized 52 more. The new bankruptcy judges were *not* to be Article III judges but were to be appointed by the courts of appeals, not the district court or the president, to 14-year terms, at a salary of $66,100, below that of a district judge. District courts were given basic bankruptcy jurisdiction but could refer civil cases related to bankruptcy proceedings to bankruptcy judges. Certain orders must be entered by district judges, after they consider bankruptcy judges' recommendations, but the parties may also consent to bankruptcy judges' decision of some matters. Appeals from bankruptcy judges' rulings go first to the district court, unless a circuit establishes a bankruptcy appeals panel of bankruptcy judges, which only one circuit (the Ninth) now has.

Additional controversy resulted from Congress' failure to agree on the compromise until 12 days *after* the expiration of the old bankruptcy courts' authority to keep operating. The Judicial Conference specifically designated U.S. magistrates to handle bankruptcy matters, and created the same number of magistrate positions as there had been bankruptcy judges, and gave district courts the option of having the bankruptcy judges serve temporarily as "consultants" until steps could be taken to appoint them as magistrates. Congress tried to handle the problem by retroactively reappointing all bankruptcy judges to serve until there was time for the new appointment process to work. However, the Director of the Administrative Office of the Courts, William Foley, probably acting at the behest of the Chief Justice, refused to pay the judges. He did so on the grounds that Congress, because it cannot appoint judges, had acted unconstitutionally in restoring bankruptcy judges' authority once it had expired. House Judiciary Committee Chairman Peter Rodino threatened hearings into the Administrative Office's action, which challenged Congress' authority, and some bankruptcy judges refused to work while their pay was being withheld. In many districts, all papers in bankruptcy cases were sent to district judges for their signature—resulting in a massive paperwork problem. After a group of bankruptcy judges sued Foley, he allowed district courts to make whatever arrangements they wished for handling of bankruptcy cases, and agreed to pay their salaries.

By late 1984, matters had worked themselves out, but not before the Department of Justice had intervened in a case brought by debtors to challenge portions of the 1984 compromise, to urge the law be invalidated. However, when a bankruptcy judge invalidated a part of the new law, the Justice Department did support the statute. In late November 1984 federal district judges upheld the constitutionality of Congress' retroactive reappointments and the Fifth Circuit upheld the law in late 1986,[15] apparently bringing matters to a close.

Other Specialized Courts

There are a number of other specialized trial-level courts. Despite the preference for general jurisdiction courts, specialized courts have been established throughout our history, when particular problems have been thought to require focused attention or there has been a large number of cases on a particular issue at one time. In the mid-nineteenth century, for example, a special court was established to settle the status of Spanish and Mexican land grants in the territory ceded by Mexico to the United States in the Treaties of 1848 and 1853. Similarly, the U.S. Court of Claims (now the U.S. Claims Court) was established in 1855 to provide for suits against the United States government and to relieve the pressure on Congress from requests for private bills to deal with claims against the government.

When it was first established, the only claims the Court of Claims could hear were those referred by the House of Representatives or the Senate; it did not have authority to award judgments against the government and could only report its findings to Congress along with a proposed bill authorizing payment. In the 1860s, however, its judgments were made final. Originally an Article I court whose judges had limited terms, the Court of Claims was made an Article III court in 1953, and the Supreme Court rejected challenges to the change.[16]

Initial determinations in the Court of Claims were made by one of 16 judges (trial commissioners), who, in addition to adjudicating cases referred by Congress, had functions analogous to those of U.S. magistrates or special masters. Only the court's Article III judges, who sat together in Washington, D.C., could enter dispositive orders; they decided major motions and appeals from trial judges' findings of fact, and handled appeals from decisions of government contract boards. The Federal Court Improvement Act of 1982 created a clearer separation between trial judges' work and that of the Article III judges, with the U.S. Claims Court again becoming an Article I court (with 16 judges) and appellate jurisdiction being lodged in the new Court of Appeals for the Federal Circuit (see page 60). The Claims Court retained the Court of Claims' jurisdiction, which encompasses claims against the United States except for tort cases; contract disputes make up the bulk of the Claims Court work.

The U.S. Tax Court was created in 1924 as the Board of Tax Appeals; it was renamed the Tax Court of the United States in 1942. It was an independent agency in the executive branch until 1969, when it became a legislative (Art. I) court, with congressional oversight vested in the House Ways and Means and Senate Finance Committees. The Tax Court has 19 judges, nominated by the president and confirmed by the Senate for 15-year terms with the same salary as district judges. They are assisted by "special trial judges" the Tax Court itself selects. Although the court is based in Washington, D.C., single judges hold hearings at 80 cities throughout the United States. The chief judge reviews opinions for uniformity; where a case appears inconsistent and the trial judge will not alter his decision, the case becomes a "court-reviewed" one, decided at a conference of the 19 judges. The Tax Court also uses the conference when it must decide how to proceed when a U.S. court of appeals has reversed it and the same issue recurs in another circuit.

The Tax Court, where over 30,000 cases are filed each year, shares jurisdiction over tax litigation with the Claims Court and the district courts. However, it is the only court to which a taxpayer can bring a case before making full payment of taxes instead of having to pay under protest and then sue to recover. Its basic jurisdiction is over cases in which the taxpayer contests the government's assertions of tax liability in excise tax cases or with respect to income, estate, or gift taxes. In 1974 and 1979, the Tax Court also was given the authority to issue declaratory judgments (statements of litigants' rights before the government takes action against them) on such matters as the tax status of organizations, employee retirement plans, and government bonds. The taxpayer who has overpaid and wishes to recover some of those funds may go either to the Claims Court or to the district courts, which also have jurisdiction over enforcement of tax levies and over liens; the districts courts, moreover, are the exclusive forum (court) for criminal tax proceedings.

The Customs Court, an administrative body that had evolved into an Article III court, was transformed in 1980 into the U.S. Court of International Trade. This court's rulings provided the uniformity concerning import transactions required by the Constitution (Art. I, Sec. 8, cl. 1). In addition to its older appellate jurisdiction over rulings and appraisals on imported goods made by collectors of customs, it now also has exclusive jurisdiction over conflicts arising under certain tariff and trade laws. Most of its work involves hearing challenges to administrative decisions of the Customs Service and the Treasury. The court has nine judges, no more than five of whom may be from one political party, appointed by the president with the advice and consent of the Senate.

Perhaps the most intriguing special court is the Foreign Intelligence Surveillance Court. It is a result of the provision of the 1978 Wiretap Act that court orders must be obtained for telephone and other electronic taps of foreign agents (individuals and embassies) in the United States—including, in exceptional cases, American citizens with information thought essential to the national security. The seven members of the court are to be appointed—to staggered terms—by the Chief Justice after consultation with the chief judges of the circuits; they are regular judges of other courts serving on the FIS Court as well when needed. What makes the court unusual is that it meets in a "secure" courtroom and conducts its work in secret, not writing opinions or publishing rulings, except in one case in which it said that the court's jurisdiction did not extend to searches of private property.

The Courts of Appeals

The U.S. Courts of Appeals are the general appellate courts for the federal judicial system; they are required to hear the cases brought to them, that is, they are mandatory jurisdiction courts. As such, they engage primarily in "error-correction," but they also engage in important "law-making" activity—much of which is not reviewed by the Supreme Court. They handle cases on all types of federal law—"traditional" areas of litigation such as admiralty and antitrust; constitutional issues that are more prominent in the Supreme Court's work; and cases appealed from federal regulatory agencies, which are in effect the trial courts for matters within their jurisdictions.

Formerly called the Circuit Courts of Appeals, the U.S. Courts of Appeals were created in their present form in 1891, as a result of increased federal court caseload and the recognition of the impracticality of having Supreme Court justices sit on circuit. The establishment of these courts—creating a basic appellate court for the federal judiciary—began the process of providing the Supreme

Court with the ability to control which cases it would hear. The courts of appeals bring some degree of uniformity to national law, providing some oversight of activities once considered primarily local. They are, however, a decentralized mechanism, exhibiting considerable diversity; they thus can reflect regional variations in needs and values. As a result of their location in the judicial system,

> they enforce national policies [but] also mediate between national law and various political and professional constituencies in regional communities. . . . As intermediates in many dimensions of responsibility, they look down to district courts and agencies, up to the Supreme Court and the central government, in to themselves, their colleagues and staffs, across to rival appellate courts, and all around to various groups and individuals who compose their attentive publics.[17]

There are now 156 authorized judgeships for the courts of appeals, 35 having been added by the 1978 Judgeship Act and 24 more in the 1984 bankruptcy legislation. (There are also 12 judges for the Court of Appeals for the Federal Circuit, a specialized court—see page 60.) Assisting the circuit judges in deciding cases are the courts' *senior* (semiretired) judges (see pages 92-93), as well as district judges and judges from other circuits who sit "by designation." There are now 12 U.S. Courts of Appeals with general appellate jurisdiction—11 numbered circuits and one for the District of Columbia—in addition to specialized appellate courts (see pages 59-62). Except for the District of Columbia Circuit, each court of appeals covers several states. The courts range in size from the First Circuit (Massachusetts, New Hampshire, Maine, Rhode Island, and Puerto Rico), the smallest with six judgeships, to the Ninth (Alaska, Hawaii, California, Oregon, Washington, Idaho, Montana, Nevada, and Arizona, plus Guam and the Northern Marianas), with 28 judgeships. Until 1980, when the Fifth Circuit (the Deep South) was divided into the Fifth and Eleventh Circuits, no new circuit had been created since the mid-1920s, when the Tenth Circuit (the Rocky Mountain states) was carved out of the Eighth Circuit, which at the time extended westward from the Mississippi River.

Division of the Fifth Circuit and failure to divide the Ninth Circuit both illustrate political aspects of structuring our judicial system. Prior to 1978, the Fifth Circuit had the largest number of judgeships (15) and it was to receive 11 more in 1978. Because a court of 26 judges was thought much too large, proposals were made to divide the circuit. However, enactment was delayed for several years—in fact, delaying passage of the Omnibus Judgeship Act until 1978—by resistance from the NAACP, concerned that a relatively liberal civil rights court would be broken up, and particularly from Senator James Eastland of Mississippi, then chairman of the Senate Committee on the Judiciary. Eastland insisted on having one circuit composed only of Texas and Louisiana, with Mississippi, Georgia, Alabama, and Florida in the other. Then came Eastland's announcement of retirement from the Senate, the appointment of some black judges, withdrawal of NAACP opposition, and support by Senator Edward Kennedy, the incoming committee chair, for a different division (adding Mississippi to Texas and Louisiana). Yet even these changes did not result immediately in a split of the circuit. The 1978 Act provided that circuits with more than 15 active circuit judges (then only the Fifth and Ninth) could create internal administrative units. When the Fifth Circuit tried to hold *en banc* courts with its full complement of 26 judges, the logistical difficulties led the court itself to ask that it be divided, and Congress agreed in 1980. Because California generates roughly three-fifths of the Ninth Circuit's caseload, the problem there remains how to divide the circuit to provide balanced caseloads without the unprecedented acts of splitting a single state or leaving a one-state circuit, so dividing that circuit has proved impractical thus far, and the Ninth Circuit's judges have worked to keep it intact.

Most court of appeals cases are heard by three-judge panels of changing membership; a panel *is* the court of appeals for the cases it decides, and a panel's ruling is not to be overruled by another panel but only by the court of appeals sitting *en banc*—that is, all of the court's judges sitting—which it does to hear particularly important cases, usually after a panel has heard the case. *En banc* sittings, developed when the Supreme Court gave the appeals courts the responsibility for producing uniformity in legal matters within a circuit, are, however, not used frequently. The 1978 Act said that large circuits could use limited *en banc* courts of some number less than the entire court, which the Ninth Circuit has done.

All members of the Supreme Court live in one metropolitan area and work in the same courthouse, but this is true of only the District of Columbia circuit; judges in the other courts of appeals reside at various and often widely dispersed locations throughout the circuit, meeting face-to-face when hearing oral argument and discussing cases immediately thereafter, while relying heavily on mail and telephone for further discussion of cases and developing of opinions. This geographic dispersion, coupled with rotation of panel membership, large caseloads, and ideological differences, can contribute to inconsistency *within* a court of appeals, limiting the courts' ability to produce uniformity in national law. [18]

The recent growth in appeals court caseload has been phenomenal and disproportionate to the growth in district court caseload. More than 25,000 cases are docketed in the U.S. courts of appeals each year, with caseload having increased 226 percent from 1969 to 1985 (compared with a 61 percent increase in judgeships). Criminal cases have grown most in recent years and now account for roughly one-third of appeals court caseload. There is no Speedy Appeal Act, but criminal appeals are expected to be handled expeditiously, helping to create a delay in reaching and deciding other types of appeals. Moreover, while increases in judges may help reduce backlogs temporarily, more decisions will be appealed as a result of new district judgeships, and proportionately more cases may be appealed by litigants whose trials are more promptly terminated by those judges, resulting in a continuing heavy appellate court caseload.

All the courts of appeals operate under the Federal Rules of Appellate Procedure but adopt separate Local Rules. They vary in reliance on oral argument, which the Second Circuit uses in almost every case while other circuits dispense with it in a significant portion of cases; in use of summary dispositions— simpler cases handled by truncated procedures; and in use of unpublished opinions, although all circuits now issue high proportions of decisions in Not-for-Publication memorandums, which cannot be cited as precedent by lawyers in other cases.[19]

Certain appeals are thought to be "frivolous," having little substance and not raising new issues. Many others are routine, and still other appeals are "ritualistic," brought because of the litigants' demands even when the likelihood of reversal of the district court is low. Only a relatively small proportion of cases involve "nonconsensual" appeals "which raise major questions of public policy and upon which there is considerable disagreement."[20] Among the nonconsensual appeals may be those in which "issue transformation" has taken place in the appeals court. Among those would be instances in which civil liberties issues were not an important part of the case at trial but became central in the appeal. Through such issue transformation, found in civil liberties cases and particularly in race relations cases in the Third, Fifth, and Eighth Circuits from 1956 through 1961, the appeals courts, which granted liberties denied in the district courts, enforced a more "national" and less local perspective.[21] However, an examination of all cases from the district courts up in the Second, Fifth, and District of Columbia Circuits in Fiscal Years 1965–67 led to the conclusion that there was very little issue transformation. Only 7 percent of the cases provided an indication that the two levels of judges defined the issues in cases differently. However, the appellate judges filtered issues as they moved up to the Supreme Court. This was part of the intermediate courts' "important functions as gatekeepers, directing traffic in the stream of federal appeals."[22]

Cases from some federal agencies may go either to the appeals court in the circuit where the controversy arose or to the Court of Appeals for the District of Columbia, the site of agency headquarters. Certain other cases—for example, radio and television station license renewal cases from the Federal Communications Commission (FCC) and certain Environmental Protection Agency (EPA) cases—must by statute be taken only to the District of Columbia Circuit, which thus has developed a particularly important role in reviewing agency decisions. This is but one example of a more general phenomenon seen also in the emphases on commercial litigation in the Second Circuit (New York) and on civil rights in the old Fifth Circuit; each court of appeals becomes "a magnet for certain subjects of federal law by virtue of location, special jurisdiction, and predilections," as well as differing propensities of attorneys and litigants to appeal different types of cases.[23]

The finality of courts of appeals' decisions is particularly significant. Because very few cases are appealed from there to the Supreme Court and it denies most petitions for review, in the great bulk of cases appeals court rulings are left as the final judicial statement. For example, in the Second, Fifth, and District of Columbia Circuits, only one in five decisions was appealed, with the Supreme Court granting review to only one-tenth of those—leaving over 98 percent of appeals court rulings as final—actually closer to 99 percent if we include cases in which the Supreme Court grants review and then affirms the appeals courts. Because most of their actions are not disturbed, the appeals courts "*make* national law," although "residually and regionally," and the Supreme Court remains largely dependent on them to "enforce the supremacy and uniformity of national law," particularly in those areas of law in which undisturbed cases tend to cluster.[24] These include such important subjects as workmen's compensation and minimum wage, Social Security, insurance contracts, and even school desegregation. This means that "Courts of Appeals are mini-Supreme Courts in the vast majority of their cases," with a division of labor—or, in the economist's term, comparative advantage—having developed between the two levels. The Supreme Court concentrates on broader policy concerns; courts of appeals, on the other hand, "concentrate on statutory interpretation, administrative review, and error correction in masses of routine adjudication."[25] Moreover, because the Supreme Court reviews selectively, paying more attention to some circuits such as the District of Columbia Circuit, it seldom supervises areas of litigation in which individual circuits specialize.[26]

Specialized Appeals Courts

There are some specialized appellate courts, just as there are specialized trial courts. Most notable was the Court of Customs and Patent Appeals (CCPA), created in 1910 and absorbed into the Court of Appeals for the Federal Circuit in 1982. The CCPA was initially an Article I court but its judges were given Article III (lifetime) status in 1948. The CCPA had appellate jurisdiction on matters of law over not only the Customs Court but also the Patent Office and Tariff Commission. That it was a specialized court may help us evaluate speculations and hypotheses that litigant interest groups, particularly if unified, have greater influence over such courts than over courts of general jurisdiction, so that specialized courts produce decisions different from those of generalist courts handling the same types of cases.

Until the mid-1950s, judges of the Court of Customs and Patent Appeals were nonspecialists not chosen from the patent bar, the lawyers who represent those seeking to obtain patents or defend patent holders against infringement of those patents. These nonspecialist judges tended to defer to Patent Office decisions denying patents because the Patent Office was an administrative agency. In the late 1950s, after the patent bar persuaded the president to appoint two patent attorneys to the CCPA, the CCPA almost immediately changed direction. The court produced substantially more reversals of the Patent Office than earlier. After having had standards of patentability roughly comparable to those the district courts applied in cases involving issued patents, the CCPA became more lenient than the district courts. Although the CCPA's nonspecialist members reversed the Patent Office more than had their nonspecialist predecessors, they continued to be more deferential to the Patent Office than were the "specialist" judges. This history of the decisions of one specialized court does not allow us to say that specialized courts will invariably behave differently from general jurisdiction courts, but it does indicate that "specialization may create conditions," such as success in obtaining nominations for certain types of people, "that cause a court to take a distinctive path."[27]

Arguments for creating any specialized court were apparent in the recent move to centralize all patent appeals in one court. A principal argument—by attorneys and federal judges alike—for creating a specialized court for patent cases was that such cases are too technical for generalist judges. One response was that patent cases are no more complex than antitrust or environment cases. Another was that judges who hear only one type of case will lose perspective as they become divorced from developments in other fields of law and will become immune to subtleties in the cases before them. (When we discuss separate courts of criminal appeals—which some states have—we talk of judges becoming "case-hardened.")

The idea that patent appeals should be centralized bore fruit in 1981, when Congress created the Court of Appeals for the Federal Circuit from the Court of Claims and Court of Customs and Patent Appeals. The new court assumed the existing appellate jurisdiction of both the Court of Claims and the Court of Customs and Patent Appeals, plus all appeals from the district courts in cases involving patents or nontax monetary claims against the United States. In addition to hearing appeals in cases involving contract and eminent domain claims against the government, the court hears appeals from the Court of International Trade (formerly the Customs Court), the Patent and Trademark Office, and the Merit Systems Protection Board (created in the recent reorganization of the federal government's personnel system). Review from the court is on certiorari to the Supreme Court.

Perhaps the most significant part of the reorganization is that, while trials in patent cases still take place in the district courts, patent *appeals*, instead of being heard in several courts (the Court of Customs and Patent Appeals, the Court of Appeals for the District of Columbia—for certain types of cases, and other courts of appeals), are now centralized in one court. This is much appreciated by the patent bar, which the Court of Appeals for the Federal Circuit has enlisted in working out its new jurisdiction. By contrast, several paths remain for tax appeals: from the Claims Court to the Court of Appeals for the Federal Circuit, and from the Tax Court to the court of appeals to which a taxpayer would have taken an appeal from the district court; the result is several diverging bodies of tax law.

There have been other specialized appellate courts, but these have been staffed by Article III judges whose full-time positions are on other courts and who are appointed to the specialized courts by the Chief Justice. These include the Temporary National Emergency Court of Appeals for cases arising under the wage-price control and emergency petroleum allocation programs of the 1970s—created in 1971 and still processing cases, so hardly "temporary"; the earlier Emergency Court of Appeals, established during World War II for wage-price cases; and a special court to handle problems under the Regional Rail Reorganization Act of 1973. (The Emergency Court of Appeals' exclusive appellate jurisdiction over decisions by the price administrator was upheld by the Supreme Court in *Yakus v. United States* in 1944.) An earlier experiment with a specialized court to hear cases from a single administrative agency—the Commerce Court, to hear cases from the Interstate Commerce Commission—was abandoned in 1913 after only a few years because the railroads preferred to deal with the ICC, shippers didn't like interference with the commission, and Congress saw a threat from the court to the commission, which it saw as more its own arm.[28]

There is also the three-judge Foreign Intelligence Surveillance Court of Review, to review applications for electronic surveillance denied by the Foreign Intelligence Surveillance Court (see page 55). Another such court is known as the Special Division of the United States Court of Appeals for the District of Columbia Circuit; one of its judges, who have two-year appointments, must be from the D.C. Circuit, with priority given to senior circuit judges and retired Supreme Court justices. That court has the task of designating independent counsel (formerly called special prosecutors) called for under the Ethics in Government Act of 1978 in cases involving the president, vice-president, and other high government officials.[29] The constitutionality of that arrangement was challenged in 1987 by former White House aide Michael Deaver and by Lt. Col. Oliver North in the Iran-Contra scandal.

There is only one Article I specialized appeals court, the U.S. Court of Military Appeals, created in 1950 under congressional power to provide for the armed forces. Its three civilian judges, of whom no more than two may be of one party, serve for staggered 15-year terms. In applying the revised Uniform Code of Military Justice (UCMJ), they must review courts-martial decisions involving general or flag officers, capital punishment decisions affirmed by the Boards of Review in the military services, and cases the service judge advocate generals (JAG) certify for review. Its principal business, however, is discretionary review of courts-martial decisions involving bad-conduct discharges and prison sentences of more than one year. It considers such cases if a Board of Review approves a petition by the convicted person, granting approximately 10 percent of the petitions and denying the others without explanation. Effective in 1984, the Supreme Court was given the authority to review decisions of the USCMA on certiorari; until then Supreme Court review was restricted to habeas corpus on the limited question of whether the military had jurisdiction over the court-martialed person, but the Court through use of that jurisdiction handed down important decisions concerning the military's authority to court-martial civilians or military personnel involved in nonservice-connected offenses.[30]

The National Court of Appeals

Problems generated by increased caseload in both the Supreme Court and courts of appeals, coupled with Chief Justice Burger's greater attention to administrative matters, led to the first serious structural examination of the national court system since the 1920s and to proposals to restructure that system. The most important proposal would create a new federal appellate court located between the U.S. courts of appeals and the Supreme Court.[31]

The first major proposal, recommended by a study group appointed by Chief Justice Burger and chaired by Harvard Law School Professor Paul Freund, called in 1973 for a National Court of Appeals, a "mini-Supreme Court," staffed by present appeals court judges on a rotating basis. The new court was to sort through the cases awaiting review by the Supreme Court and select roughly 400 each year most worthy of the Supreme Court's attention. From these, the Supreme Court was to select 120 to 150 cases to which it would give full-dress treatment. The new court's denials of review and its determinations of legal conflicts between the courts of appeals would have been final. This hotly contested proposal was shelved, largely because it would have deprived the Supreme Court of considerable power through its finality of denials of review.

Then in 1975 the Commission on Revision of the Federal Court Appellate System, created by Congress, made recommendations based on its examination of the national court system's capacity for "declaring and defining the national law." If such capacity was to be increased without simultaneously increasing the diversity of legal interpretations, the commission thought such methods as appointment of additional judges, creation of new appeals court circuits, a changed basis of federal court jurisdiction, and new methods for disposing of caseload would be insufficient. Thus it proposed a National Court of Appeals of several judges to be appointed by the president. The new court would receive cases in two ways. The Supreme Court could send cases before deciding them ("reference jurisdiction") and the courts of appeals could send them when a rule of federal law was applicable to recurring factual situations or when federal courts had reached inconsistent decisions on a rule of federal law ("transfer jurisdiction"). The new court could refuse to accept cases, a decision that would not be reviewable, but its decisions of cases on the merits could be reviewed by the Supreme Court on certiorari. This proposal received more substantial support than the Freund Study Group proposal had received. However, it—and more recent versions—have not been enacted, in part because the negative reaction to the screening portion of the Freund Study Group proposal has continued to "follow" subsequent revised versions. Creation of the Court of Appeals for the Federal

Circuit, discussed previously, did come as part of an effort to salvage some part of the proposal.

Justices continued to speak out for or against the idea of a National Court of Appeals; some took issue with colleagues' suggestions while agreeing that some thing had to be done about workload (see page 195). In 1983 and thereafter, Chief Justice Burger, in a number of forums, including his State of the Judiciary addresses to the American Bar Association, renewed his call for the new tribunal, even suggesting that it be established on an experimental basis for five years. Before being nominated, Justice Rehnquist advocated it but without claiming the Supreme Court is overworked or suggesting the Court would shed cases. Neither Burger nor Rehnquist was able to persuade the ABA of the value of the proposal, with the organization rejecting it in 1986.

In its more recent versions, the new court would obtain cases only if the Supreme Court referred them, and review of its rulings would be on certiorari to the Supreme Court. Bills to establish such an Intercircuit Tribunal of the United States Courts of Appeals were approved by subcommittees in both houses of Congress, and by the full Senate Judiciary Committee in 1986, but no legislation has passed both houses. Although one proposal had a court of 26 circuit judges (two each from the courts of appeals, including the Federal Circuit) and a "Chancellor of the United States," with cases heard by five-judge panels drawn by lot, a more recent version has only nine judges sitting, with four held in reserve; one judge would come from each court of appeals. The method of selecting judges has been a bone of contention: Chief Justice Burger wanted them selected by the Chief Justice or the Judicial Conference, while the circuits have opted for selecting their own members of the new court. During his confirmation hearings to be Chief Justice, Justice Rehnquist recognized that allowing the Chief Justice to appoint would give that individual too much power, but he also felt that the primary loyalty of judges chosen by the circuits would be to the circuits, not the new court. He thus would have given the appointment power to the president, although that would not be palatable to senators whose party was not in control of the White House.

Knowledgeable lawyers and scholars continue to express the view that such a significant structural change not be made before other methods of reducing the Supreme Court's caseload—like eliminating remaining mandatory appeals or removing federal courts' diversity-of-citizenship jurisdiction—are attempted and before other concerns are addressed. One is that the Supreme Court's work will be increased to some extent if, in addition to deciding whether to grant review in a case, the justices have to decide whether a case is of sufficient importance to be heard by the new court but not by the Supreme Court; adding a choice to those available to any decision-making body increases the opportunities for conflict.[32] In addition, critics suggest that the amount of unresolved intercircuit conflict with which the new court is supposed to deal may be overestimated.

Judicial Administration

Judicial administration—"the direction of and influence on the activities of those who are expected to contribute to just and efficient case-processing, except legal doctrinal considerations insofar as they dispose of the particular factual and legal claims presented in a case"[33]—is a low-visibility activity, yet neither any single court nor the judicial system as a whole could function without it. It encompasses activities related to processing cases, the judicial branch's personnel needs, budgeting for the judiciary, planning, and research. The federal courts' increasing caseload and Chief Justice Burger's efforts have focused more attention on judicial administration and have helped produce a greater desire to shift from haphazard, inefficient management to more organized and "professional" administration. From the early years, the Chief Justice "received information on the State of judicial business in the far-flung districts,"[34] but only in the twentieth century has serious and protracted attention been given to problems of judicial administration, particularly by Chief Justices Taft and Burger.

Particularly important among aspects of judicial administration has been budgeting for the court system, given greater importance by efforts to reduce the nation's budget deficit. Even though the judiciary's budget is *one-tenth of one percent* of the total federal budget, the judicial branch was affected by the Gramm-Rudman-Hollings Budget Reduction Act's targeted reductions in budget deficits and provisions for automatic cuts if Congress did not reach the targeted amounts. For Fiscal Year 1986 (ending September 30, 1986), the across-the-board 4.3 percent reduction meant that $42,000,000 had to be saved from a $1.1 billion budget. Federal courts began to feel the pinch in mid-1986, with a reduction in the number of security guards at federal courts and elimination of parking fees for federal jurors. Because funds to pay basic juror fees were depleted, the Administrative Office of the Courts ordered that no new civil jury trials be started. Congress provided funds for this purpose in a supplemental appropriations bill, but not before two federal courts had declared the action a violation of the constitutional right to a jury trial. Other cuts, in staffing levels at the courts and for lawyers appointed to represent indigent defendants, as well as in judges' travel allotments, were made, and additional cuts will have to be made as long as the budget deficit-cutting effort continues. (For further discussion of judicial-legislative interaction concerning the judicial budget, see pages 300-301.)

For many years, little attention was given even to the selection, retention, and supervision of personnel necessary to make the courts operate effectively, despite the number of people working in the federal judicial branch—in 1979 over 12,500 people, an increase of well over 100 percent since 1960. Hiring of administrative personnel was essentially a matter of judges' patronage and was unsystematic. This was certainly true with respect to clerks of court, who generally focus on day-to-day aspects of processing of cases and who until recently were fully responsible for administering court activities. Similarly, court reporters, who record and transcribe what is said in court, were not hired by the courts on a uniform basis until 1944; before then, most courts left it to the litigants to arrange for private reporters. Although most court staff positions are now filled through regularized hiring procedures, executive branch civil service mechanisms are not used.

Other personnel involved in the courts' work are probation officers and U.S. marshals. The former, originally under the supervision of the Bureau of Prisons, are now responsible to the Administrative Office of the Courts (A.O.). The U.S. marshals, nominated for each district by the president and confirmed by the Senate, are executive branch employees formally responsible to the Attorney General but who work closely with the courts. Under an agreement between the A.O. and the General Services Administration (GSA), they are responsible for courtroom security—a matter of increasing concern, particularly in larger cities. They also enforce judicial orders. Their working relations with the courts are usually smooth, but the question of whether marshals must transport state prisoners to testify in federal court cases ended up in the Supreme Court, which ruled that federal courts had no authority to order the marshals to perform that task. [35]

Before attention was paid to administrative personnel who serve the court as an institution, some concern was shown about law clerks, recent top-ranked law school graduates who serve a judge for a year or at most two years. Judges use several methods to select their clerks: many have open competitions, while some depend on law school professors to make selections for them, and others enlist former clerks to screen candidates while making the final selection themselves. Clerks perform a variety of tasks for judges. They examine briefs and court records in cases, research matters of law, and draft opinions; at the Supreme Court, they also summarize petitions for review (see pages 207-8). The extent of their input depends on the judge or justice for and with whom they work; some clerks are able to offer ideas in addition to performing more basic research and writing tasks.

Despite their importance to the performance of judges' tasks, law clerks, who appeared at the Supreme Court early in this century, did not appear on a salaried basis in the district courts until the mid-1940s; now each district judge has two law clerks. In the courts of appeals, where each judge has three law clerks, for the last 20 years the courts have also hired staff attorneys, who perform legal tasks for all the judges of the court rather than being assigned to individual judges. Each of the Supreme Court's nine justices is assisted by four clerks, except for Justice Rehnquist, who as an associate justice used only three, and Justice Stevens (two). To provide expertise and continuity, Justice White has adopted a practice of keeping one of his four clerks for a second year.

The basic units involved in administering the federal judicial system are the Judicial Conference of the United States, the Administrative Office of the United States Courts, and the circuit councils. All were established relatively late in the national judicial system's history, largely as a result of judicial and administrative politics. Perhaps the primary reason was that federal judges wished to retain their independence both of each other and of any central authority. This can be seen in the problems faced by chief judges of districts and circuits: getting the judges of a court to work together and to work with or under a chief judge can be difficult, particularly if the "chief" is strongwilled. Conflict in the Northern District of Ohio between Chief Judge Frank J. Battisti and his colleagues in 1985 led the Sixth Circuit to rule that, while Battisti could remain chief judge, policy for the court's operation would be set by a majority of the district's judges.

Because the position of chief judge is filled on the basis of seniority, there is no guarantee that a chief judge will be good as either an administrator or leader. Until recently, the chief judge of a circuit or district has been the most senior judge of the court under the age of 70, at which time the chief judge must give up the position. Under legislation adopted several years ago, someone cannot become chief judge after his or her sixty-fourth year unless no one else is eligible and, in any event, may serve for only seven years.

Judges' insistence on independence and their resistance to central authority, which includes their lobbying of members of Congress to seek support for their own policies, has made it difficult to establish even something seemingly as simple as uniform personnel and salary systems for the federal courts. Pressure has nonetheless been substantial to make the court's internal operations administratively efficient so that the courts might be more effective in performing their functions. Reformers have sought to improve court administration through "centralization, bureaucratization, and professionalization of judicial administration . . . at the expense of judicial informality and autonomy." Such trends, "accelerated by the law explosion," are "rooted in external demands for efficiency, fiscal accountability, and professional standards of personnel management."[36]

The difficulty in bringing about effective, rational management of the federal court system is demonstrated by the problems in developing methods for assignment of judges to handle cases where their help is needed. Until 1850, a federal judge could not sit outside his district. After 1850, he could be assigned only to a court within his own or a contiguous circuit—and only to help a sick or disabled judge. In the early twentieth century, the Chief Justice could ask that a judge serve elsewhere, but the chief judge of the judge's circuit could refuse the request—and did so. Judges, as a result of their primarily local or state orientation, did not see themselves as part of a national judicial system.

Problems surrounding intercircuit assignment of judges have changed—it is not as easy to block a requested transfer—but have not disappeared. If all courts have crowded dockets, it is difficult to find anyone except senior judges, who are willing to be assigned around the country, not just in their own circuit, to assist with particularly overloaded districts. Yet, despite Chief Justice Taft's support for the idea, a "pool" or "flying squadron" of federal judges available for assignment anywhere in the system has never been established on a *regular* basis, although, after elimination of the Commerce Court, its five judges were available for assignment to trial or appellate work throughout the country. Assignments between the circuits must now be cleared by the Intercircuit Assignment Committee, closely responsive to the Chief Justice's wishes; fear of congressional objection to the expenditure of funds for judges to travel from one part of the country to another—even before Gramm-Rudman—has led the Chief Justice to be chary about approving intercircuit assignments.[37] (The Chief Justice has authority to select judges from another circuit when all the judges of a court of appeals withdraw from a case because a defendant has filed a complaint against them or when they are colleagues of a judge involved in some way in a case. There are no statutory directives about how the Chief Justice can select the replacement judges, giving rise to the claim that selections might be made to produce a desired result.[38])

Circuit Councils

The basic administrative unit of the federal judicial system is supposed to be the judicial *council* in each circuit, created in part to decrease the chance of political attacks on the central judicial establishment in Washington, D.C. (There is also a *circuit judicial conference* in each circuit, which includes all circuit and district judges and lawyer representatives and meets once a year to consider a wide range of matters.) Until 1981, the circuit council was composed of all circuit judges on active-duty status, in effect, the *en banc* court of appeals wearing administrative rather than judicial hats. Legislation effective in 1981 affected the councils' responsibilities for judicial conduct (see pages 94-95) and also changed their structure by adding district judges. No longer are all the circuit judges automatically members of the council, although all active-duty circuit judges by majority vote determine council membership. They decide the number of circuit judges and, within a statutory formula, the number of district judges who together will compose the council, which is chaired by the circuit's chief judge. Nine of the 12 circuits chose to have all circuit judges serve on their new councils. The number of district judges ranges from two to six; specific arrangements for their choice vary among the circuits, with membership usually being rotated among a circuit's districts.

The council's wide range of powers, in addition to its role in judicial discipline, includes approving judicial accommodations, directing where court records should be kept, and performing other "housekeeping" tasks; consenting to the assignment of judges to courts in other circuits and dividing judicial business in the districts if the district judges cannot agree among themselves; and the far more sensitive business of certifying to the president that because of disability a judge is unable to discharge his or her duties. The council also receives reports from the Administrative Office on the dockets in the circuit's courts and is supposed to take appropriate action on the basis of those reports.

The circuit councils are assisted in carrying out their tasks by the *circuit executives,* who assist the chief judge and the circuit council with general administration of the circuit and with special projects. Some circuits have made substantial use of their circuit executives, but experience over 10 years shows clearly that more than appointing someone with such a title is necessary to solve administrative problems. Chief judges' inability to delegate responsibility to circuit executives, the executives' involvement in detail, and conflict between the executive and clerk of court—who increasingly is also likely to be well trained—are principal difficulties.[39]

Judicial Conference

Diffusing responsibility among all a circuit's judges serving as the circuit council often led to a lack of willingness to act on important matters or to exercise authority. For this reason and because the councils are more attached "to the ideal of local self-government and an independent judiciary,"[40] they have played a less important role than the Judicial Conference of the United States; indeed, the circuit councils blocked the trend toward a centralized administration for the judiciary, "an executive-centered administrative apparatus" presided over by an "executive" who was a judge.[41]

Establishment in 1922 of the Judicial Conference (originally the Conference of Senior Circuit Judges) was the first official manifestation that authority in the federal judicial system was being centralized. Chaired by the Chief Justice, the Judicial Conference consists of the chief judges of the courts of appeals, a district judge from each circuit except the Federal Circuit, and the chief judge of the Court of International Trade. District judges were not part of the original membership. (The subsequently invalidated bankruptcy statute would have placed two bankruptcy judges on the Conference.) The Conference meets twice a year, with a six-member executive committee acting for the Conference between meetings. The Chief Justice has wielded significant authority in the Conference's work. That authority, initially enhanced because he had to speak for the Conference between meetings, was later strengthened because only he, and not the other justices, participated in the Conference. The other justices have generally not wanted to be involved in such administrative matters, are busy, and, with few exceptions (Justice Tom Clark, the former attorney general), lacked an administrative background.

The Conference was created to be the chief administrative policymaker for the federal judiciary but "constituted only a first step toward a more integrated administrative system." At first it operated mainly by tying the senior circuit judges into a national communications network. However, it never developed the predominance for which it was intended. Its potential strength was reduced by its infrequent meetings and the later development of committees, which proliferated and became more important under Chief Justice Stone. The Chief Justice's position is strengthened by the fact that the more than 20 standing and ad hoc committees attached to the Conference report to him.[42] Development of the committees left the Conference largely a ratifying body for committee-recommended policies. Such policies covered a wide variety of matters, such as rules of evidence and procedure for the federal courts, the intercircuit transfer of judges, and the need for additional judges to deal with the ever-growing caseload of the federal courts.

The authority of the Conference itself has remained substantial, and it has dealt with such matters as ethical standards for judges and other court personnel, qualifications for those personnel, bankruptcy administration, and most important, the budget for the federal judiciary. Because of the importance of the issues with which the Conference and its committees deal, pressure has recently been brought to bear to open up the process by which Conference policy is made, and to require the Conference and its committees and subcommittees, as well as circuit judicial councils, to hold public meetings to transact business, but such efforts have thus far been unsuccessful.

Encompassed in the committees' work is the development of legislation to be submitted to Congress. The judges representing the Conference and its committees and the Director of the Administrative Office present legislative proposals to Congress. This allows the Chief Justice to stay away from a direct role in that area, which can cause trouble. When Director of the Administrative Office Rowland Kirks, in the company of an interest group lobbyist, visited Speaker of the House Carl Albert in late 1972 about a bill concerning product safety, Chief Justice Burger was accused of sending a lobbyist to argue against the bill. Denying the charge, the Chief Justice said his only concern was the bill's possible effect on the court system—part of his desire for "court impact statements." Another example of the difficulty into which the Chief Justice can get himself in acting for the Conference occurred in 1978 during final stages of consideration of the new bankruptcy statute. Before either House or Senate passed its version of the bill, Chief Justice Burger reportedly made telephone calls to several legislators asking that consideration of the bills be delayed until certain issues could be explored further and the Judicial Conference's opinion on compromise legislation heard. Although his position was based on Conference opposition to giving bankruptcy judges Article III status and having bankruptcy appeals go directly to the courts of appeals, Burger's reported anger—for example, in a call to the Senate subcommittee chairman in charge of the legislation—particularly irritated some members of Congress, who felt that the Chief Justice was going far beyond his proper role and exceeding the powers of the judicial branch. However, this is not the only instance when "Chief Justices . . . have cast aside the judicial robe long enough to press their Court's case before coordinate branches of the national government and even to mobilize public opinion." In so doing, they have at times sought legislation of assistance to the Supreme Court or the judiciary more generally; they have also "entered the political arena to fend off legislation they have perceived as potentially harmful to the Court."[43]

The Administrative Office and the Department
of Justice

From its creation in 1870, the Department of Justice performed day-to-day administrative tasks for the federal courts. The department's involvement was not ended by the formation of the Judicial Conference. Pervasive conflict over administration has taken place between the department and individual judges. Department field auditors visiting judicial districts to look over books, records, and accounts performed "a communication function as well as an investigative one."[44] However, clerks of court resisted department demands for the reporting of financial transactions. Despite such opposition, the department increased its control over district court clerks and their deputies in 1919, courts of appeals clerks in 1922, and the probation service in 1925. Yet obtaining statutory authority over particular functions did not lessen the need for the department to fight to obtain actual control, and its failure to submit recommendations of the Conference of Senior Circuit Judges to Congress or to support them when submitted did not win the judges' favor.

Considerable change in the administrative center of gravity for the federal judicial system occurred in 1939. In his "Court-packing" plan, President Roosevelt, proposing to reform judicial functioning, had suggested that a proctor (court administrator) be appointed for the Supreme Court. Although the plan to "pack" the Court was defeated, Congress did establish the Administrative Office of the Courts (A.O.). The A.O. is *not* part of the executive branch, and its creation within the judiciary reinforces separation of powers by allowing the judges to handle the administration of their own branch of government. At the same time, integrating administrative functions for the judiciary in the judiciary itself has increased friction between the branches, perhaps a natural result of separation of powers, in part because administration of the judiciary was cut off from the political power base on which it rested while in the Department of Justice.[45]

The A.O.'s director is appointed by the Supreme Court. The provision that the director perform duties assigned by the Supreme Court and the Judicial Conference acting together has, however, served to reduce the administrative role of the Supreme Court as a whole, although the Chief Justice has continued to be important after the director is named. This is true even when a Chief Justice like Earl Warren gives the director a relatively free hand, and is particularly true where there is a close working relationship, as there was between Chief Justice Burger and the directors who served during his tenure. There is no one to deal with the A.O. on the Chief Justice's behalf; the Chief deals directly with the director.

When the A.O. was first established, members of the Judicial Conference acted to limit the authority of the office and its director. It was the Conference's intent that the A.O. be "an executive office with strictly limited power," dealing with judges and other court personnel only upon authorization of the Conference, circuit councils, or individual courts, and performing housekeeping functions for the courts without employing the courts' personnel. However, the A.O. has often initiated policies later considered by the Conference and its recommendations have carried great weight.[46] It has even been suggested that judges show considerable deference to the Administrative Office, even for legal advice, instead of having their own clerks provide research on such matters or asking the staff of their own courts.

The Administrative Office took over most functions the Justice Department had performed plus others that the department had not performed. The A.O. has the duty to compile suggested budgets and prepare vital statistics, examine dockets, determine personnel needs and procure supplies, and carry out additional tasks the Supreme Court or the Judicial Conference assigns, for example, establishing federal public defender systems to implement the Criminal Justice Act. The A.O. also serves as the secretariat for the Judicial Conference and its committees and as the liaison between the judiciary and Congress, individual judges, professional organizations, and other government agencies. As a result of the establishment (in 1976) of a Legislative Affairs Office, the A.O. has been able to focus its responsibilities for legislation better and to go beyond information gathering to supplying of information and helping to resolve problems that develop during the process of enacting legislation affecting the judiciary.

The *Federal Judicial Center* is the most recently created (1967) element in federal judicial administration. It was set up to meet research and educational needs of the judiciary. Among the tasks that it has undertaken have been testing calendaring procedures and means of transmitting judicial documents. The Center has studied elements of the court system such as magistrates and circuit executives and such matters as case-screening, delays in the filing of transcripts, case management, and adoption by a court of administrative innovations. It has prepared a manual for complex and multidistrict litigation and a "bench book" for judges, and has conducted seminars and other training programs for newly appointed judges, magistrates, and probation officers.

The Supreme Court

We are so accustomed to a United States Supreme Court of nine justices that altering that number would be extremely difficult. The Constitution provides for a Supreme Court but does not designate its size, which was six at first. The number of justices fluctuated until well after the Civil War as presidents left seats vacant (Lincoln did so with three seats) and Congress ordered positions not to be filled (during Reconstruction) or increased the number (to 10 during the Civil War). In his Court-packing plan of 1937, President Franklin Roosevelt would have added a justice for each one over the age of 70 who did not retire. Chief Justice Hughes helped defeat the proposal with a statement to Congress that a Court of more than nine justices would be unwieldy and that the Court could not divide into panels or "divisions" to hear cases, as some state high courts do, because the Constitution speaks of "one Supreme Court." Chief Justice Burger suggested in 1984 that the Court have a tenth justice, but the "Associate Justice for Administration," chosen by the Chief Justice from among sitting federal judges, would have no judicial duties.

Original Jurisdiction

Only the Court's original jurisdiction—cases brought to it directly—is detailed in the Constitution. (See Art. III, Sec. 2.) The Court's original jurisdiction accounts for only a very small proportion of its workload; there have been only approximately 150 such cases decided in the Court's history. The Court itself said in *Marbury v. Madison* that original jurisdiction was limited to the subjects designated in Article III. More important, the Court often changes its original jurisdiction into appellate jurisdiction by sending cases brought as original jurisdiction cases to the district court first. The Court exercises "substantial discretion to make case-by-case judgments as to the practical necessity of an original forum in this Court for particular disputes within our constitutional original jurisdiction" and there has been disagreement about whether that discretion should be exercised.[47]

When the justices do accept an original jurisdiction case and it cannot be resolved on the pleadings alone, they appoint a special master (often a senior federal judge) to hear testimony and to make findings and recommendations, which the justices decide to accept, modify, or reject after hearing from the lawyers. In this way, the justices act, as usual, in an appellate capacity, with the master really serving as a trial judge, but the Court has not always agreed about how much weight is to be given to the master's findings.

> In all cases affecting ambassadors, other public ministers and consuls, and those in which a state shall be a party, the supreme court shall have original jurisdiction. In all the other cases before mentioned, the supreme court shall have appellate jurisdiction, both as to law and fact, with such exceptions and under such regulations as the Congress shall make. (Art. III, Sec. 2)

The Court's avoidance of original jurisdiction cases leaves for its original jurisdiction only cases between two states, for example, over boundaries or water allocation, that would be a "cause of war" if the states were sovereigns or between a state and the national government. The suits by states to test the validity of the 1965 and 1970 Voting Rights Acts (*South Carolina v. Katzenbach* and *Oregon v. Mitchell*) are examples of the latter. Yet even when two states are involved, the Court may try to send cases elsewhere, particularly if the parties' interests would be adequately protected in those courts.[48]

Appellate Jurisdiction

The Constitution makes the Supreme Court's appellate jurisdiction, which accounts for the bulk of the Court's work, relatively open-ended and subject to modification by Congress (see pages 308-9). The Supreme Court long had to hear all cases appealed to it that came within its jurisdiction, but it is important to remember that large classes of cases were outside the Court's appellate review. For example, until 1914, only state court decisions *denying* federal rights could be heard by the Supreme Court; only then, in order to provide uniform interpretation of federal law, did the high court get the authority to review those state court rulings *favoring* the federal right. Likewise, only decisions of the U.S. courts of appeals in civil cases could be appealed to the Supreme Court—if the case involved more than $1,000 and did not arise under the federal courts' diversity of citizenship, admiralty, patent, or revenue jurisdiction; only then were criminal cases from those courts subject to the Court's appellate jurisdiction. Indeed, while we are accustomed to assuming that criminal cases can be appealed, for much of our history federal criminal cases were not subject to appeal to the Supreme Court.

When the Supreme Court had to hear all the cases within its appellate jurisdiction, cases came to the Court on a *writ of error*, which allowed only review of the law, not of the facts in a case as a present-day appeal would. One way in which cases came to the Court was when there was a "division of the court" in the lower court: with only two judges (a justice and a judge) sitting, they could split evenly. Now almost all cases come to the Court in one of two ways—*appeal* and *certiorari*. After the present courts of appeals were established, the Supreme Court was provided authority to pick and choose the cases it would hear, that is, its certiorari jurisdiction, which now accounts for the great majority of its cases. Litigants with cases in the Court's certiorari jurisdiction that they wish the Supreme Court to hear file a petition for a writ of certiorari, which is an order to a lower court to send up the records in a case; when the Court issues the writ, it has accepted the case.

Certiorari jurisdiction was initiated in 1914 and was first restricted to state court decisions favoring rights claimed under federal law. Two years later, the Court's writ of error jurisdiction for appeals from state court decisions denying federal rights was somewhat curtailed, with some of those cases shifted to the Court's certiorari jurisdiction. Then the full growth of the certiorari jurisdiction came in the Judges Bill of 1925. Among the categories of cases within that jurisdiction are state court "federal question" decisions favorable to the federal claim, for example, when a state law is invalidated under the Supremacy Clause, and decisions by the U.S. courts of appeals interpreting or applying the Constitution, treaties, and federal laws or holding that state laws or constitutional provisions are *not* contrary to federal law.

The other principal category of the Supreme Court's appellate jurisdiction, cases brought on *appeal*, is in theory mandatory, that is, the Court must hear all cases in this category. However, the justices have made this jurisdiction largely discretionary (see page 202). Cases eligible for appeal encompass decisions in which:

- the highest state court invalidates a federal law or treaty as unconstitutional or upholds a state law or state constitutional provision against a challenge that it violates a federal law, treaty, or the U.S. Constitution;
- a U.S. court of appeals declares a state law or constitutional provision unconstitutional or declares a federal law unconstitutional when the federal government is a party to a case;
- a federal district court declares a federal law unconstitutional, again when the United States is a party; or
- a three-judge district court (see pages 47-48) has granted or denied an injunction in cases required to be brought before such a court.

There have been calls by the justices themselves for eliminating all the Court's mandatory jurisdiction; were that to be done, the above classes of cases would, like all others, come to the Court on petition for certiorari. Among the objections to mandatory jurisdiction is that the Court is sometimes forced to deal with an issue before it would prefer to do so and that, even when a mandatory jurisdiction case is given a summary disposition (see page 202), the Court nonetheless must spend more time with the case than it would with a certiorari petition. [49]

Quite infrequently, the Court receives a case on *certification*. Here a lower court faced with a new legal qustion, instead of resolving the case, "certifies" the question for answer by the Supreme Court. The justices have three basic choices: (1) they can refuse the certificate, forcing the lower court to decide the question on its own; (2) they can provide an answer, which the lower court applies; or (3) they may simply take the case and decide it directly without the extra step of returning it to the lower court, as the Supreme Court did with the Japanese Relocation Cases during World War II (see page 320). [50] (We might call this type of certification "upward" certification, to distinguish it from "downward" certification, a procedure for federal courts to send cases to state courts; see page 184.)

Supervisory Power and Rule Making

As the highest court in the federal court system, the Supreme Court affects rulings of the lower courts not only through its interpretations of statutes or the Constitution but also by exercising *supervisory power* over the lower federal courts. Some of the Court's decisions on procedural matters are based on this power, which is implied from the Constitution's providing for a Supreme Court and the reference to other federal courts, to be established by Congress, as "inferior" (that is, lower). A well-known example of the Court's use of its supervisory power is *Mallory v. United States* (1957), holding that a suspect must be taken before a magistrate for arraignment rather than being held by the police so that they can obtain a confession; another is *United States v. Hale* (1975), ruling that a defendant's silence after being given *Miranda* warnings cannot be used against him. Because rulings like *Mallory* were based on the supervisory power rather than the Constitution, they were not applicable to the states through the Fourteenth Amendment; because it involved the interpretation of the Federal Rules, it could also be revised by Congress. (The *Hale* ruling was, however, later given constitutional footing.[51])

Such exercises of the supervisory power are related to another, and separate, element of the Supreme Court's work: its role in the development of the rules of procedure for the federal judiciary. Rules are developed only occasionally through cases. More complete sets of rules (the Federal Rules of Criminal Procedure, Civil Procedure, Evidence, Appellate Procedure, and Bankruptcy) are promulgated by the Court under a grant of authority from Congress, the Rules Enabling Act (28 U.S.C. §2072). The Court does not itself develop the rules; an advisory committee, and, more recently, a committee of the Judicial Conference, itself aided by several advisory committees, prepares them, the Conference adopts them, and the Supreme Court then issues them. Even the Court itself knows that it is "in truth merely a conduit" for the transmission of the rules, although the justices are "nominally the promulgators" of them.[52] The Supreme Court develops its own Rules without use of an advisory committee or proceeding through the Judicial Conference, simply announcing Rules changes when it is ready to do so.

Justices Black and Douglas often criticized the Supreme Court's involvement in the promulgation of the rules. They felt that the Court should restrict itself to deciding cases, and that because the Court could not give full consideration to the Conference-proposed rules, the Conference itself should have full power to promulgate them. There have also been occasional disagreements by some of the justices with the substance of the Rules transmitted to Congress. For example, when amendments to the Federal Rules of Civil Procedure affecting pretrial discovery were transmitted to Congress in 1980, Justices Powell, Stewart, and Rehnquist stated that the proposed changes were insufficient to bring about needed changes in civil lawsuits; they feared that acceptance of these rules would deter consideration of more thorough and more effective reforms.

The Rules Enabling Act provided that the rules go into effect unless disapproved by Congress (a legislative veto); now Congress must pass a bill to defer the Rules' effect and the president must sign the bill. Ninety days has been the period usually designated for congressional action. For years, Congress accepted new Court-announced Rules without debate. However, when the Supreme Court announced new Federal Rules of Evidence in 1972, Congress, because of substantive disagreement over a number of the rules that embodied noticeable change from the past, delayed the effective date, subjected the rules to section-by-section reconsideration, and enacted them only in 1975. At the same time, Congress doubled the 90-day "waiting period" for congressional consideration of the evidence rules and provided that each house of Congress could extend that period for a specified time or until the rules were specifically approved by legislation. Congress also postponed for a year the effective date for the Federal Rules of Criminal Procedure, and in 1983 almost delayed changes in the Federal Rules of Civil and Criminal Procedure, but an agreement to extend consideration of them fell victim to legislative attention to other business. Congress, which granted the courts the authority to develop and promulgate the Rules, can itself change them, as it has done from time to time when considering, for example, issues of criminal procedure or, more recently, sentencing.

Judicial Review

What makes the Supreme Court particularly important is the power of *judicial review*—the power to invalidate acts of Congress, the executive branch, and state and local governments. The Court itself developed this power, which is not mentioned in the Constitution. All courts in the United States may exercise judicial review, but the Supreme Court, because of its position, has the final judicial word on matters of judicial review concerning the United States Constitution.

Judicial review in the United States had several sources; the idea was not wholly original. Its establishment and development were affected by philosophical views on such matters as the distribution and separation of powers that influenced the Founding Fathers. Also relevant, although not determinative, was the practice concerning the review of decisions made in the American colonies. "Conformity clauses" in state charters required acts of the colonial legislatures to conform to the laws of England. They gave the king's Privy Council and its Committee on Appeals the power to disallow the legislation—power exercised in fact by the Board of Trade. Such action was, however, review without a written constitution, which England did not have, so that it did not lead those in the colonies to associate judicial review with a written constitution. Decisions of the courts in the colonies could also be appealed to the Privy Council when the royal governor granted a request to appeal. Here the Committee on Appeals often based its decisions on the colony's local law.

The Articles of Confederation did not establish judicial review, as the Articles contained no provision for a separate national judiciary. Congress became the court of last appeal, or the board of arbitration, for controversies between the states and for a limited number of cases involving individual rights. The Constitution's Supremacy Clause was anticipated, however, in the stipulation that the Articles and acts of Congress be accorded the status of law within the states:

Every State shall abide by the determination of the United States in Congress assembled, on all questions which by this Confederation are submitted to them. And the Articles of this Confederation shall be inviolably observed by every State. (Art. XIII)

No plan submitted to the Constitutional Convention of 1787 conferred directly upon the judiciary any power of passing on the constitutionality of congressional acts. Under one major proposal—the Virginia Plan—there would have been a national court system whose judges would have been chosen by Congress. Congress would have had the right to disallow state legislation; a council of revision composed of the executive and a "convenient number" of the judiciary would have had a suspensive veto over national legislation. The major alternate plan made acts of Congress and treaties the "supreme law of the respective States." The state judiciary would be bound by congressional acts, notwithstanding state constitutional provisions. Because state courts would initially decide federal cases, the need for lower federal courts would be eliminated and the strength of the national government thus decreased. There would, however, be a supreme national tribunal, appointed by the executive. This court would have appellate jurisdiction in certain classes of cases coming from the state courts.

The Convention eliminated congressional disallowance of state legislation and judicial participation in the veto. Establishment of a Supreme Court was indicated, with Congress having the power to create lower federal courts. Although the jurisdiction of the courts generally and of the Supreme Court in particular was spelled out, and although supremacy of national law was established, not a word was said regarding the power of these federal courts to invalidate laws contrary to the Constitution. As with much of the rest of the document, the language was left general—perhaps a necessity if approval of the Constitution was to be obtained.

> This Constitution, and the Laws of the United States which shall be made in Pursuance thereof and all Treaties made, or which shall be made, under the Authority of the United States, shall be the supreme Law of the Land; and the Judges in every State shall be bound thereby, any Thing in the Constitution or Laws of any State to the Contrary notwithstanding. (Art. VI, cl. 2)

The leaders of the Constitutional Convention may not have foreseen that judges would engage in general expounding of the Constitution's meaning. However, they apparently did believe that the federal judiciary had the right to refuse to recognize unconstitutional federal law. Hamilton, Madison, and Jay, who wrote *The Federalist* papers to secure ratification of the Constitution in New York, argued strongly for judicial review. (They dealt summarily with the Supreme Court's right to overrule state legislation, thus indicating it was less of an issue, at least for them.) According to *The Federalist*, the Constitution as fundamental law was to be preferred when there was an irreconcilable variance between it and a legislative act, and the courts had a duty "to declare all acts contrary to the manifest tenor of the Constitution" void. There was, however, no direct empowerment to construe laws according to the Constitution's *spirit*. Judicial review was not an exercise of judicial power over the legislative branch. Instead, through judicial review the intention of the people—who ratified the Constitution—would be enforced against the intention of their agents, the legislators; the prior act of a superior authority would be preferred to the subsequent act of an inferior one.

The authors of *The Federalist* also noted that state judges were to be incorporated into the operation of the national government and would be bound by oath to support federal laws when those laws concerned legitimate and enumerated objects of federal jurisdiction. The Supremacy Clause was deemed imperative in helping produce needed uniform interpretation of federal law and treaties, as was national court jurisdiction and a supreme tribunal of last resort, because without appeal and review, state courts of final jurisdiction would produce an endless variety of decisions on the same point. So that all matters of national law would receive original or final determination in the national courts, appeal would run from state courts to either the federal district courts or the Supreme Court. However, in an appeal to states' rights interests, it was pointed out that the state courts—which would look beyond their own law in making decisions and would recognize relevant federal court rulings—would retain their former jurisdiction unless specifically limited by Congress, and that this system of initial state court determination with appeals from the state court to the federal courts would actually diminish the number of federal courts.

Judicial review of state decisions occurred before judicial review of national actions and, despite controversy, became firmly established earlier. In 1797, in *Ware v. Hylton*, the Court held our treaty of peace with Great Britain superior to Virginia's statute sequestering property; the next year, in *Calder v. Bull*, the Court reviewed a state action challenged under the Ex Post Facto Clause, although it did not invalidate the statute in question. Twelve years later, in *Fletcher v. Peck*, stemming from the Yazoo land fraud case, the Court ruled a Georgia statute in violation of the Constitution.[53] The most severe early test of judicial review of state *court* decisions came when Virginia courts declared unconstitutional a provision of the federal Judiciary Act establishing appeal of state decisions affecting federal rights. Responding in *Martin v. Hunter's Lessee* (1816), Justice Joseph Story ruled that the U.S. Supreme Court had a right to review the decisions of state courts in order to produce uniform intepretation of the nation's "supreme law." Five years later, Virginia's claim that a criminal defendant's appeal from a state ruling violated state sovereignty—part of the early battle over "states' rights"—was rejected in *Cohens v. Virginia*. Chief Justice Marshall stated that the Supreme Court had the right to appellate jurisdiction over decisions of highest state courts in all questions of national power.

The need for uniform national interpretation of constitutional provisions has led to the feeling that the Supreme Court's power to review state decisions may be more important than its power over national government actions. As Justice Holmes put it, "I do not think the United States would come to an end if we lost our power to declare an act of Congress void. I do think the Union would be imperilled if we could not make that declaration as to the laws of the several states."[54] Throughout our history the Court has invalidated state laws more frequently than federal laws. Until the end of the Civil War, only 2 federal laws—but 60 state laws—were struck down. In the period from 1888 to 1937, over 400 state laws were invalidated, while only 70 national statutes were declared invalid. In the post-1937 period, well over 1,000 state laws were declared unconstitutional, but, under the legislative veto case, only a few more than one hundred had received such treatment; in invalidating the legislative veto, the Court struck down portions of over *two hundred* statutes at once. (See page 305 on continuing use of legislative vetoes.) (The Warren Court invalidated 19 acts of Congress in 16 years; before the Gramm-Rudman budget ruling and not counting the multiple statutes affected by the legislative veto decision, the Burger Court struck down 29 acts of Congress in the same period.)

The exercise of judicial review of state laws may be more readily accepted now than in the Court's earliest days, although particular rulings may be disputed. However, resistance to such judicial review *itself* still occurs at times. During the height of resistance to the Court's 1954 desegregation decision, Arkansas Governor Orval Faubus asserted that state governments were not bound by Supreme Court decisions because those decisions were not part of the "supreme law of the land." In the famous Little Rock case, *Cooper v. Aaron* (1958), the Supreme Court rejected this contention and stressed the supremacy of national law, *including* the Supreme Court's interpretation of it. More recently, when a federal judge's efforts to gain compliance with his orders concerning Native Americans' rights to their share of spawning fish (steelhead and salmon) encountered serious resistance from Washington State officials, the Supreme Court had to reiterate that a state's prohibition against compliance with a federal district court's decree could not survive under the Supremacy Clause.[55]

Judicial review of national government actions has been far more controversial. *Marbury v. Madison*, an 1803 case, was the first instance in which the Court invalidated a national statute, but the Court had earlier upheld a federal statute, an implicit recognition of judicial review. In 1796, in *Hylton v. United States*, the Court had reviewed an act of Congress imposing a carriage tax but, by ruling the tax not a direct one that would have had to be apportioned among the population, the Court did not have to rule on the statute's constitutionality. Four years earlier, in *Hayburn's Case* (1792) Chief Justice John Jay and four other justices, ruling in Circuit Court decisions, said that a statute subjecting Circuit Court decisions on individuals' eligibility for pension benefits to review by the Secretary of War and Congress was invalid because the courts' decisions were not final and thus were mere advisory opinions. The justices, this time sitting as the Supreme Court rather than as circuit justices, ruled to the same effect in *United States v. Todd* in 1794. Nonetheless, it was the *Marbury* decision that established judicial review. In the waning hours of the Federalist administration, Marbury had been appointed to a minor judicial position but had not received his commission. He sought a writ of mandamus from the Supreme Court to make the new Secretary of State, James Madison, hand over the commission. Chief Justice John Marshall, himself one of the last of the Federalist appointees, found that Marbury had a right to his commission and thus was entitled to a remedy. However, he ruled that the Court could not issue the requested writ because the Judiciary Act of 1789 unconstitutionally added to the Court's original jurisdiction:

> If congress remains at liberty to give this court appellate jurisdiction, where the Constitution has declared their jurisdiction shall be original; and original jurisdiction where the Constitution has declared it shall be appellate; the distribution of jurisdiction, made in the Constitution, is form without substance. . . .

Marshall insisted that the language of the Constitution be taken seriously. "It is a proposition too plain to be contested," he asserted, "that the constitution controls any legislative act repugnant to it; or that the legislature may alter the constitution by an ordinary act"; there were no other alternatives. The Constitution had to be either a "superior paramount law, unchangeable by ordinary means" or it was like any other law. But, Marshall said,

> Certainly, all those who have framed written constitutions contemplate them as forming the fundamental and paramount law of the nation, and consequently, the theory of every such government must be that an act of the legislature repugnant to the constitution is void.

From this he concluded that the courts should invalidate the "repugnant" acts, giving the courts power over the other branches of government when constitutional questions were at issue.

In ruling as he did, Marshall gave himself an opportunity to lecture the Jeffersonians and established judicial review over acts of Congress, perhaps putting the administration on notice that future legislation might be declared unconstitutional. It is quite important to recognize *Marbury* as a decision founded in large measure on political prudence. Although Jefferson's administration was lectured, "the actual holding of the case worked to the advantage of the . . . administration" because there was no order for it to disobey; in that sense, it could be seen as "a conciliatory gesture on the part of the Supreme Court" toward the administration.[56] More important, had Marshall *not* acted as he did, it would have been seen as a retreat by the judiciary. Thus "a brief opinion simply denying jurisdiction would not have been a 'neutral' act without important political effects" but "would have been interpreted as the act of a fearful judiciary bending before a triumphant and hostile party that was dominating the legislative and executive branches."[57] As Chief Justice Burger has observed, if Marshall had mandamused the administration and the order had been ignored, the Court would have faced "ridicule, and the ale houses would rock with hilarious laughter."[58] Because Marshall was Chief Justice before we had a stable political system and while there was still a lack of agreement about our fundamental principles, it was crucial that Marshall defend the Constitution to the nation, as he did in his opinion, where he engaged in examination of the Constitution "to support the general argument from the nature of the U.S. government."[59]

Marshall's opinion is open to considerable criticism. Under today's standards, he would have withdrawn from the case because of his earlier involvement; as secretary of state, he had failed to deliver Marbury's commission. Had he followed usual procedure and looked first at whether the Court had jurisdiction, he could have invalidated the statute but could not have lectured the administration about not giving up the commission. More important, Marshall could have followed a rule of judicial self-restraint and construed the Act of 1789 to save its constitutionality by saying the items of original jurisdiction enumerated in the Constitution need not be exclusive but could be supplemented by Congress, a view generally accepted in the 1790s.

Nor was Marshall's conclusion the only one he could have reached. Judge Gibson of the Pennsylvania Supreme Court was later to say in *Eakin v. Raub* that the courts were limited to looking to see whether the legislature, in passing a law, had used the proper procedures because "the legislative organ is superior to every other, inasmuch as the power to will and command is essentially superior to the power to act and to obey." Judges implementing a law properly passed but in violation of the constitution were not, Gibson said, themselves committing an unconstitutional act but only doing what they were required to do.

Moreover, there are other arguments aimed at limiting the force of judicial review. One is that each branch of government should decide for itself what is constitutional and then should act on the basis of its own conclusions. President Andrew Jackson, saying he had to make his own judgment, vetoed legislation for a national bank even though Chief Justice John Marshall, in *McCulloch v. Maryland*, had earlier sustained the validity of such a bank. President Jefferson thought Supreme Court determinations about statutes' validity were entitled to respect but were not binding on him as president. Similarly, after *Dred Scott*, President Lincoln said he would again vote to ban slavery in the territories: a ruling not embodying what he conceived to be the Constitution's basic or fundamental values was not a "political rule" he had to follow nor did it command permanent obedience but was to be challenged.[60] Such a position—based on the idea that legislators and executives as well as judges take an oath to support the Constitution and can be thought to be as committed as judges to that oath—is close to that taken by President Nixon's lawyer when he told the justices that the question of whether the Watergate tapes had to be surrendered was being submitted for the Court's "guidance and judgment with respect to the law."

Most recently, Attorney General Meese said in a 1986 Tulane University speech that Supreme Court interpretations of the Constitution were not "the law of the land" and that officials' own views of the Constitution should guide their acts. In so doing, he was only repeating what earlier officials had stated, and was restating the view that the Supreme Court and the Constitution are not one and the same. However, he went on to say that a Supreme Court ruling "does not establish a 'supreme law of the land' that is binding on all persons and parts of the government, henceforth and forevermore." The Court's own overturning of precedents takes care of the "henceforth and forevermore" but the Court's rulings *are* supposed to bind "all . . . parts of government," including the states, not simply "the parties in the case and the executive branch for whatever enforcement is necessary." Given Meese's previous attacks on specific Supreme Court rulings (see page 315), it is no surprise that his statement produced an uproar and an outcry, not much lessened by a subsequent modification in which he talked of the general applicability of the Court's rulings. Moreover, his willingness to encourage extension of Supreme Court rulings consonant with the adminstration's position suggested a selectivity in the rulings to which he did not want broad adherence given.

The position that each branch should look to its own views would make judges' rulings potentially persuasive but not determinative for the other policy-making branches, and would not prevent them from taking actions they thought appropriate or from trying to enforce laws without the courts' assistance, but it would still allow judges to refuse to *enforce* policies they thought unconstitutional when those policies came before the courts in "cases and controversies." However, even under this view, the Court's ability to rule effectively on challenges to acts of the other branches might not be severely limited because the executive needs to seek judicial assistance in enforcing the law.

In another, related version of judicial review, each branch should have the final word about matters directly affecting it or "naturally" falling within its respective special competence. In this view, we would have "judicial supremacy" only about matters within the judiciary's particular bailiwick. Examples are the jurisdictional question in *Marbury*, the advisory opinion aspect of *Hayburn's Case*, and judicial remedies for constitutional violations, such as desegregation orders. Chief Justice Marshall, of course, went further, to establish judicial review over the acts of the legislative and executive branches affecting the entire government, not simply the judiciary, although after *Marbury* the Court took no further such action for more than 50 years—a time lapse that has, however, been "attributed to lack of provocation rather than to judicial self-restraint" because judicial review "had long since won general public acceptance."[61]

The criticisms of *Marbury* ignored the case's long-term implications for judicial review, and it was Marshall's position, not Gibson's or that of unhappy political executives, that won the day. *Marbury* came to stand for the Supreme Court's power—and by extension the power of other courts—to invalidate acts of

Congress and the president. As Marshall asserted, in language the Court was again to use in *United States v. Nixon* in ruling that the president was not the sole judge of when he could invoke executive privilege:

> It is, emphatically, the province and duty of the judicial department, to say what the law is. Those who apply the rule to particular cases must of necessity expound and interpret that rule. . . . If a law be in opposition to the constitution; if both the law and the constitution apply to a particular case, so that the court must either decide that case, conformably to the law, disregarding the constitution, or conformably to the constitution, disregarding the law; the court must determine which of these conflicting rules governs the case; this is of the very essence of judicial duty.

Although judicial review was extended the year after *Marbury* to executive orders, in *Little v. Barreme*, the power was not used again until 1857, when the Court struck down congressional action concerning slavery in the territories in *Dred Scott v. Sandford*, only the first instance of national judicial review not dealing with strictly judicial matters. Perhaps in part because of the bad name given to judicial review of other branches of the national government by Chief Justice Taney's ruling in *Dred Scott* that slaves were not citizens and thus could not bring lawsuits, it became common only at the end of the nineteenth century. Because of this and the fact that it was not used frequently until the 1930s, we should remember Justice Cardozo's words: "The utility of an external power restraining the legislative judgment is not to be measured by counting the occasions of its exercise":[62] judicial review has become fully established.

Notes

1. *Stuart v. Laird*, 1 Cr. 299 (1803). See Wythe Holt, "The First Federal Question Case," *Law and History Review* 3 (Spring 1985): 169–89.

2. Julius Goebel, Jr., *History of the Supreme Court of the United States: Antecedents and Beginnings to 1801* (New York: Macmillan, 1971), p. 565.

3. See Joel Grossman and Austin Sarat, "Litigation in the Federal Courts: A Comparative Perspective," *Law & Society Review* 9 (1973): 321–46.

4. *Thermtron Products v. Hermansdorfer*, 423 U.S. 336 (1976).

5. Published district court rulings, a very small proportion of all those decided, may be found in the *Federal Supplement*, cited as "F.Supp.," as in 535 F.Supp. 234 (E.D.Va. 1986).

6. J. Woodford Howard, Jr., *Courts of Appeals in the Federal Judicial System: A Study of the Second, Fifth, and District of Columbia Circuits* (Princeton, N.J.: Princeton University Press, 1981), p. 39.

7. Ibid., p. 34.

8. Ibid., p. 41.

9. This section draws on Steven Puro, "United States Magistrates: A New Federal Judicial Officer," *Justice System Journal* 2 (Winter 1976): 141–56; two monographs by Carroll Seron: *The Roles of Magistrates in Federal District Courts* (Washington, D.C.: Federal Judicial Center, 1983), and *The Roles of Magistrates: Nine Case Studies* (Washington, D.C.: Federal Judicial Center, 1985); and Christopher E. Smith, "Who Are the U.S. Magistrates?" paper presented to Midwest Political

84   Elements of the Federal Judicial System

Science Association, Chicago, 1987. See also Seron, "Magistrates and the Work of Federal Courts: A New Division of Labor," *Judicature* 69 (April–May 1986): 353–59.

10. *United States v. Raddatz*, 447 U.S. 667 (1980).

11. *Mathews v. Weber*, 423 U.S. 261 at 272 (1976).

12. *Pacemaker Diagnostic Clinic v. Instromedic, Inc.*, 725 F.2d 537 (9th Cir. 1984) (en banc), overruling a Ninth Circuit panel holding to the contrary, 712 F.2d 1305 (9th Cir. 1983). See also *Wharton-Thomas v. United States*, 721 F.2d 922 (3rd Cir. 1983).

13. *Northern Pipeline Construction Co. v. Marathon Pipe Line Co.*, 458 U.S. 50 (1982).

14. Another famous instance was the Court's postponement of school desegregation, after its initial ruling in *Brown v. Board of Education* (1954), first by asking for further argument on implementation of the ruling and then, in its 1955 ruling in the case, allowing implementation to proceed "with all deliberate speed." *Brown v. Board of Education* (1955).

15. *In re Koerner*, 800 F.2d 1358 (5th Cir. 1986).

16. *Glidden v. Zdanok*, 370 U.S. 530 (1962).

17. Howard, *Courts of Appeals*, pp. 20–21.

18. See Stephen L. Wasby, "Communication Within the Ninth Circuit Court of Appeals: The View From the Bench," *Golden Gate University Law Review* 8 (1977): 1–25; and "Inconsistency in the United States Courts of Appeals: Dimensions and Mechanisms for Resolution," *Vanderbilt Law Review* 32 (November 1979): 1343–73.

19. Published opinions of the courts of appeals appear in *Federal Reporter*, now in its second series; it is cited as "F.2d" (when speaking, "Fed Second") so a court of appeals case would be 624 F.2d 325 (5th Cir. 1986).

20. Richard J. Richardson and Kenneth N. Vines, *The Politics of Federal Courts* (Boston: Little, Brown, 1970), pp. 118–19.

21. Ibid., pp. 127–29.

22. Howard, *Courts of Appeals*, p. 42.

23. Ibid., p. 55.

24. Ibid., pp. 3, 78.

25. Ibid., pp. 58, 76.

26. See Harold Spaeth, "Supreme Court Disposition of Federal Circuit Court Decisions," *Judicature* 68 (December–January 1985): 245–50; Gerald F. Uelmen, "The Influence of the Solicitor General Upon Disposition of Federal Circuit Court Decisions: A Closer Look at the Ninth Circuit Record," *Judicature* 69 (April–May 1986): 360–66.

27. Lawrence Baum, "Judicial Specialization, Litigant Influence, and Substantive Policy: The Court of Customs and Patent Appeals," *Law & Society Review* 11 (Summer 1977): 845–46; see generally 833–46.

28. See Ellen R. Jordan, "Should Litigants Have a Choice Between Specialized Courts and Courts of General Jurisdiction," *Judicature* 66 (June–July 1982): 14–27, for a discussion of this and other specialized courts.

29. For a thorough discussion of the "independent counsel" provisions, see Mark Bertozzi, "Separating Politics from the Administration of Justice: The Role of the Federal Special Prosecutor," *Judicature* 67 (May 1984): 486–98.

30. See *Reid v. Covert*, 354 U.S. 1 (1957) (no courts-martial of wives of servicemen stationed overseas); *United States ex rel. Toth v. Quarles*, 350 U.S. 11 (1955) (ex-servicemen); *O'Callaghan v. Parker*, 395 U.S. 298 (1969) (nonservice-connected offense). See also Norma G. Cooper and John S. Cooke, "Military Justice: Marching to a Different Drumbeat," *American Bar Association Journal* 64 (September 1978): 1363–65.

31. See also the proposal for a National Court of State Appeals to review state court decisions in which federal questions were raised. James Duke Cameron, "Federal Review, Finality of State Court Decisions, and a Proposal for a National Court of Appeals—A State Judge's Solution to a Continuing Problem," *Brigham Young University Law Review* 1981: 545–78.

32.   See Arthur Hellman, "Caseload, Conflicts, and Decisional Capacity: Does the Supreme Court Need Help?" *Judicature* 67 (June–July 1983): 41, where Hellman thoroughly presents other arguments against establishing the new court.

33.   Russell R. Wheeler and Howard R. Whitcomb, "What Is Judicial Administration: A Tedious Effort to Explain Some Basic Concepts," *Judicial Administration: Text and Readings*, eds. Wheeler and Whitcomb (Englewood Cliffs, N.J.: Prentice-Hall, 1977), p. 8.

34.   Peter Graham Fish, *The Politics of Federal Judicial Administration* (Princeton, N.J.: Princeton University Press, 1973), p. 8. Fish's book is the source of much material for this section.

35.   *Pennsylvania Bureau of Correction v. United States Marshals Service*, 106 S.Ct. 355 (1986).

36.   Howard, *Courts of Appeals*, p. 275.

37.   See Peter G. Fish, "Politics Rides the Circuits: State and National Itineracy," *Justice System Journal* 5 (Winter 1979): 115–69.

38.   This was raised in the Claiborne case (see p. 96). See *United States v. Claiborne*, 781 F.2d 1327 (9th Cir. 1986) (Reinhardt, J., dissent from denial of rehearing en banc).

39.   See John T. McDermott and Steven Flanders, *The Impact of the Circuit Executive Act* (Washington, D.C.: Federal Judicial Center, 1979); and Steven Flanders, "Court Executives and Decentralization of the Federal Judiciary," *Judicature* 70 (February–March 1987): 273–79.

40.   Fish, *The Politics of Federal Judicial Administration*, p. 408.

41.   Peter Graham Fish, "The Office of Chief Justice of the United States," *The Office of Chief Justice* (Charlottesville, Va.: University of Virginia, 1984), p. 135.

42.   Fish, *The Politics of Federal Judicial Administration*, p. 39.

43.   Fish, "The Office of Chief Justice," p. 59.

44.   Fish, *The Politics of Federal Judicial Administration*, p. 93.

45.   See Fish, "The Office of Chief Justice," p. 36.

46.   Fish, *The Politics of Federal Judicial Administration*, p. 191.

47.   *Texas v. New Mexico*, 462 U.S. 554 at 570 (1983); see the opinions in *South Carolina v. Regan*, 465 U.S. 367 (1984).

48.   See *Arizona v. New Mexico*, 425 U.S. 794 (1976) (parties' interests would be protected by state court lawsuit).

49.   See Arthur Hellman, "The Proposed Intercircuit Tribunal: Do We Need It/Will It Work?" *Hastings Constitutional Law Quarterly* 11 (Spring 1984): 389–91.

50.   See Peter Irons, *Justice at War: The Story of the Japanese American Internment Cases* (New York: Oxford University Press, 1983), p. 183.

51.   *Doyle v. Ohio*, 426 U.S. 610 (1976).

52.   *United States v. Abel*, 105 S.Ct. 465 at 468 (1984) (Justice Rehnquist).

53.   See C. Peter McGrath, *Yazoo: Law and Politics in the New Republic* (Providence, R.I.: Brown University Press, 1966).

54.   Oliver Wendell Holmes, in *Collected Legal Papers* (New York: Harcourt, Brace, and Howe, 1920), p. 295.

55.   *Washington v. Washington State Commercial Passenger Fishing Vessel Association*, 443 U.S. 658 (1979). Quoting the Ninth Circuit's opinion, the Court observed that, "except for some desegregation cases, . . . the district court has faced the most concerted official and private efforts to frustrate a decree of a federal court witnessed in this century." At 697.

56.   Richard Ellis, "The Impeachment of Samuel Chase," *American Political Trials*, ed. Michal R. Belknap (Westport, Conn.: Greenwood Press, 1981), p. 62.

57.   Christopher Wolfe, *The Rise of Modern Judicial Review* (New York: Basic Books, 1986), p. 87.

58.   Warren Burger, "The Doctrine of Judicial Review: Mr. Marshall, Mr. Jefferson, and Mr. Marbury," *Views from the Bench*, eds. Mark Cannon and David O'Brien (Chatham, N.J.: Chatham House, 1985), p. 14.

59.   Wolfe, *Modern Judicial Review*, p. 84. It also appears that Marshall selectively used precedent in *Marbury*, combining several cases into one to support a position and then ignoring that same precedent when it did not support his position. See Susan Low Bloch and Maeva Marcus, "John Marshall's Selective Use of History in *Marbury v. Madison*," *Wisconsin Law Review* 1986: 301–37.

60.   Don E. Fehrenbacher, *The Dred Scott Case: Its Significance in American Law & Politics* (New York: Oxford University Press, 1978), pp. 4–5, 442–43.

61.   Ibid., p. 232.

62.   Benjamin Cardozo, *The Nature of the Judicial Process* (New Haven: Yale University Press, 1921), p. 92.

3   Judicial Selection

F<small>EDERAL JUDGES</small>—<small>NOMINATED BY</small> the president and confirmed by the Senate—
are chosen by a political process involving both formal procedures and relatively
well-defined patterns of participation by nongovernmental groups. Most nominees for federal judgeships are confirmed, but the process, particularly prior to
nomination, and even after submission of the nomination to the Senate, can be
far from routine, and rejections of nominations, even to the Supreme Court,
indicate the importance of the process's nonformal aspects.

The Constitutional Convention debated several methods of selecting the
justices. These included selection by the Senate alone, by the entire Congress,
and by the executive alone. The method ultimately adopted was the one already
in use in Massachusetts—nomination by the chief executive with the advice and
consent of the Senate. However, the Constitution specifies no formal process by
which the president is to choose those to be nominated. This leaves it to the
executive, working with members of the Senate, to develop the process by which
the name of a person reaches the stage at which it is to be sent to the Senate.

Usually a nominee to a federal judgeship does not assume office until after
Senate confirmation. However, when a judgeship is vacant, and certain conditions are met, the president may make a *recess appointment* to a vacant judgeship,
allowing the person to take office immediately. This has happened over 300 times
and included the appointments of Chief Justice Earl Warren and Justices Brennan, Stewart, and Marshall. A recess appointment is valid only under certain
circumstances, designed to prevent the president from naming as a recess appointee someone whose nomination has been rejected by the Senate or from carrying
over a recess appointee from before one Senate term to after its conclusion. The

constitutionality of recess appointment was recently questioned after President Carter gave the first such appointment in twenty years to someone on whose nomination (to a district judgeship in Hawaii) the Senate had not acted. Deciding an appeal from a conviction in that judge's court, a court of appeals panel ruled he had not been properly appointed because a recess appointee, subject to political pressures during subsequent Senate consideration of his nomination, would lack proper judicial independence. However, the full court of appeals upheld the president's authority to make recess appointments.[1]

The Judges, both of the Supreme and inferior Courts, shall hold their Offices during good Behaviour, and shall, at stated Times, receive for their Services, a Compensation, which shall not be diminished during their Continuance in Office. (Art. III, Sec. 1)

Attracting, Retaining, and Removing Judges

In the Supreme Court's early years, presidents at times had difficulty obtaining men to serve as justices because of the job's lack of prestige. Some who did serve left the Court after brief service or simultaneously held other government jobs. Now, however, the position of justice of the Supreme Court is thought to be the highest to be attained in the legal profession and is likely to be accepted readily when offered—although apparently President Johnson's initial offer of a position was refused by Abe Fortas. Justices now only rarely leave the Court for other positions, and then only at the president's urging, for example, when James Byrnes became the president's special assistant during World War II and Arthur Goldberg became ambassador to the United Nations.

There are somewhat greater problems in attracting lower court judges and particularly in retaining them. The recent frequency of departure is certainly higher than it had been. Between 1970 and 1981, 30 federal judges, most of them from the district courts, resigned their positions, and another baker's dozen did so by mid-1986. Most of them entered private practice, although several took major government positions—senator, FBI Director, Secretary of Education, Solicitor General, Attorney General. (One, G. Harrold Carswell, resigned after his nomination to the Supreme Court was rejected, and Otto Kerner did so after being convicted for bribery, mail fraud, and income tax evasion for events occurring prior to his judgeship.) Most had from five to 10 years' service, and several of the appeals court judges had more than 10 years' service.

What might be the reasons for the departures of district judges or the reluctance of others to become judges? Despite the high prestige of the job, some say its status has been diminished by the increased number of judgeships: there are now more U.S. court of appeals judges than U.S. senators and more district judges than members of the House of Representatives. For the politically active, a judgeship may mean too much isolation. Danger may also play at least a small part. The number of serious threats against federal judges has increased in the last few years and reductions in security guard positions as a result of Gramm-Rudman have increased judges' concern about their safety. In 1979, a federal judge in west Texas, John H. Wood, Jr., was shot and killed, apparently as a result of the severity of his sentences in drug cases; in 1982 two men were charged with conspiring to murder a district judge in California (also in connection with a drug case); and someone seeking revenge against a Maryland federal judge abducted the judge's wife (she was quickly released). In 1986, a federal judge in North Dakota who had presided over some controversial trials was the intended target of a pipe bomb that was defused.

Supreme Court justices have also been subject to potential or actual violence. In 1982, a man angry at the Court's rulings struck Justice Byron White several times while White was about to deliver a speech to a bar association meeting in Utah, but the Justice was not injured. There have been death threats against Justice Blackmun, some by a radical, antiabortion group, and a shot was fired into his home in February 1985, although the shot was later thought to be random or a wandering distant shot.

Salary

The principal difficulty in attracting and retaining judges—cited as at least one reason for departure by many of those who left during the 1970s and 1980s—is salary, because the double-digit inflation of that period resulted in a decrease in federal judges' real income and because most could earn high six-figure incomes in major corporate law firms. Fringe benefits could also be a problem: an appellate judge resigned in 1981 because of limited annuities for judges' survivors, a problem subsequently remedied.

Federal judges did not receive raises for more than six years until 1975. The raise that year placed salaries of district judges at only $42,000 and that of court of appeals judges at $44,600. These salaries led over 80 federal judges to pursue litigation. They asserted that the Compensation Clause (Art. III, Sec. 1)—the provision that their pay shall not be reduced during their term in office—had been violated by the erosion of their pay by inflation since 1969 to the equivalent of $27,510 for a district judge and $29,230 for a court of appeals judge. (By 1985, inflation reduced a district judge's salary to $26,032 in 1969 dollars.) Some judges proceeded with their lawsuit despite a $12,000-plus pay increase in early 1977, only to have the Court of Claims rule that the Constitution provided no protection against inflation-caused "indirect" reduction in judges' salaries.[2]

New litigation was initiated when Congress in four successive years (1976–79) either stopped or reduced statutory automatic cost-of-living increases. In two of the years, the stop or reduction became law before the start of the fiscal year, but in the other two years, because of congressional delay, the fiscal year had already begun, resulting in a temporary increase followed by a reduction. When the case (*United States v. Will*, 1981) reached the Supreme Court, the justices first had to face the problem that with all judges affected by a ruling, no judge could decide it without being involved in a conflict of interest. On this point, the Court ruled that, when every judge has a conflict, some judge nonetheless has to hear a case (the Rule of Necessity) to assure that plaintiffs' complaints could be heard. Then, underscoring the Compensation Clause's importance for judicial independence, the Court ruled that Congress, which had the authority to set judges' salaries, could change an already-adopted salary formula *only* if the change were made before the beginning of the fiscal year. Thus judges were entitled to increases (of 4.8 percent and 12.9 percent) for two years, but not for the other two years when Congress acted in time. This litigation affected only Article III judges, as others, such as bankruptcy judges and magistrates, are not protected from salary reductions, and a lower court upheld Congress' reduction of proposed salary increases enacted ten days into the fiscal year.

Under the present arrangement for setting judicial salaries, the Commission on Executive, Legislative, and Judicial Salaries recommends a figure to the president, who makes recommendations to Congress; those recommendations are to go into effect after 30 days unless Congress, by joint resolution (which requires a presidential signature), overturns the resolution, or overrides a presidential veto of the joint resolution. Prior to 1985, a negative vote by either house was sufficient to reject the recommendations. In addition, the Comptroller General has issued a ruling that cost-of-living increases for judges require specific congressional approval, and cannot be automatic, but a reconsideration of that ruling has been requested by Judicial Conference members.

By late 1982, district judges' salaries reached $73,100 and appeals court judges were receiving $77,300 as a result of the Supreme Court's ruling, further congressional delays in reducing proposed salary increases, and an additional increase granted by Congress. A 3.5 percent pay increase in 1985 brought salaries for the district courts and the Court of International Trade to $78,000, and for the courts of appeals to $83,200. Supreme Court justices, who had received $63,000 in 1977 ($65,600 for the Chief Justice), now receive $104,100 ($108,400 for the Chief Justice). Some members of Congress objected to further increases. They said the pool of those both competent and willing to serve is quite adequate, so that making judges' salaries so much higher than those of the "common person" to attract candidates is not necessary. However, inflation, increased costs of college education for judges' children, and availability of far higher compensation in private law practice (at least $200,000—and likely much more—in major corporate law firms) led to recommendations for even higher salaries, and some judges, frustrated about the Judicial Conference's apparent inability to convince Congress of their salary needs, formed a group, the Federal Judges Association, to lobby Congress concerning pay and fringe benefits, although Chief Justice Burger strongly disapproved of such an organization.

In early 1987, the president severely reduced the commission's recommendations of $130,000 for district judges, $135,000 for appeals court judges, and

$165,000 for Supreme Court justices ($175,000 for the Chief Justice), recommending to Congress increases of approximately 10 percent for lower court
judges—$89,500 for the district courts, $95,000 for the appeals courts—and less
than 3 percent for the Supreme Court ($110,000 for associate justices, $115,000
for the Chief Justice). Although the Senate voted in time to cancel even these
increases, the House, which also voted negatively, did so one day late, and the
changes in justices' salaries went into effect (subject to possible judicial challenges to the salary-increase process).

Also relevant to judges' salary complaints is their outside income. The 1978
Ethics in Government Act requires high-level government officials, including
judges, to file annual financial disclosure statements, indicating stocks or bonds
worth more than $1,000 or savings accounts of $5,000, the threshold figures for
reporting, which is only within very broad categories. When several judges
argued that, as applied to judges, the law violated separation of powers and
allowed intrusions on judicial independence, the Fifth Circuit upheld the law
and the Supreme Court refused review.[3] Examination of lower court judges'
statements for 1980 showed that only two had no outside income—including
honoraria for speeches, book royalties, and pensions from previous positions—
and only 16 had less than $5,000 such income, while more than 20 earned more
than $100,000 from investments or the sale of property. The range at the Su-
preme Court was great, from Justice Thurgood Marshall, with no outside income and no reportable stocks, bonds, or savings accounts, to Justice Lewis
Powell with outside income of over $90,000 plus stock, bond, real estate, and
trust holdings worth at least $1,600,000. In 1981, Chief Justice Burger had assets
of at least $500,000, and Justice O'Connor showed assets of at least $840,000;
according to 1978 forms, Justice Stewart had been the wealthiest member of the
Court until then.[4]

Discipline and Removal

A problem of potentially greater dimension than retaining judges is getting
others—old, ill, or not functioning effectively—to leave the bench. Within the
period of the Burger Court, there were problems with Black (loss of memory),
Harlan (failing eyesight), and Douglas (a serious stroke), with Douglas being
particularly reluctant to leave the Court even after he had formally resigned and
a replacement (Stevens) had been named.

In earlier years, judges and justices died in office—some, it was said, long
after they had become senile. The U.S. Constitution, unlike some state constitutions, makes no provision for judges' retirement at a certain age, and the en-
treaties of other colleagues seldom proved successful in getting eligible judges to
retire on the pension in effect until the late 1930s: their then not-very-generous
salary. In 1937 Congress provided that after 10 years of service, on reaching age
70, judges could opt for partial retirement, with full pay *and* any subsequent
salary increases. The law now provides that a judge may take senior status at age

65 after 15 years of service or with any combination of age and years of service equaling 80 (66 + 14, 67 + 13, etc.). These *senior judges* can continue to hear cases if they wish—an incentive for older judges to reduce their workload without having to quit the bench completely—and are available to travel to courts that are temporarily in need of additional judges. Because a judge taking senior status formally vacates a judgeship, a new judge is appointed and both the new judge and the senior judge can work on cases; senior judges' assistance to the federal courts is essential in dealing with the courts' substantial caseloads. The federal courts almost lost the services of many senior judges in early 1986 when their salaries for the first time became subject to deduction of Social Security taxes and, for those under age 70, to reduction in Social Security benefits and possible loss of Medicare coverage if they earned more than a certain amount. Roughly half the senior judges stopped working, with deleterious effects on court calendars in some districts, until Congress permanently exempted them from Social Security taxation.

Senior status is also available to those with serious disabilities even if they are not yet eligible for regular senior status; with 10 years or more of service, these judges receive full pay, but only half-pay if they have less service. They may seek such status voluntarily, receiving it if properly certified by the chief judge of the circuit, or they may be certified for it by their colleagues; the constitutionality of the latter (forced) use of disability senior status has apparently not been tested by any judges, although in some situations the circuit councils have pressed fairly hard for them to leave the bench via this route. A judge who resigns from a judgeship—that is, leaves the court completely—after age 70 with at least 10 years of service gets the full salary received at the time of the resignation but no subsequent increases. A Supreme Court justice who wishes to step down—such as Potter Stewart in 1981 or Tom Clark, who left the Court so that his son, Ramsey Clark, could become attorney general without creating conflicts of interest for both—can sit on the lower courts, as Clark, Stewart, and Justice Stanley Reed all did. They can also resign outright, as Justices Whittaker (1962), Goldberg (1965), and Fortas (1969) did for different reasons.

Because it cannot be forced on a judge who is not physically or mentally disabled, senior status is not a solution for the "difficult" judge who continues to serve, and further action is also necessary to terminate the judicial activity of senior judges who wish to continue hearing cases. For example, Judge Julius Hoffman, the Chicago Seven trial judge, had finally taken senior status in 1972 at age 77. Although he was no longer hearing criminal cases or complicated litigation, in 1980 the Court of Appeals for the Seventh Circuit ordered that he not be given cases expected to take more than 35 hours of trial time; in 1982, amid complaints that his behavior was increasingly erratic, the court refused to allow any new cases to be assigned to him.

The difficulties of dealing with a problem judge before the present discplinary system was enacted are perhaps best illustrated by the controversy between the

Tenth Circuit's Judicial Council and District Judge Stephen Chandler (W.D. Okla.).[5] The council had removed Chandler—a defendant in civil and criminal lawsuits and the object of attempts to disqualify him from sitting in several cases—from deciding any pending or future cases. Chandler, not wanting to acknowledge the council's authority, did not appear at a council hearing on the matter. The council then left Chandler his pending cases, but distributed new cases to other judges in the district. Chandler objected to the council's action, arguing that the Constitution provided nothing short of impeachment, which was thus the only way to proceed against a judge. Chandler's efforts to obtain relief from the Supreme Court were turned away on the procedural grounds that he had failed to seek relief from either the council or some other court. Although the Court did not deal with the substance of Chandler's claim, Chief Justice Burger, speaking for the Court, did make the statement,

> There can . . . be no disagreement among us as to the imperative need for total and absolute independence of judges in deciding cases or in any phase of the decisional function. But it is quite another matter to say that each judge in a complex system shall be the absolute ruler of his manner of conducting judicial affairs.

Justices Douglas and Black, however, argued both that the Court was being unfair in forcing Chandler to recognize the council's authority in order to get relief and that impeachment was the only way to remove a judge. They also spoke out against the circuit council's methods:

> It is time that an end be put to these efforts of federal judges to ride herd on other federal judges. This is a form of "hazing" having no place under the Constitution . . .
> If they break a law, they can be prosecuted. If they become corrupt or sit in cases in which they have a personal or family stake, they can be impeached by Congress. But I search the Constitution in vain for any power of surveillance which other federal judges have over those aberrations.

Some federal judges have been impeached, convicted, and removed from office, and in times past others have resigned under certain threat of impeachment. Impeachment efforts began with friction between Federalists and Jeffersonian Democrats, which led to the sole impeachment of a Supreme Court justice, the Federalist Samuel Chase, for his highly partisan charges to grand juries while on circuit; Chase was, however, not convicted. In the same period, New Hampshire district judge John Pickering, also a Federalist, was impeached and convicted, but he was senile, so his removal expanded the grounds for impeachment to cover that situation.[6]

An unresolved question concerning impeachment is whether indictment of a federal judge on criminal charges could precede or only follow impeachment. Because Judge Kerner did not raise the question at his trial but only on appeal, a court ruled he had waived his claim. When Judge Alcee Hastings, a district judge in Florida, was indicted in 1982 on bribery charges, he raised the issue prior to his trial, but lower courts ruled against him; when he was acquitted, the question was again left unanswered. In the case of Judge Harry Claiborne (see below), judges also ruled against him on the impeachment-before-prosecution question and he was in fact impeached and convicted, but no Supreme Court ruling on the question resulted from his case, nor on the question of whether he could be imprisoned before impeachment.

A number of devices other than impeachment have been used to deal with judges' ethics. One effort aimed at dealing with questions of federal judges' proper behavior, intended to supplement earlier bar association Canons of Judicial Ethics, is the Code of Judicial Conduct for United States Judges, adopted by the Judicial Conference. The Code indicates more clearly to judges what is expected of them, for example, when it is appropriate for them to disqualify themselves from hearing cases because of potential conflicts of interest; it serves as well to provide guidelines against which judges' conduct can be evaluated. The promulgation of the Code has not, however, served to still all concerns about judicial behavior, and leaves unresolved the problem of dealing with noncriminal, recalcitrant, erratic, or possibly unbalanced judges within the confines of the Constitution without seriously eroding judicial independence.

The Chandler case and another Tenth Circuit controversy involving Chief Judge Willis Ritter (D. Utah), embroiled in conflict with the Mormon Church, led to serious congressional attention to providing judicial discipline, including removal, short of impeachment. Proposals were based on the proposition that appointment during "good behavior" did not necessarily mean "for life" and permitted discipline for misbehavior. One proposal that passed the Senate covered all federal courts, including the Supreme Court, provided for filing complaints with a Judicial Conduct and Disability Commission, and allowed removal—except for Supreme Court justices, concerning whom recommendations would be made to the House of Representatives; another provided for review of circuit council actions by a separate Court of Judicial Conduct and Disability. Other proposals, including those made by the Judicial Conference, provided for filing of complaints with the circuit judicial councils, which argued forcefully for a further chance to deal with the problem.

The Judicial Conduct and Disability Act, passed in 1980, reaffirmed the circuit councils' central place in the disciplinary process and did not provide for a separate conduct court; because councils could discipline district judges, district judges were added to council membership (see pages 67-68). Under the procedures established by the statute, any person may file complaints against a judge with the clerk of the court of appeals. Complaints then proceed through a three-tier arrangement, going first to the chief judge of the circuit, then to a panel of judges, and finally to the judicial council. The chief judge may dismiss a complaint if it simply concerns a ruling in a particular case (likely to be sour grapes), is frivolous, or does not allege "conduct prejudicial to the effective and expeditious administration of the business of the courts" or inability "to discharge all the duties of office by reason of mental or physical disability." The chief judge may also close a complaint upon finding that "appropriate corrective action" had been taken. If a complaint survives this review, the chief judge must appoint an investigating committee—the chief judge and an equal number of circuit and district judges—to report to the judicial council. The council may remove magistrates or bankruptcy judges; as to Article III judges, the council may issue a public or private reprimand, certify disability, request voluntary resignation, or prohibit further case assignments for a fixed period. If the council thinks the judge's conduct "might constitute" grounds for impeachment, the matter is to be transmitted to the Judicial Conference of the United States, which may in turn transmit the case to the House of Representatives. Any unsatisfied complainants and accused judges may petition the Judicial Conference or its appropriate standing committee to review judicial council actions on their complaints.

At least as measured by the number of complaints filed, the new disciplinary system has received considerable use. Although less than 100 complaints were filed in 1982, there were close to 200 in 1985. Most concern alleged bias in a judge's handling of a case, although one against Chief Judge John Feikens (E.D. Mich.) was for "racially patronizing and biased" remarks in a newspaper interview. Most go no further than the circuit's chief judge, who dismisses them as unfounded. Dismissal may also occur because the underlying issue has been dealt with elsewhere. For example, when the U.S. Court of Appeals for the Eighth Circuit rebuked District Judge Miles Lord (D. Minn.) for his chastisement in open court of company officials for putting profit ahead of women's health and ordered the remarks struck from the record, nothing further was done with the discipline complaint against Lord. Even when a complaint is formally dismissed, the attendant publicity such as that from the dissent by four judges (including two black appellate judges) over the dismissal of the complaint against Judge Feikens, undoubtedly affects judges' behavior. A judge under attack may, however, add to the publicity, as Chief Judge Frank Battisti (N.D. Ohio) did in criticizing judicial discipline councils, "ethical zealots," and the media, after a grand jury inquiry produced no indictments and complaints against him were dismissed. Actual action against a judge has occurred, for example, censure of District Judge Allan Sharp (N.D. Ind.) for interfering with an investigation of his wife, and a recommendation for impeachment of Judge Alcee Hastings (see page 96). In addition, some judges have resigned after being investigated.

The use of the new disciplinary process for ideological reasons can be seen in the complaint, filed by the Washington Legal Foundation, a conservative public interest firm (see page 150), against Judge Abner Mikva of the D.C. Circuit for chairing and recruiting for the "activist" and "politicized" Section of Individual Rights of the ABA. This matter was resolved when Judge Mikva accepted a recommendation from the Judicial Conference Committee on Codes of Conduct that he refrain from participation in membership drives for the section.

Events in 1986 demonstrated that, despite the belief that impeachment was too difficult to accomplish and too severe for most judicial ethics infractions, it could be used—against Chief Judge Harry Claiborne (D. Nevada), initially indicted for bribery and obstruction of justice and convicted on two tax counts and sentenced to two years in jail. Claiborne refused to resign from the bench as Judge Kerner (see page 88) had done and became the first sitting federal judge to go to prison. Appalled by Claiborne's continuing as a federal judge, drawing his full salary although a convicted felon, and by his promising to return to the bench after his prison term, legislators moved to impeach him. The House Judiciary Committee recommended four articles of impeachment, the Judicial Conference stated its belief that there might be grounds for his impeachment, and the House unanimously voted the impeachment articles.

The Senate, faced with its first impeachment trial since it convicted Judge Halstead Ritter in 1936, instead of having the entire Senate hear the case, appointed a 12-member committee to take testimony. Acting on the basis of the committee transcript, the Senate refused to hear witnesses. After Judge Claiborne's lawyers were turned down both in the lower federal courts and by Chief Justice Rehnquist in their efforts to get a full-blown Senate trial, the Senate rejected Claiborne's defense that he had been careless and was the target of a government vendetta, and convicted him by overwhelming margins, thus removing him from office. However, some senators were troubled by the abbreviated procedures used, and another senator (a former state judge) was ready to propose a constitutional amendment to allow an independent commission to impeach and try federal judges, thus removing the Senate from the process.

The Claiborne case and that of Chief Judge Walter L. Nixon (S.D. Mississippi), convicted of perjury and sentenced to five years in prison, involve judges convicted in a criminal trial. However, as the matter of Judge Alcee Hastings, a Carter appointee and the first black federal judge in Florida, illustrates, acquittal does not end the use of the new judicial discipline procedure to produce impeachment. After Hastings' acquittal on bribery counts, other judges filed complaints against him, including obstruction of justice in his trial and making false claims that he was prosecuted because he was black. The circuit's investigating committee concluded he should be impeached, and sent that recommendation to the Judicial Conference, which told Congress that impeachment of Hastings "may be warranted." Judge Hastings' attacks on investigatory procedures and the discipline statute's constitutionality were rejected by the courts and further action is pending. The House Judiciary Committee has, however, made clear it would not be an appellate court to which people could turn with disliked decisions when they rejected petitions from over 100,000 Georgia residents to have three Eleventh Circuit judges removed from office for overturning murder convictions because of excessive and inflammatory pretrial publicity. In so doing, the committee reinforced the conduct statute's provision that complaints could not be based on rulings in particular cases.

Selection: The Lower Courts

Selection: President and Senate

The Constitution does not specify a formal process for the president's selection of judicial nominees and also fails to provide eligibility requirements or selection criteria. Different administrations have given varying weights to factors such as prior judicial experience, age, American Bar Association ratings, "affirmative action" to increase the number of women and minority judges, and ideology. In the first half of the twentieth century, patronage considerations dominated in appellate court nominations in administrations not concerned about the court's policy-making possibilities, but a mix of patronage and concerns about professionalism occurred where government's role was limited but judges' role in policy-making was recognized. When administrations, including FDR's later terms, sought to increase the role of government and also saw judges' possible effects on those efforts, they paid more attention to judges' policy views (what we now refer to as "ideology").[7]

In the century's second half, the Eisenhower administration explicitly stressed previous judicial experience, particularly for appeals court positions; age; and the ABA's ratings. The Kennedy administration said less about the age factor, and indeed had far less interest in judicial appointments than in social programs, despite judges' potentially great impact on those programs. The Carter administration gave substantial emphasis to nominees' "demonstrated commitment to equal justice" and to affirmative action, with the president promising to appoint at least one black federal judge in each state in the South. However, the administration also emphasized "stringent age and experience requirements," at least for the courts of appeals: only under unusual circumstances would those with less than 15 years legal experience or over 60 years of age be considered. Most important, President Carter altered the structural process by which nominees were chosen for all appeals court seats and for many district judgeships as well (see pages 101-3).

President Reagan has paid particular attention to the political philosophy of potential nominees, although other factors like age (preference for younger people) and intelligence are also considered. Attorney General Meese has said the adminstration seeks "the highest standards of integrity"; "intelligence, competence [and] appropriate judicial temperament"; and those with "the proper judicial philosophy and approach to the bench, which precludes judicial activism, or substituting the courts for the legislature."[8] The Nixon administration paid close attention to ideology in its Supreme Court nominations but less so for lower court appointments than does the Reagan administration. It is not fully clear whether, as charged, the administration uses a "litmus paper test" in which a potential nominee must adopt the "proper" position on specific issues. Meese has said he doesn't think "any single test should be a disqualifying factor," but a potential nominee's views on the Supreme Court abortion ruling "might be indicative of the way in which that judge would generally approach the whole subject of judicial activism." Solicitor General Fried, at about the same time, told a group of judges that it would be "crude" to screen potential judges on their views about abortion and the death penalty. (At the same conference, Justices Rehnquist and O'Connor expressed discomfort about selection focused on specific issues.)[9]

The Reagan administration, far more than its predecessors since Franklin Roosevelt, has paid more attention to the views of judicial nominees, perhaps because of its lack of success in getting "social policy" agenda items (abortion and church-state concerns) enacted by Congress or submitted as constitutional amendments. Another reason may be that Reagan, like Franklin Roosevelt, felt that the judiciary had blocked his goals and therefore needed to be altered. The administration's emphasis has produced much criticism that "merit" should instead be the primary criterion for selecting judges. However, many critics are liberals, perhaps jealous that the president did his job more systematically and successfully than Democratic presidents.

Vacancies occur in judgeships as judges resign, die, or assume senior status, and as new judgeships are created to keep up with increasing caseload. Particularly signficiant is the creation of a large number of new judgeships at one time, a highly political issue because a president of one party thus is able to name many judges of similar ideology and party background. Such conflicts go back to the early years of the Republic. The Judiciary Act of 1801, which provided for 16 circuit judgeships (and also provided that the next Supreme Court vacancy not be filled), was passed during the lame-duck session of the Federalist-dominated Congress before Thomas Jefferson assumed the presidency; the judgeships would, of course, have been filled by Federalists. However, in March 1802, Congress repealed the 1801 Act, with the circuit judges losing both their offices and salaries. In recent times, omnibus judgeship bills were enacted in 1961 and 1966 by a Democratic Congress, with judgeships to be filled by a Democratic president. The 1970 judgeship act was somewhat unusual in that a Democratic-controlled Congress provided new judgeships to be filled by a Republican president. Despite repeated requests from the Judicial Conference for more judgeships, the Omnibus Judgeship Act of 1978, creating 35 court of appeals and 117 district court judgeships, came only after delay by a Democratic Congress unwilling to have a Republican president name a large number of judges, and it was not passed until there was a Democratic president. In 1984, in providing for the addition of more than 80 new federal judges, Congress directed that only 40 could be nominated in 1984, with the remainder not to be selected before the start of the new presidential term in 1985, so that, if the Democratic candidate had won, all the positions would not already have been filled.

The addition of large numbers of judges at one time means that a president, particularly one who serves more than one term, can name a large proportion of the federal judiciary. Most notable is Franklin Roosevelt's selection of over 80 *percent* of the federal judges. Eisenhower was able to name over half the judges (56.1%) and Nixon almost half (45.7%) but others were able to name smaller proportions—John Kennedy (32.8%) and Lyndon Johnson (37.9%) because of shorter time in office, and Gerald Ford (13.1%). Because of the 1978 Omnibus Judgeship Act, President Carter was able to name 40.2 percent of the federal judges in only one term. President Reagan may well be able to have named a majority by the end of his second term, in part by getting "both halves" of the numbers added in the 1984 legislation.[10] Despite his choice of many young nominees, done in the hope that their ideological position will be evident on the bench for several decades, it is unclear how long they will remain. The opportunity to obtain much higher salaries in private law practice may become increasingly appealing to these judges as their children approach college age; moreover, judges appointed in their 30's or early 40's might not wish to serve for 25 years or more to be eligible for senior status, and departure after 10 or 15 years on the bench would put them, then in their 50's, in a position to have an extended career as a private attorney.

Congress' delays in adding judgeships that the Judicial Conference claims it needs led Chief Justice Burger to propose in 1980 that the Judicial Conference be given the authority to establish federal judgeships as they are needed, subject to congressional veto. Although the Conference's recommendations, once made every four years but now done every other year, do carry some weight, such a proposal is politically unacceptable. The Conference's Judicial Statistics subcommittee considers a number of factors, including the district court's weighted caseload per authorized judgeship (the most important factor), the complexity of a district's cases, its backlog, utilization of magistrates, and presence of senior judges. A judgeship created for a judicial district when caseload demands it but when the permanent need is not clear is considerd *temporary*. Although filled by an Article III (lifetime) judge, the position is created on a nonpermanent basis. In some instances, the temporary judgeship lapses with the first vacancy in that judicial district, with the judge sitting in the temporary judgeship moving to the vacancy; in others, the position remains until its incumbent departs.

The basics of the process now used to select nominees were put in place during the Eisenhower administration, although important alterations in selection of names for the president's consideration occurred during the Carter and Reagan administrations. Prior to formal nomination by the president, the Department of Justice, usually through the Deputy Attorney General, identifies and screens candidates for the president's consideration. For both district and appeals court positions, the Justice Department works as the president's surrogate with the appropriate senators. The president himself is seldom directly involved in the selection process except for Supreme Court vacancies or other matters staff brings to his attention, but the involvement of White House staff can be great. The FBI conducts an intensive investigation of those being seriously considered, and other Department of Justice officials evaluate FBI reports. Prior to the Nixon administration, a background check was run only on the person already selected, but it is now usually performed earlier to ensure sufficient information and to avoid embarrassment. (In part because the announcement of Justice O'Connor's nomination was made earlier than the president first planned to make it, the FBI field check on her was not performed until after the anouncement.)

The president has the formal constitutional power to make judicial nominations. However, under the practice of *senatorial courtesy*, judicial selection is shared with the senator(s) from the president's party in the state in which the appointment is to be made; if there are no senators from the president's party, the state party organization may be consulted. Under President Reagan, in states without Republican senators, Republican members of that state's House delegation submit recommendations, perhaps after consulting with Republican officials in the state; they may also consult with the Democratic senators, part of a pattern in which minority party senators interact with the president and his representatives about appointments. In states without senators from the president's party, members of the Cabinet may also serve as contact points for judicial appointments, and judges appointed by the president (or by a previous president of his party) may suggest names for judgeships; at times they volunteer those names, and at other times they are invited by the president, senators, or the Department of Justice to suggest names.

Senatorial courtesy operates most fully for district court vacancies. Because informal allocation of appeals court judgeships within a circuit may have been necessary to obtain congressional approval of courts of appeals judgeships, some seats "belong" to particular states, making senatorial courtesy also operative in the courts of appeals—except for the D.C. Circuit because the District of Columbia has no senators. For Supreme Court nominations, however, senatorial courtesy is virtually never operative, although the sponsorship or at least acquiescence of the senators from the nominee's state is helpful in achieving confirmation. Most senators take senatorial courtesy seriously, feeling they should designate the nominee, and "some even take the proprietary view that they own the job."[11] Others, however, play only a minor role in the selection process, perhaps to avoid owing the president a favor; they may do no more than submit a list of acceptable nominees, leaving the final choice to the president's staff, and at least one senator sends forward the names of *all* who wish to be considered. Many senators also do not wish to trade a vote on an issue to obtain approval of a nomination. The executive regularly consults the appropriate senators and seldom challenges senatorial choices because either the nominations are noncontroversial or the president will later need senators' votes for his program.

There can, however, be conflict between the White House and senators, even those of the president's party. Conflict between Senator John Warner (R-Va.) and the White House, when Warner objected to the proposed nomination of Kenneth Starr, a former partner in Attorney General William French Smith's law firm, to the Fourth Circuit, led the president to nominate Starr to the D.C.

Circuit. When Senator Warner submitted three names for the Fourth Circuit vacancy, the president chose none of them, nominating someone else instead. In another notable instance, probably because the nominee was thought too liberal, the Reagan White House refused to nominate someone New York's senators had agreed upon under their arrangement in which the party not in control of the White House gets a proportion of the judgeships. In that case, there was considerable delay, used in the past to pressure senators; recess appointments have also been used for that purpose, but not recently. Delay was used effectively by the Kennedy administration in one-fifth of its judicial nominations. It was used again in the Carter administration, when southern senators failed to nominate blacks, but it did not prove an effective tool then. The Reagan administration's delay in "moving" senators' preferred choices provided a bargaining chip for use when a nomination desired by the administration encountered difficulty; some senators voted for the nominee (Daniel Manion) in return for White House promises to advance the senators' preferences to the nomination stage (see page 107).

Considerable time can elapse from the creation of a judgeship—and certainly from the Judicial Conference's recommendation that one be created or the occurrence of a vacancy through death or a judge's assuming senior status—to the filling of that judgeship. Agreement on the nominee a senator will submit may take time, which may be further stretched out by White House staff consideration and other far from perfunctory investigations. Consideration by the American Bar Association and then by the Senate Judiciary Committee further extends the process, which can be stretched even further if Congress is entering an election period when senators wish to get home to campaign. Because caseloads justifying a position have already been exceeded when a judgeship is created (see page 301), not filling a position creates serious caseload problems in some districts, particularly those with few judges where the absence of a single judge is felt more.

Selection Commissions. President Carter's belief that judges should be chosen through "merit selection" and his emphasis on affirmative action brought about a significant change in the way many senators selected those whose names were to be forwarded to the president, leading to more formal consultative and screening devices. The president had spoken of using merit selection for both district courts and courts of appeals, but Attorney General Griffin Bell and Senate Judiciary Committee Chairman Eastland "struck a deal" in which appeals court nominees would be produced by selection commissions established by executive order, with senators continuing to choose nominees for district judgeships.

The change in the selection process initiated by President Carter for vacancies on the courts of appeals was significant both structurally and in the results produced. The new process was put into effect in 1977 and 1978 by executive order. [12] Thirteen selection panels were established—one for each circuit, with two each for the not-yet-divided Fifth Circuit and the Ninth Circuit—with each panel to have equal numbers of members of the bar and laypersons, with representation of women and minorities. The panel members were predominantly white and Democratic, with "a disproportionate number of Carter activists." Opening up the selection process by seeking out potential nominees instead of relying on those who volunteered their candidacies, panel members did not, however, place much importance on a candidate's political activity or on partisan recommendations, instead ranking mental health and "character and personality traits" most important.[13] Lawyers and lay members did differ, the former giving *less* weight to bar association recommendations.[14] Panels initially had 60 days to submit nominations—no less than three names or more than five for each position. Although later given more flexible time periods in which to work, their principal complaint was of inadequate time to screen and interview candidates and to debate their qualifications.[15]

The 1978 Omnibus Judgeship Act (OJA) also gave a push to the use of commission selection mechanisms for district judgeships, which were to be filled on the basis of merit selection guidelines. President Carter's implementing executive order encouraged use of selection commissions and active recruitment of qualified minorities and women, but no nomination could be blocked for failure to comply with the executive order's standards. Indeed, a majority of senators felt that the selection process used by their Senate colleagues from other states was not a proper basis for voting against a nominee to a judgeship.[16] The idea of special selection panels for district judgeships took hold. By 1979, senators in 29 states had established either ad hoc or permanent judicial nominating commissions, with 20 of them where both senators were Democrats.[17] Yet, even with the president's encouragement, some senators refused to set up commissions; Senator Lloyd Bentsen (D-Tex.) was known as "I am the Judicial Commission for Texas" Bentsen; and Senator Adlai Stevenson III (D-Ill.) attacked the new device. Stevenson said the commissions isolated senators from candidates and placed responsibility for recommending nominations "in the hands of a 'sanitized' committee" made up of various categories of persons (lawyers, nonlawyers, men, women, minorities) without regard to merit.[18]

Commission size and procedures varied, as did the sponsoring senators' role in designating candidates.[19] Perhaps more important were variations after the panels produced names: some senators sent the full commission-generated lists directly to the executive branch; others, giving themselves greater control over the nomination, reduced the lists first. Newer members of the Senate were more likely to accept a greater executive role in the process, undoubtedly a function of their use of the selection commissions; senior senators were more likely to assume a greater role in the selection process.[20]

President Carter's efforts at "affirmative action" in the judiciary, although successful in terms of the numbers of women and minorities placed in the federal judiciary (see pages 115–16), indicate problems a president faces in trying to increase the number of federal judges from groups who do not constitute a large proportion of the legal profession, such as blacks or Hispanics, or who are disproportionately "junior" in legal experience, such as women. Because there is only a small initial "pool" of nontraditional candidates from which to select, finding appropriate candidates within that pool may not be easy. The pool becomes even smaller if ABA guidelines are used and nominees are submitted to usual evaluation processes. Moreover, there are relatively few alternative nominees available if questions are raised about any particular nontraditional nominee. This situation allowed the white southern establishment, which had refused to handle civil rights cases, opportunities to question the qualifications of black attorneys whose principal legal work was in the civil rights field, and to force withdrawal of some nominations. (It was President Reagan, in one of his few appointments of blacks, who named the first black federal judge in Virginia.)

Use of the selection commission device had some definite effects. Some were structural: the executive branch and the Judiciary Committee played larger and more independent roles than under the earlier, more traditional selection mechanism. The number and variety of participants in the selection process—particularly persons from outside the government—increased. Scrutiny of applicants was greater and also more repetitive. Perhaps of particular significance is that commission-selected candidates thought the process was more open than it had been: half of those surveyed "believed they would not have sought or been considered for appointment under the traditional system," in large part because they did not know senators, were politically inactive, or were not "traditional" candidates (older, white males).[21] This view may have resulted because most senators defined their affirmative action obligations in terms of search and outreach, for example, expanding the candidate pool with women and minorities, but not doing so to produce a certain proportion of black, Hispanic, or female judges.[22]

There were, however, some other differences: panels selected a higher proportion of nominees with teaching experience and panel nominees were also more likely to have been government attorneys than those selected in other ways. (At times they were relatively conservative, at least compared to what one would have expected a Democratic president to nominate.) After President Reagan terminated panels for U.S. Court of Appeals vacancies in May 1981 and ended presidential encouragement for district judgeship panels and after the 1980 change in Senate party control, there were commissions in only 15 states by 1983. The senators who did retain panels without presidential mandate or statutory exhortation really wanted to use them. That may explain why there were greater differences between panel and nonpanel-generated district court nominees in 1981–82 than there had been during the Carter administration. In 1981–82, panel selections were much more likely to have had judicial experience, all those with teaching experience were chosen from panels, and panel nominees were much more likely to be rated Well Qualified and Exceptionally Well Qualified by the ABA.[23]

Selection under Reagan. The Reagan administration eliminated circuit selection commissions. It also revised and formalized the executive branch structure for selecting nominees. There has been more intensive Justice Department examination of possible nominees, including long interviews, and increasing involvement of the president's office. Assisted by a Special Counsel for Judicial Selection, the Assistant Attorney General, for the Office of Legal Policy, rather than the Deputy Attorney General, became the principal executive branch official for judicial selection. With the attorney general, these officials meet to make recommendations to the nine-person President's Committee on Federal Judicial Selection, which also includes the president's counsel, the White House chief of staff, and some assistants to the president. That group, because it creates a more active White House role in selecting nominees, provides the greatest difference from previous practice. Not merely a "check" on Justice Department suggestions, the President's Committee plays an independent role; new names of potential nominees enter the process at that stage and the committee provides a further mechanism for review of a potential nominee's ideology even when such considerations have entered into the Justice Department's earlier examination.

The Senate. The executive's consultation with senators over nominations stems from senatorial courtesy. However, senatorial courtesy does not operate formally until a nomination is submitted to the Senate and is not publicly invoked until the Judiciary Committee has sent the nomination to the floor. However, there is an equivalent of senatorial courtesy when a nomination is referred to the Judiciary Committee. Senators from the nominee's state are sent a *blue slip*; failure to return the slip is supposed to kill a nomination automatically. However, most senators seldom have used the blue slip except to comment or to sign off, or have delayed returning it to obtain more information or to negotiate over, rather than kill, nominations. When Senator Edward Kennedy (D-Mass.) took over the committee chairmanship in 1976, he decided that a nomination would not automatically be killed when someone failed to return the blue slip; instead, the committee would vote on whether to proceed. Although not necessarily willing to defer to colleagues' use of the blue slip, a majority of senators supported continuing the mechanism; Republicans, the minority party at that time, showed greater support.[24] In 1981, on assuming the chairmanship, Senator Strom Thurmond (R-S.C.) retained the rule that committee consideration of a nomination could not be delayed indefinitely by use of the blue slip. When Senator Alan Cranston (D-Cal.) used the blue slip for the first time in the Reagan presidency, the committee approved the contested nomination on party lines (and the Senate confirmed). In addition to the blue slip, individual senators, saying they wish more time to consider nominations, place "holds" on them. Because of senators' deference to each other, this allows a senator to hold disliked nominations hostage—or to delay them sufficiently at session's end to ensure that they are not approved.

Apart from the senators from the nominee's state, the members of the Judiciary Committee are the most important senators in the nomination process.

The power of the committee's chair can be substantial. A particularly stubborn chairman like Senator Eastland can force a hard bargain, delaying consideration of a much-wanted nomination until the president submits others the chairman wants. The committee as a whole can test the president's will by delaying action on nominations. The committee holds hearings—although often by subcommittees of only a few senators—to take testimony from the nominee, supporters, and opponents. Through these hearings, at which the committee can decline to let someone testify, relegating objections to the less visible printed record, and can control the sequence in which witnesses appear and the hostile or friendly treatment they receive, the entire Senate, the media, and the general public can be attuned to objections against the nominee.

Because the committee chairman can set the tone of the committee's questioning and can either encourage or discourage committee members' aggressive approach to nominees, control of the committee—by the majority party in the Senate—is quite important. This control makes elections to the Senate, such as those of 1986 when party control changed hands and put Senator Joseph Biden (D-Del.) in the chairmanship, quite important in the judicial nomination process. When the Democrats gained control of the committee in 1987, they established their own screening panel to give particular attention to the president's nominees, and its head, Senator Patrick Leahy (D-Vt.), attacked the competence of the administration's previous nominees as well as its failure to nominate more women and blacks.

The Judiciary Committee at times is able to affect selection criteria. In recent years, the committee became involved in issues concerning the ABA's age guidelines (see page 109) and judges' memberships in clubs without minority group members. After a controversy when a nominee felt that resigning from an all-white group would be admitting that his membership was improper, Senators Kennedy and Thurmond, then chairman and ranking minority member of the committee, agreed on a statement that "it is inadvisable for a nominee for a Federal judgeship to belong to a social club that engages in invidious discrimination." Although the statement led a number of nominees to resign from such clubs, it did not settle the question about sitting judges, many of whom belonged to such clubs.

In the late 1970s, because it was not satisfied with the FBI's investigations, the committee began to conduct its own, with committee investigators using FBI files and financial information about the nominees, and under Senator Kennedy the committee began to send its own questionnaire to all nominees to supplement information obtained by the administration. When Republicans controlled the committee, conservative Senators Hatch, Denton, and East sent a questionnaire to a district court nominee asking views on abortion, school prayer, the right to bear arms, the Equal Rights Amendment, and the death penalty. The conservative ideology embodied in this set of issues and the request for specific answers rather than views on broad topics like federalism or a general discussion of the role of judges was too much for chairman Thurmond, who said he didn't want such a questionnaire used in the future and that senators were to question nominees only during committee hearings. (The senators who had sent the questionnaire, although calling their questions relevant, said they would support the nominee.) When Democratic committee members, who believed that more marginal nominations—requiring greater investigation—were being sent to the committee, began to focus more attention on them, a bipartisan agreement reached within the committee in late 1985 gave the Democrats more time to investigate, with no hearings to be held for two weeks after the nominations. To prevent delay for delay's sake, a vote on noncontroversial nominations was to take place within five weeks of the nomination, but no timetable was specified for controversial nominations.

After hearings are concluded, the committee makes a recommendation to the full Senate. That recommendation is usually positive, but the Judiciary Committee's more independent examination of nominees resulted in rejection in 1980 of a nominee for a North Carolina district judgeship, the first time in 42 years the committee had taken such action, and in 1986, the committee refused to recommend confirmation of Daniel Manion to the Seventh Circuit, sending the nomination to the Senate without a recommendation. (See below.) Shortly thereafter, the committee rejected the nomination of Jefferson B. Sessions III to an Alabama district judgeship. Sessions, U.S. Attorney in Mobile, had unsuccessfully prosecuted blacks for vote fraud in what critics thought was an effort to intimidate black voters, and had made disparaging remarks about the NAACP and a white civil rights lawyer.

When a nomination goes before the full Senate, often there are only some laudatory comments, little debate, and approval by voice vote. However, senators at times debate before voting on the nomination. Judiciary Committee members lead any debate, which provides senators with another opportunity to embarrass the president by questioning an appointment. Anticipating that such questions will be raised, a president may prefer to avoid a particular nomination or even, despite the resulting embarrassment, to withdraw it once made. It is at the floor stage that senatorial courtesy operates officially. Formerly a senator could invoke senatorial courtesy with little challenge simply by stating that, whatever the reason, an opposed nominee was "personally obnoxious," but expectations have developed that a senator has to substantiate rather than merely assert objections. Senatorial courtesy is used defensively to try to block a presidential nominee, not always successfully, but even its effective exercise does not ensure acceptance of a senator's nominee. Senators have generally lost battles with the president over nominations, often because the successful appointee was sponsored by the state's other senator of the same party. Moreover, although not inclined to interfere regularly with district court nominations in other states, other senators may become involved—or may be pressured by interest groups to get involved—in nominations seen as affecting the federal judiciary's quality and image, illustrating that senators do not accept either the president's or their colleagues' assessments totally at face value and also look both at a nominee's professional competence and at policy views or ideology. In part because of the increased assertiveness by Democratic members of the Judiciary Committee, those instances became more frequent in Reagan's second term.

The most serious and protracted battle occurred over Daniel Manion's nomination to a Seventh Circuit judgeship. The son of a John Birch Society leader, the younger Manion had relatively limited legal experience as a member of a small law firm and had never argued a case before the Seventh Circuit, although he had been a state deputy attorney general. The combination of his conservative ideology and lack of professional qualifications made his nomination an obvious target for the Democrats, the more so when they learned that, as a state senator, he had sponsored legislation that the Ten Commandments be posted in public school classrooms—despite a Supreme Court ruling striking down similar legislation from another state. More than 40 law deans signed a statement saying he was unqualified, and a Seventh Circuit senior judge wrote that confirmation would be a disservice to the court. President Reagan criticized Manion's critics in one of his weekly radio speeches, and Attorney General Meese expressed continuing support. After complicated voting maneuvers, the nomination was approved, 50-49, with the vice-president casting the deciding vote.

The ABA's Role

The American Bar Association (ABA), lawyers' principal national interest group, has assisted in selecting federal judges since 1946. Its Committee on the Federal Judiciary initially suggested names of candidates but sought to review nominations before they were made public. President Eisenhower's emphasis on "quality" in the federal judiciary led to increased ABA involvement. By 1953, instead of only making recommendations, the committee was evaluating the names of those under "active consideration." The ratings used by the ABA are Exceptionally Well Qualified, Well Qualified, Qualified, Qualified/Not Qualified, and Not Qualified; the rating Not Qualified by Reason of Age has been dropped. (The split Qualified/Not Qualified rating is given when a majority of the ABA committee rates a possible nominee Qualified and a minority gives the Not Qualified rating.) The Eisenhower administration's practice made it difficult for later administrations to avoid the ABA, despite objections to the ABA's special access and its alleged conservatism, masked by its claim to be interested only in judicial competence.

The weight given to ABA recommendations by subsequent administrations has, however, varied; ABA participation in judicial selection has been more significant in Republican administrations than in Democratic ones. In Eisenhower's last two years, for example, the ABA committee "had a virtual veto power" so that only those the committee rated Qualified or better were nominated. The Kennedy administration tried to limit the ABA's role. Top Justice Department personnel were unwilling to give in to the ABA when they differed with its committee. Indeed, using "argument and cajolery," the administration was able to get the ABA to change some of its ratings. Almost one-third (29 percent) of the ABA's informal ratings differed from formal ratings finally announced. In 30 percent of the changes, the rating was *up*graded, perhaps as a result of the ABA's desire to appear successful when the administration was intent on a particular nomination.[25] Although President Lyndon Johnson's initial relations with the ABA were strained, extremely negative reaction to some of his nominations made him more sensitive to the bar's views. The ABA committee ranked six of Johnson's first 56 appointments to the district and appeals court Not Qualified, but by 1966 the committee thought the administration's appointments quite good.

During the Nixon presidency, the ABA's position again strengthened. The president said he would not name someone considered Not Qualified, but late in his administration he broke his word over an appointment to the court of appeals. The ABA's importance in lower court nominations continued into the Ford administration, and the bar group seemed quite pleased, at least publicly, with its relations with the administration.

The ABA also seemed satisfied with the district judge selection commissions during the Carter administration. A higher proportion of commission-selected nominees than of nominees not chosen through the commission mechanism were rated better than Qualified. Overall, however, ABA ratings of Carter district court nominations compared favorably with those in previous administrations. Friction between the Carter administration and the ABA did, however, occur. Most serious was conflict over the nomination of Donald O'Brien to be a district judge in Iowa. The ABA rated him Not Qualified not once but twice on the basis of his poor preparation for trials and some questionable conduct as a prosecutor—only the fourth instance in which the ABA had rated a candidate unqualified and had gone public with its opposition.

Because many women have become lawyers at an older age than men and have been limited in the trial work available to them, the Carter administration's emphasis on appointing women conflicted with the ABA's preference that nominees have considerable trial experience. Not directly disagreeing with the ABA, Attorney General Civiletti said that certain standards, adopted years earlier, "ought not to be mandatory," although they would be given serious consideration. He felt there ought to be "room for an outstanding or qualified exception under certain conditions."[26] The friction between the ABA and the administration on this matter and the ABA's influence could be seen when a woman solicitor in the Labor Department was nominated to be a district judge in the District of Columbia: the ABA rejected her because of lack of trial experience, and the administration withdrew her nomination. Also noteworthy is that in

1977-79, the only nominees to be rated Exceptionally Well Qualified (72 of 157) were white males, and, although 62.5 percent of all Carter judicial nominees were rated Well Qualified or Exceptionally Well Qualified, only 30 percent of the women were so rated, and only one was rated Exceptionally Well Qualified.[27] Beginning in 1979, the Carter administration allowed the Federation of Women Lawyers Judicial Screening Panel to review nominees for their "commitment to equal justice under law" and sought similar input from other organizations, practices terminated by the Reagan administration, although in early 1987 the Justice Department took up the Federation of Women Lawyers' offer to help the administration find women candidates for judgeships.

Controversy over another appointment—to the Court of Appeals for the First Circuit—led to reevaluation of another ABA standard. Initially, Archibald Cox, Harvard Law School professor and former Watergate prosecutor, was proposed for nomination. He was rejected by the administration ostensibly for being over 65, although friction between President Carter and Senator Edward Kennedy may also have played a part. (The position eventually went to another, 40-year-old Harvard law professor who had been a Kennedy assistant.) Critics soon attacked the ABA's age policy, under which in no event would anyone not already a federal judge be considered for an appeals court judgeship if over 64, and those 60 and over had to be in excellent health and rated Well Qualified or better; a district judge could not be elevated to the court of appeals if over 68. In April 1980 the Senate voted unanimously in favor of a resolution calling for an end to the guidelines, and the House followed with a similar resolution in November 1980. Shortly thereafter, the ABA committee announced it was discontinuing its age guidelines and its Not Qualified by Reason of Age rating. The ABA has not had guidelines for *minimum* age, increasingly relevant as President Reagan nominates people in their 30's, but ABA expectations concerning trial (or judicial) experience would apply.

Although President Reagan is a Republican, the friction between his administration and the ABA has been obvious. Because of its more thoroughly developed selection process and greater concern for ideology, the administration does not consult the ABA prior to nomination—"the first Republican Administration in 30 years" not to do so.[28] However, decreased reliance on the ABA Standing Committee on Federal Judiciary originated not with the Reagan administration but with the Carter administration's use of selection commissions. President Reagan's counsel "expressed concern that the ABA's screening process . . . takes too long and may delay appointments unnecessarily." ABA ratings should be given "due weight" but the ratings, even Not Qualified, should not bind the president.[29] Nonetheless, the administration succeeded in having its nominees receive high ABA ratings. Seven percent of Reagan's first-term appointees to the district court were rated Exceptionally Well Qualified—"the best record since the Johnson administration." The same was true of appellate court nominees during the same period. However, such appointments did not preclude low-quality appointments (as measured by ABA criteria): Reagan appellate appointees had the highest proportion of the lowest favorable ratings (Qualified) in five administrations, perhaps in part because such ratings were given to appointees who were law professors despite their distinguished records as legal scholars and because the ABA committee made increasing use of the Qualified/Not Qualified rating. [30]

This picture is, however, only for judges actually confirmed; other nominees encountered difficulties with the ABA or state or local bar associations, and some of those nominations were withdrawn. For example, after the ABA said it would oppose an appellate judgeship for University of Texas law professor Lino Graglia, criticized for urging parents in Austin, Texas, to avoid a school-busing order, the Justice Department asked former (Carter administration) attorney general Griffin Bell to conduct an investigation, and then withdrew the nomination. And after the New York City Bar Association, one of the nation's most prestigious, said that James L. Buckley, about to be nominated to the Second Circuit, had failed to prove his qualifications—he failed to meet with the bar group or to answer their questionnaire—the administration instead nominated him to a position on the D.C. Circuit.

The ABA's ratings process was brought into public and negative scrutiny when the administration nominated J. Harvie Wilkinson III to the Fourth Circuit. Wilkinson, then a University of Virginia law professor, had no trial experience, but had been a clerk to Justice Lewis Powell. Under straightforward application of ABA criteria, Wilkinson would not have been rated Qualified. When the ABA rating was thought in difficulty, ABA committee members were lobbied—by Justice Powell, the Justice Department, and by Wilkinson himself. Although a committee member contacted by Powell voted against Wilkinson, questions were raised about the pressure's effect, particularly when the committee voted 11-5 in favor of a Qualified rating. Some thought the committee had improperly waived its standard that judicial nominees be lawyers for at least 12 years and have "substantial" trial work—standards the committee had generally been unwilling to waive for women. Wilkinson's lobbying in his own behalf did not stand him in good stead at the confirmation stage, but his nomination was confirmed, 58-39.

Attacks on the ABA from another direction came in 1985 and 1986 when the Washington Legal Foundation, which felt the ABA was obstructing and delaying nominations of conservative candidates and was giving lists of nominees to liberal groups like the American Civil Liberties Union and People for the American Way, sued the ABA Committee on the Judiciary to obtain its lists of prospective nominees and investigation records and to attend its closed meetings and sued the Justice Department for its connections with such a group. The suits did not succeed in court but the ABA may well have heard the message.

Judicial Backgrounds

Correlations between federal judges' votes and their background characteristics have not been particularly consistent; positive correlations appear to be time-bound.[31] The party of the appointing president does make a difference, however. More than nine of every ten times, the selection process for the lower federal courts produces judges of the president's political party. This affects outcomes because when political party is taken into account, relationships between other factors and judges' voting disappear, leaving party affiliation the single most helpful explanatory factor;[32] however, party affiliation does not have a uniform effect, having affected civil liberties decisions of district court judges more "in the wake of the transition from Warren to Burger" when the Supreme Court's cues were changing and more ambiguous than earlier.[33] The importance of political party in the selection process was no less true of the Carter administration's "merit selection" mechanisms than of earlier methods of selection, although in states where senators from opposite parties jointly sponsored a selection commission, a portion of the available judgeships went to the party not in the White House. With the Reagan administration, we find the highest level of partisanship in district court appointments since Woodrow Wilson; Reagan appointed *no* Democrats to the courts of appeals, the first time since Warren Harding that had occurred.

Voting records of U.S. courts of appeals judges show that appointees of Democratic Presidents Kennedy, Johnson, and Carter cast votes supporting criminal defendants and prisoners over half the time, while those appointed by Presidents Nixon and Ford did so less than one-third of the time. On sex discrimination and racial discrimination cases, differences were in the same direction but were not as great in racial discrimination cases, although differences were greater in nonunanimous cases. Comparison of only Carter and Reagan appointees for 1983–84 cases showed that in nonunanimous cases, the former were more than two times as liberal as the latter in most categories of cases. When Carter- and Reagan-appointed judges sat on the same cases and disagreed, Carter's nominees were liberal in 95 percent of the cases, Reagan's more ideologically homogeneous nominees, who vote much like Nixon and Ford appointees, only 5 percent.[34] Also of interest is the extent to which judges support the power of the presidents who appoint them. We find that from 1940 through 1984, Republicans were more supportive of presidential power than were Democratic appointees in nine of ten policy areas (the spending power was the tenth area). The president's law enforcement powers were supported by almost two-thirds of Republican judges (63.1%), but by only slightly more than one-third of the Democrats (36.4%). Overall, presidents obtained their strongest support from judges whom they had appointed and who were from their own party.[35]

Whatever their minimal effects, the personal and social characteristics of judges—their race, gender, and religion; where they received their legal education; and their prior occupations—have received much attention, stemming basically from the feeling that in a democratic system judges should be roughly representative of the general population in a statistical sense. There is also an important symbolic element to this concern—that, in a government of all the people, an all-white male judiciary is a slight to women and racial minorities. Few argue for appointment of women or black judges, so those judges can serve as representatives of a point of view arguing "black" or "feminist" positions, although, as we will see, the possible relation between judges' background characteristics, such as race or religion, and certain types of cases has caused some litigants to raise questions about the judges' ability to be impartial in those cases. Yet some argue for broader representation on the judiciary because they feel that judges who are women or from minority backgrounds, because of their personal experiences, will be more sympathetic to concerns of those who share their characteristics—just as former business lawyers have been—or that, at a minimum, their very presence will serve to remind their white male colleagues of the concerns of such people.

Federal judges' formal education and their parents' occupations have always been somewhat unrepresentative. During the nation's first century, both the nation's elite and particularly the "common man" were underrepresented in the lower federal courts: two of three judges were from middle-class homes.[36] Despite the small number of federal judges then, many appointees had other family members in the judiciary and even more had kinfolk in public service. Those appointed to the (Article III) district courts were usually of higher social status than territorial judges, who were "ambitious and generally successful middle-class lawyers" often not from the territories.[37]

Prior Occupation. The contemporary period has seen three basic paths to the federal judiciary: private legal practice and national party service or a local sponsor; in-service promotion from a position as U.S. attorney or from a district judgeship to the court of appeals; and lateral entry at an older age, such as from service as U.S. attorney after a career in private practice.[38] The Carter administration's new selection methods and affirmative action efforts meant additional paths to judgeships from public interest or civil rights law practice and from law schools. "Nontraditional" nominations were more likely when senators sent President Carter a list without designation of a preferred nomination than when senators exercised the nomination choice themselves.

Nominees to judgeships often have been judges or prosecutors. During the Johnson administration and Nixon's first term, only one-fifth of the appeals court nominees and a comparable proportion of district court nominees outside the South had neither type of experience.[39] Statements emphasizing the selection of people with prior judicial experience are not always matched in practice, however. Thus the Eisenhower administration, which stressed this factor, did not do as well in this regard as had the Truman administration. The Hoover administration had a particularly good record in rewarding prior judicial experience: eleven of sixteen appeals court appointees came from the district courts. Because a president is not likely to elevate district judges appointed by a president of the opposite party, efforts to promote district judges to the courts of appeals are limited when the presidency changes hands. Generally, district judges who move to the courts of appeals are likely to do so within a short time of their district court appointment or not at all.

District judges are also more likely to be elevated when patronage considerations are central in judicial nominations; not only can senators recognize "one of their own" through the elevation, but they can also create a district court vacancy they can fill. When professionalism is central, nominations go not only to present district judges but also to state judges. The lowest rate of elevation of district judges to the appellate courts comes when policy considerations dominate: in that situation, even district judges appointed by a president of the same party are not likely to be promoted.[40]

The Carter and Reagan administrations both drew heavily on prior judicial experience, state or federal, in selecting their nominees. For district court appointments, the Carter administration had the highest proportion of former judges, followed by the Reagan administration; roughly half the Reagan appellate appointees were in judicial service when the president named them. If we look at prior judicial and prosecutorial experience combined, we find it predominant among Reagan district court appointees, more than 70 percent having one or the other. Of particular note is that "nontraditional" appointees of the Carter administration were particularly likely to be judges (three-fifths compared to two-fifths of white males), so that it appears that a judgeship may substitute for other, absent credentials.[41]

Nomination of a member of Congress can present a special problem—possible violation of Article I, Section 6 of the Constitution, prohibiting appointment of members of Congress to any position "the Emoluments whereof shall have been increased" during their term in office. When Hugo Black's appointment to the Supreme Court was challenged on this basis in 1937, the Supreme Court ruled the plaintiff lacked standing (*Ex Parte Levitt*, 1937). A similar challenge arose when President Carter chose Rep. Abner Mikva (D-Ill.) for the Court of Appeals for the District of Columbia, prompting much conservative opposition. Shortly after Mikva's confirmation, Congress passed a law granting standing to members of Congress specifically to challenge judicial appointments to the D.C. Circuit on eligibility grounds. Senator McClure (R-Idaho) then filed suit, financed by the National Rifle Association, based on an automatic pay raise that went into effect during Rep. Mikva's term (but after he had resigned his House seat). Notwithstanding the statute, a three-judge district court denied the senator standing to challenge an approved nomination, and the Supreme Court affirmed without comment the lower court's ruling that Congress itself had to decide the eligibility of nominees.[42]

In terms of judges' prior law practice, Eisenhower's nominees were particularly likely to be from relatively large private law firms or from government practice; high-ranking Justice Department officials—likely candidates for federal judgeships—accounted for roughly 10 percent of his nominations. More of Kennedy's choices had been either in elective positions or some form of government administration; the private lawyers he nominated were more likely to have been in small firms or individual (solo) practice. The same differences occurred between the (Democratic) Johnson and (Republican) Nixon administrations; 40 percent of Nixon's district court appointees were partners in large law firms, with only 10 percent from small firm and solo practice, while roughly one-fifth of Johnson's appointees came from the latter sources. The higher socioeconomic status of Republicans was perhaps not, however, reflected in their differing educational backgrounds. The pattern has not changed since. In the Carter administration, half the white males moved to judicial positions from private practice, although only one-fourth of nontraditional nominees did so.

Religion. Differences in religion also existed between Republican- and Democratic-appointed judges. Over three-fourths of Eisenhower's appointees were Protestant, more than Kennedy's district court (three-fifths) and appeals court (two-thirds) appointees. Similarly, proportionately more Nixon than Johnson appointees were Protestant; Johnson, like Kennedy, appointed proportionately more Catholics and Jews. It is interesting that President Reagan had a pattern more like a Democratic administration, as he named more Catholics and Jews and fewer Protestants than earlier Republican presidents, and even more than Presidents Carter and Johnson.[43]

Continued active participation as a church official caused problems for a judge hearing a lawsuit challenging the extension of the deadline for ratifying the Equal Rights Amendment and raising the question of whether states could rescind earlier ratification of ERA. Judge Marion Callister (D.Idaho) was a regional representative of the Church of Jesus Christ of Latter Day Saints (the Mormon Church), which actively opposed the ERA. The Justice Department, acting on the basis of a statute providing that a judge "shall disqualify himself in any proceeding in which his impartiality might reasonably be questioned," asked the judge to stand aside, but he refused, noting that his legal judgment would not be affected even if he sat in high church councils. (Shortly thereafter, the church relieved him of his regional representative duties.)

Race. Race and gender are of greater current concern than religion. President Eisenhower appointed no blacks to federal judgeships; Kennedy named five—four to the district court and one (Thurgood Marshall) to the court of appeals. Johnson, in addition to appointing Marshall to the Supreme Court, making him the first black to sit there, appointed five black district judges and two black court of appeals judges. (One Johnson district court nominee, not confirmed, was later appointed by President Ford and elevated to the appeals court by President Carter.) Nixon named only four black district judges.

Blacks and Hispanics accounted for a higher proportion of nominations in President Carter's administration—roughly one-fifth—than in previous administrations, and Carter also appointed some judges of Oriental background in California. More important, President Carter appointed more blacks and Hispanics to the federal bench than the *total number* appointed by all previous presidents. If President Carter greatly increased the number of blacks on the federal bench, President Reagan's record was "the worst since the Eisenhower administration" in the district court and about the same for the appellate courts, with only one black appointee among the first 59 appellate judges and only four black district judges appointed in the president's first 208 selections. Reagan's record in appointing Hispanic judges is better, being slightly behind Carter's,[44] with one Hispanic appellate judge and 12 Hispanics at the district court level. Although most Hispanic judges were appointed in places where there is some concentration of Hispanic population (Arizona, California, Florida, New Mexico, Texas, and Puerto Rico), they have also been appointed in Connecticut (by Carter) and New Jersey (by Reagan).

Some black judges' right to preside over race relations cases has been challenged because of their prior civil rights involvement. Third Circuit Judge Leon Higginbotham, asked by litigants to excuse himself from a civil rights case, refused because to agree would mean that only white judges could hear such cases. Former NAACP lawyers Judges Constance Baker Motley (S.D.N.Y.) and Nathaniel Jones (Sixth Circuit) have taken the same position. However, when Judge U. W. Clemon, a black, refused to disqualify himself in a Justice Department suit against racial segregation in Alabama higher education, the Eleventh Circuit appointed another judge to decide the disqualification issue and he issued a disqualification order against Judge Clemon, relying not on his race but his friendship with the lawyer for one of the black institutions in the case. In view of such concerns, does a judge's race make a difference? Appellate judges' voting records show that black male judges were more liberal on criminal defendant and prisoner cases than white males and more liberal as well on sex discrimination cases, although by a smaller amount; they were *not*, however, more liberal on race relations cases.[45]

Gender. The first woman federal judge was Florence Allen, appointed to the Sixth Circuit in 1934. After her retirement in 1959, there was no new woman appeals court judge until Shirley Hufstedler was named to the Ninth Circuit nine years later. When she became President Carter's Secretary of Education, women were sitting on a majority of the courts of appeals; by mid-1980 there were ten women court of appeals judges. Presidents Johnson and Ford each appointed two women to the district court. When President Carter took office, there were only three women district judges, but by mid-1980, there were 31 plus three on the Tax Court and one on the Claims Court. President Carter appointed twice as many women judges—roughly one-fifth of his appeals court nominations and 14 percent of his district court nominations—as had been appointed by all previous presidents. These women were not likely to have reached the bench by the same career paths as did "traditional" (white male) candidates. They were less likely to have been judges, or to have worked for large, corporate law firms, and had less previous political activity than male nominees, but were more likely to have been law professors. Nonwhite females were particularly likely to be younger than most nominees.[46] In short, women lawyers could become federal judges if they were "exceptional"—which they became "by escaping their stereotyped legal roles" (such as working in trust departments of banks rather than litigating in court) "and, perhaps, by being at the forefront of professional developments which were altering those very roles during the decade of the 1970s."[47] Just as with his appointment of members of racial minorities, it was somewhat easier for President Carter to appoint so many women because he could often nominate women and men simultaneously for the multiple vacancies that occurred in a district or circuit under the Omnibus Judgeship Act; appointing a woman or minority group member to a judgeship in a single-judge district is more difficult.

Women's groups were concerned that President Reagan would appoint only traditional nominees. He did name only six women to district judgeships and none to appellate judgeships by mid-1983, and made only 23 such appointments (20 to the district bench, 3 to the appeals courts) in his first 287 appointees (roughly 9 percent overall), but that meant he had appointed more women than any other Republican president. Reagan's female appointees have differed from Carter's. For example, they were more likely to have been prosecutors—and were more so than male Reagan appointees—with only one having neither prosecutorial nor judicial experience. Reagan's appointees were also twice as likely as Carter's to have been politically active. Of particular note is that women Reagan appointed to federal judgeships are *less* likely to feel conflict between their careers and roles as wives and to rank their spouses negatively on support on matters of childcare and housework than are women judges appointed by Carter; whether this is a result of their spouses being different or of the two sets of judges having different expectations is unclear.[48] As with race, it was not clear that sex strongly affected judges' voting. President Carter's white female appointees were more liberal than white male judges on both sexual and racial equality, although not by substantial amounts, but showed no difference in criminal defendant and prisoner cases; a match of female with male Carter appointees showed no significant differences.[49]

The Supreme Court

The Justices' Qualifications

The qualifications of Supreme Court justices can be categorized as representational, professional, and doctrinal.[50] One element of representation is geography. There have been more justices whose home states were in the East (the older part of the nation) than in the West, although some effort is made to avoid overrepresentation of any region; that does not prevent two justices being from the same state or even same city (Rehnquist and O'Connor are from Phoenix) or the same court: Justice Scalia and nominee Bork both served on the U.S. Court of Appeals for the District of Columbia.

The principal representational qualification is political party. As with lower court judges, the great majority (90 percent) of the more than one hundred justices have been of the appointing president's party. Nonetheless, explicit partisanship is played down and could act as a disqualification. Party affiliation was a much better predictor of voting in the nineteenth century than it is now, because then the parties were more clearly divided on some issues, particularly regional/sectional ones like slavery.[51] A recent study has indicated that in cases involving presidential power where the decisions went one way or the other, the hypothesis that "a greater proportion of the judges from the president's party are likely to decide for him than are the judges for the opposition party" was confirmed in 64 percent of the cases.[52]

Representation of minorities has been apparent, although whether it has been purposeful in every instance is disputed. As far as racial minorities are concerned, no black reached the Supreme Court until Lyndon Johnson's appointment of Thurgood Marshall and no one of Hispanic or Oriental background has served. A "Jewish seat" seemed to exist with the appointment of Louis Brandeis, opposition to whose nomination was infused with much anti-Semitism. In succession, Felix Frankfurter, Arthur Goldberg, and Abe Fortas served on the Court. Yet asserting existence of a "Jewish seat" is difficult because Benjamin Cardozo served with Brandeis, Frankfurter was appointed before Brandeis resigned, and Fortas was not replaced by another Jew. There has been less conscious attention to a "Catholic seat," and Catholics who served on the Court have usually been chosen for a reason other than their religion. For example, William Brennan was selected by Eisenhower when the president needed a highly qualified "sitting judge" to quiet criticism of the "political" appointment of former Republican vice-presidential candidate Earl Warren and New Jersey Chief Justice Arthur Vanderbilt was unavailable because of age. Antonin Scalia was chosen because of his judicial experience and ideology, although his religion and ethnic background (he is the first justice of Italian-American heritage) may have made some difference.

Most of the justices have come from upper-middle-class or upper-class surroundings; very few have been of "essentially humble origin." Into the nineteenth century, justices came from "socially prestigeful and politically influential" families of the gentry class; later, professional family backgrounds predominated, and economic rather than political prominence was likely.[53] The nation's more open political system resulting from Jacksonian democracy was not directly reflected in the Court's membership. Members of justices' families were often active in public life, and more than one member of the same family has served on the Court, for example, Stephen Field and his nephew David Brewer (some said this gave Field two votes) and the two John Marshall Harlans, one at the end of the nineteenth century and his grandson in the 1950s and 1960s.

Justices' ages increased as the nineteenth century progressed; this was a result of our political development and the concomitant growth of informal career lines. The likelihood that justices would be older was reinforced by formal law training and greater specialization in the legal profession, so that it took longer to become established in the profession and receive appropriate recognition. Although Justice Douglas was 40 and Justice Rehnquist in his forties when appointed, appointment to the Court in an individual's late fifties, as with John Paul Stevens, or sixties, true of three of the Nixon nominees, is more typical. At the time of their appointments, Justice O'Connor was 51 and Justice Scalia, 50.

Professional qualifications mean prior judicial and governmental service. The state courts provided most of the Supreme Court justices in the last century, although at the end of the century justices were more likely to have had national rather than local experience. A nominee's judicial experience has always been taken into account, although lack of it has not been a bar to appointment, as in the case of Hugo Black, who had served briefly as a police magistrate but whose primary activity had been as a U.S. senator. The American Bar Association focused more attention on this factor and criticized nominees who lacked judicial service, such as Earl Warren—criticism compounded by his being chosen Chief Justice, but diminished by his experience as a prosecutor and state attorney general as well as governor.

Most other recent appointees either had judicial experience, had held important government jobs, or were distinguished lawyers. Eisenhower appointees John Marshall Harlan, Potter Stewart, and Charles Evans Whittaker, Johnson appointee Thurgood Marshall (solicitor general at the time of his appointment), Nixon appointees Burger and Blackmun, Ford appointee Stevens—a former Supreme Court law clerk—and Reagan appointee Scalia were federal appeals court judges, as were unsuccessful Nixon nominees Clement Haynsworth and G. Harrold Carswell, earlier a district judge. Burger, Rehnquist (also a former Supreme Court law clerk), Kennedy appointee Byron White, and Scalia all had held major Justice Department positions. Both Arthur Goldberg and Abe Fortas were distinguished attorneys, as was former ABA president Lewis Powell. Although Sandra Day O'Connor was a member of the Arizona intermediate appellate court, she had not been in the national positions common to other recent appointees.

Counter to the bar's expectations, past judicial performance does not produce a greater reliance on precedent. Instead justices who had significant pre-Supreme Court judicial experience or who came from families containing judges were more likely to depart from precedent than were justices without such experience or without judges among their relatives.[54] Perhaps those familiar with the judicial role could understand that a judge has to depart from precedent in order to resolve disputes, but those without such experience would be more likely to follow the law school taught norm of following precedent. Those with prior judicial experience and those from "judicial families" have also been less likely to dissent, maybe because they have accepted the norm of minimal dissent, quite strong in the lower federal courts and state courts. Judges from the more liberal party, who were more likely to have prior judicial experience, were more prone to abandon precedent, but the liberals were also more likely to dissent than conservative judges. Those most likely to dissent were most often those adhering to an earlier status quo and unwilling to abandon it.

Presidential Expectations

Generally, justices consistently support the policies of the presidents who select them. Such results stem from ideological affinity or "doctrinal qualifications" that the president attempts to ascertain through individuals' professional qualifications because presidents lack personal knowledge of most of those they nominate. Considering this lack of personal knowledge and the fact that some nominees are without extensive judicial records that could be examined, presidents have been quite successful overall in identifying their nominees' doctrinal proclivities; roughly three-fourths of the justices "for whom an evaluation could be made conformed to the expectations of the presidents who appointed them."[55] However, as Justice Rehnquist noted in a 1984 speech, presidents' expectations are not always met. For example, for justices appointed by Presidents Eisenhower through Nixon, there is only "limited support for [the] hypothesis that there would be a strong relationship between the civil rights support scores of presidents and those of the justices they appointed." This and the divergence among appointees of each president except LBJ mean that these presidents were "only moderately successful in appointing justices who would later take positions consistent with the appointing president's public statements on civil rights."[56]

Some presidents appear to have had few expectations of their nominees, but others have placed justices on the Court to do a specific job. Thus Lyndon Johnson put Thurgood Marshall on the Court to do more about social justice, Warren Burger was nominated to implement President Nixon's "law 'n order" concerns, and William Rehnquist can be said to have been put there because the trend toward social justice had gone too far. President Franklin Roosevelt's focus in selecting justices was on overturning the Court's rulings on economic regulation. His concentration on that topic and on choosing people for their opposition to or criticism of the conservative Supreme Court, their support for his Court-packing plan, and their divergence from what the "Establishment Bar" would have chosen, meant that discord developed among his appointees when the political context and types of cases changed from the late 1930s to the early 1940s. Although FDR's justices tried to apply the lessons they had learned about the "old Court," they diverged considerably in their applications, further dividing the Court.[57]

Some presidents have expended much energy to ensure that those they have nominated will vote the "right" way on key questions. This may explain inclusion of appellate judges among potential nominees, because their records on some issues likely to come before the Supreme Court can be checked. Whether nominees have agendas when they reach the Court is not always clear. However, both Justice Rehnquist and Justice Scalia—whose agenda could be determined from his law review writings and lower court rulings—appeared to have the same agenda: minimalist government. On the other hand, Justice Powell, appointed on short notice, and Justice Blackmun appeared not to have agendas. Yet, whatever their personal values, those who wish to be selected must deny having an agenda they would implement on the Court, as Justice Scalia did during hearings on his nomination. However, in addition to trying to learn a nominee's agenda, others may use the selection and confirmation process to try to shape a potential justice's agenda: "Where there are gaps in a nominee's agenda, the Justice-Makers try to provide their preferred items (and directions)." In the case of Justice O'Connor, who did not have strong ties to women's organizations, abortion was an issue placed on her agenda; indeed, "This change in her agenda was . . . the price of her selection."[58]

Even when care has been taken to appoint the "right" person, the president's expectations may be disappointed. The best-known story involves President Theodore Roosevelt, who selected Oliver Wendell Holmes for the Supreme Court after assuring himself that Holmes would vote "correctly" on antitrust matters. Yet Holmes, in his first antitrust case, voted the "wrong" way, provoking Roosevelt to say he could make a judge with a stronger backbone out of a banana. And the Nixon nominees failed to reflect the president's position on electronic surveillance (a criminal procedure issue), important aspects of desegregation, aid to parochial schools, and abortion—although abortion may not have been on anyone's minds at the time the justices were appointed. In the end, of course, Nixon's appointees joined in handing down the Watergate Tapes Case that led to his departure from office.

Prior Judicial Experience. A good example of prior judicial service facilitating a president's choice is Chief Justice Warren Burger. In the policy area in which Nixon was most interested, criminal procedure, Burger's decisions as a court of appeals judge showed a "judicial philosophy . . . generally described in terms of strict construction, conservatism, and judicial restraint." Burger had decided against the criminal appellant in 25 of 26 nonunanimous arrest and search and seizure cases during the 1956–69 period, and in 14 *en banc* criminal procedure rulings between 1965 and 1969 had not once voted in favor of the appellant. His opinions on the question of "probable cause" to arrest or search reflected a "proprosecution orientation which reject[ed] legal technicalities in criminal procedures that restrict the police in conducting their business."[59] Although Antonin Scalia and Robert Bork did not serve on the D.C. Circuit as long as Burger, their opinions there also provided a guide for those wishing to nominate them.

A general risk in choosing someone with prior judicial service is that it provides an easy basis for criticism of disliked opinions. During consideration of Fortas' nomination to be Chief Justice, his presence on the Court facilitated criticism of the Court's civil liberties decisions, such as those on obscenity. Justice Rehnquist's extremely conservative record likewise upset groups advocating greater protection for civil liberties and civil rights. The National Organization for Women (NOW) objected to John Paul Stevens' nomination because of some of his Seventh Circuit opinions, and Scalia's D.C. Circuit opinions likewise drew criticism from feminist groups, which felt he was not sufficiently sensitive to their concerns. The records of the three Supreme Court nominees rejected in the twentieth century—Parker, Haynsworth, and Carswell—were attacked by labor and civil rights groups.[60] The defense of Parker that his criticized labor rulings only properly implemented Supreme Court decisions did not persuade his attackers, nor were Haynsworth's detractors convinced by the view that his school desegregation decisions, some of which were later overturned by the Supreme Court, reflected Supreme Court rulings accurately at the time he made them. Far more serious were criticisms of Carswell, said by former Yale Law School Dean (and later federal judge) Louis Pollak to have had "more slender credentials than any nominee for the Supreme Court put forth in this century," the statement that provoked Senator Hruska (R-Neb.) to proclaim the need to have mediocrity represented on the Supreme Court. Carswell's service as a district judge produced complaints that he had handled civil rights cases with hostility and had treated black lawyers and black defendants rudely. His professional competence was also questioned, because the Fifth Circuit had reversed him more frequently than all but a few other district judges in the circuit.

Even if prior judicial service assists the president in making choices, there are reasons why it does not provide a basis for selecting a Chief Justice from within the Court. Such a choice tends to expose animosities and has provoked threats of resignation, as when Justice Jackson was considered as a replacement for Chief Justice Stone. This may help explain why only four nominees to be Chief Justice—Edward White, Harlan Fiske Stone (neither from the president's party), Abe Fortas (not confirmed), and William Rehnquist—have come from within the Court; Charles Evans Hughes, earlier a member of the Court, was not on the Court when named Chief Justice. Rehnquist's ability to get along with his colleagues—who stated that they would all be able to work with him—may well have helped him, while what administration officials may have perceived as Justice O'Connor's "streak of independence" on some issues, at least compared to Rehnquist's more consistent position, in addition to her lesser experience, served to sidetrack the possibility of her being named Chief Justice. (There have been only 20 nominations to be Chief Justice, with 16 confirmed.)

Ethics. Prior judicial service may also reveal a judge's ethical sense, a matter that has received much attention in recent years, starting with Justice Fortas' resignation upon the disclosure that he had temporarily retained money from

Louis Wolfson, a financier in trouble with the government, as part of a contract to be a foundation consultant to Wolfson. This action created the appearance that Fortas was practicing law for Wolfson while on the Court or perhaps—and worse—trying to influence the government's prosecution of Wolfson. The ABA's ethics committee found that Fortas had violated provisions that a judge should avoid "impropriety and the appearance of impropriety" and that a judge should not undertake work inconsistent with his judicial duties.[61]

Ethics was at the heart of the Senate's rejection of Judge Haynsworth's nomination. His not having recused (withdrawn) from a case in which he appeared to have a financial interest was said to be improper, as was his purchase of stock in a company that had been a litigant in a case before him; the purchase was made after the case was decided but before the decision was announced, something Haynsworth attributed to inadvertence. Haynsworth had been cleared of charges of unethical conduct relating to the first matter,[62] but the second matter hurt his cause, particularly in the aftermath of Fortas' conduct. Although ethics issues were also raised during consideration of Fortas' nomination to be Chief Justice and Carswell's subsequent nomination, "only in Haynsworth's case did ethics seem to have an important influence on the final vote."[63] An indication of the closer attention paid subsequently to ethics matters was the close questioning of John Paul Stevens about corporations in which he had held stock or been an officer, even though he had resigned as officer on joining the Seventh Circuit and had later sold most of the securities.

Because it is considered more acceptable to focus on a nominee's ethics than political philosophy, ethics concerns were central to the debate over Rehnquist's nomination to be Chief Justice. Some concerned nonjudicial matters, such as whether he had acted properly in helping to administer a trust fund for an ill brother-in-law. One of the most important issues did, however, involve judicial action: Rehnquist's refusal to recuse from participation in the case testing Army surveillance of civilian activity, *Laird v. Tatum* (see pages 221-22), despite his Justice Department involvement as a congressional witness and policymaker on the topic.

Political Activity. Doctrinal qualifications may be revealed not only by prior judicial service but also by previous political involvement, which is said to show "judicial temperament" or lack of it; the term is usually left undefined. Quite likely because he had advocated minimum wage and maximum hours legislation, Louis Brandeis was said to lack judicial temperament. Had Hugo Black's membership in the Ku Klux Klan been known before rather than after the confirmation of his nomination, it would have been used against him. However, he probably would have been confirmed in any event because of his overall liberalism and the norm of Senate approval of judicial nominations of its own members. (Moreover, his judicial defense of civil rights led to the comment that "Hugo Black used to go around in white sheets, scaring black people; now he goes around in black robes, scaring white people.") In the 1950s, John Marshall

Harlan was questioned about his membership in the Atlantic Union, which supposedly indicated a diminished commitment to United States sovereignty, and about his attachment to the liberal faction of the Republican party. Carswell's alleged racism probably produced the defeat of his nomination; unlike Judge Parker's campaign statement that Negroes shouldn't vote, apparently an isolated incident that occurred in the political climate of 1920, a comparable campaign statement by Carswell came after World War II and was followed by his helping the Tallahassee, Florida, municipal golf course become a private club to avoid desegregation—action he took while U.S. Attorney.

Prior political activity also produced opposition to the Powell and Rehnquist nominations. Powell's membership on the Richmond, Virginia, School Board and the Virginia State Board of Education led Congress' Black Caucus to oppose him. Opposition to Judge O'Connor, whose position on federalism, stated in a law review article,[64] seemed quite compatible with contemporary Republican views, was not based on her past judicial record. However, some religious and antiabortion groups did not feel her votes as a state senator indicated sufficient antiabortion sentiment. Her unwillingness to say how she would treat legal aspects of abortion as a judge further inflamed this opposition.

Complaints about Rehnquist, whose initial nomination was opposed by the Leadership Conference on Civil Rights and the American Civil Liberties Union, centered on his 1964 opposition to a Phoenix public accommodations ordinance, his Justice Department work on policy concerning electronic surveillance and mass demonstrations—raised again in 1986—and his defense of Carswell's nomination as the administration's spokesman. During the nomination proceedings on his becoming Chief Justice, a memo he wrote while in the Justice Department stating objections to the proposed Equal Rights Amendment (ERA) also received attention. So did claims that he had directly challenged black and Hispanic potential voters in Phoenix, a matter that had arisen in the 1971 hearings but had not been aggressively pursued by his opponents. At that time, in written responses to Senate Judiciary Committee questions, although saying he had participated in a voter eligibility (not disqualification) program, he had denied any direct involvement in challenging voters, but in 1986 that claim was flatly contradicted by several direct witnesses.

As these examples suggest, a nominee's past political participation is likely to produce opposition by a variety of interest groups—particularly labor and civil rights groups. Those groups have probably been more interested in protecting interests they thought the nominees would injure or in demonstrating their ability to block a nomination than in the particular individual involved, although opposition to Carswell as a person was quite severe.

American Bar Association

Largely as a result of actions by the executive, the American Bar Association's relationship to the executive concerning Supreme Court nominations has not been consistent over the last two decades. However, ABA actions have led to problems for itself. In 1962 it had decided to use only the ratings Qualifed and Not Qualified for Supreme Court nominees, who, unlike nominees to lower court positions, were not cleared with the ABA before being announced. Prior to the Haynsworth nomination, the ratings Highly Acceptable, Acceptable, or Not Acceptable were adopted, but the ABA later readopted the Qualified–Not Qualified standards. The shift damaged Carswell, who was rated only Qualified, but it would have hurt more had people known it was by a majority, not a unanimous vote. A further change in the rating scale was made after the Carswell defeat—to "high standards of integrity, judicial temperament and professional competence," "Not Opposed," or "Not Qualified."

Probably because of embarrassing information about Haynsworth and Carswell not uncovered by its own investigations, the administration agreed to allow the ABA committee to evaluate not only the person already selected but all those being considered for a Supreme Court position. This arrangement lasted only a short time, however. After the committee rated one potential nominee Not Qualified and another Not Opposed, President Nixon (unfairly) accused the committee of having "leaked" the nominees' names to the press, and dropped the ABA's prior screening of nominees. The ABA thus knew no more than anyone else (nothing) about the Powell and Rehnquist nominations when they were announced.

The vacancy created by Justice Douglas' resignation provided the ABA its desired prior involvement in screening for the first time. Attorney General Edward Levi sent a list of potential nominees to the ABA, which could add to the list. Fifteen names were screened over a two-week period, and after interviewing lawyers and judges and reviewing over 200 of his opinions, the ABA gave John Paul Stevens, the ultimate choice, its highest rating. When Sandra O'Connor was nominated, the ABA—not consulted before the nomination—found that she had "the professional qualifications required of an Associate Justice of the Supreme Court of the United States." Neither the nomination of Rehnquist to be Chief Justice nor the Scalia nomination encountered objections from the ABA, which gave Rehnquist its highest evaluation, Well Qualified. Most lawyers and law professors found Scalia to be of the highest caliber, but some law professors objected to Rehnquist after the Judiciary Committee hearings and before floor debate on his nomination because they did not feel he had been sufficiently forthcoming about important issues during the hearings, thus raising questions about his qualifications to be Chief Justice. Of particular concern to lawyers was whether he had been aware of religious and racial restrictive covenants on his properties and why he had not acted to remove them. His response, that he had not been aware of them because lawyers had handled the transaction, was contradicted by one of the lawyers. That he was Assistant Attorney General at the time of one of the transactions, said his critics, raised a question of his sensitivity to minorities.

Judges' Involvement

Supreme Court justices themselves at times get involved in selection politics. Chief Justice William Howard Taft frequently exerted pressure on behalf of people he wanted nominated.[65] More recently, Chief Justice Warren attempted to exert some pressure on behalf of Arthur Goldberg and Byron White for the Frankfurter and Whittaker vacancies. In connection with the latter, when President Kennedy sought Warren's advice (through Attorney General Robert Kennedy), Warren strongly opposed two potential nominees because they would be aligned with Justice Frankfurter as "self-restrained" justices.[66] Warren also tried to exert some pressure on behalf of Abe Fortas to succeed him as Chief Justice, but apparently also paid a visit to his old political enemy Richard Nixon to comment against Justice Stewart's effort to succeed him. Chief Justice Burger was apparently not silent concerning Supreme Court nominations, but appears to have been less active than Taft.

The most frequent method used in these efforts by the justices has been a letter of recommendation or comparable statement (as in the case of their supporting Rehnquist's nomination to be Chief Justice), followed in frequency by personal visits to either the president or the attorney general. Next most frequent has been a presidential request to the justices, in responding to which they are able to supply information and recommendations. Intense lobbying has been used only infrequently. Efforts in favor of a candidate appear to be less successful than those against, although judges' intervention is, of course, only one factor among many affecting the ultimate nomination.[67] Moreover, too much pressure from a Supreme Court justice can drive the president away from a potential nominee, not toward him, as appears to have been the case with Justice Frankfurter's efforts to obtain a Supreme Court appointment for Circuit Judge Learned Hand.[68]

Lower court judges may also try to play a role in the selection of Supreme Court justices. For example, the judges of the District of Columbia Circuit supported Burger's nomination to be Chief Justice, and all the judges of the Fourth Circuit supported Judge Haynsworth's nomination. Carswell's supporters in the lower federal judiciary also tried to gain additional support for his nomination, with 50 of 58 district judges and seven of 13 senior district judges in the Fifth Circuit sending the White House a statement endorsing the nominee after the press noted a lack of support for the nomination among Carswell's Fifth Circuit colleagues.

President and Senate[69]

The president's position when he deals with the Senate is stronger for Supreme Court nominations than for those to the lower courts. That the president's position is not absolute is shown by the Senate's successive rejections of President Nixon's nominations of Judges Haynsworth and Carswell—the first formal rejections of a nominee since 1930 and the first "double rejection" since 1894. Despite these rejections and the Senate's failure to confirm the nomination of Justice Fortas to be Chief Justice and the nomination of Judge Homer Thornberry that accompanied it (both withdrawn), presidents have done far better in the twentieth century than earlier. Including those of 1894, seven nominations were rejected before 1900 and 19 others have not been confirmed—for example, withdrawn after the Senate's extended delay in acting on them.

Most nominations sail smoothly through the confirmation process. Usually less than two months is necessary from submission of the nomination to the Senate to final Senate vote, and the time was less than three weeks each for Harry Blackmun and John Paul Stevens. Most of the time is consumed in the period between committee hearings and release of the committee's report; once it receives the nomination, the full Senate votes promptly. In Justice O'Connor's case, two months elapsed between the nomination and the hearings, with a Senate vote coming promptly thereafter. With the Rehnquist and Scalia nominations in 1986, several months elapsed between nomination and September confirmation, but that included Congress' summer vacation. Judiciary Committee hearings are perfunctory in most instances, with one-day hearings the pattern in the past, although those for Brandeis occupied 19 days. Roughly half the post-1950 hearings have occupied at least two days, but in only two instances were they more than four days: Haynsworth (eight days) and Abe Fortas to be Chief Justice (11 days). Negative votes have occurred in committee on only one-fourth of the nominations, with Rehnquist's nomination to be Chief Justice attracting five negative votes (13-5). There have been close committee votes (margins of four or fewer votes) in only three of 55 nominations in this century: Parker (6-10), Brandeis (10-8), and Haynsworth (10-7).

The nominee's actions during the confirmation process, particularly at the committee hearings, may have some effect on the outcome. When under fire from Senator Walsh of Montana, Harlan Fiske Stone offered to appear before the Judiciary Committee—not the custom at the time. His offer was accepted, and he handled himself quite successfully, an indication of the importance of the nominee's candor with the committee. Sandra O'Connor's prehearing visits with individual senators apparently aided her. On the negative side, although in 1971 Rehnquist provided affidavits to the committee chairman dealing with questions that arose after his hearing, his failure to reappear angered some senators, and the lack of candor charged by his critics in his 1986 appearance as well as his earlier misrepresentation of his Justice Department role concerning military surveillance of civilians provided senators ammunition to use against him. More damaging, however, was Judge Haynsworth's failure to deal with ethical conduct charges, and Carswell's chances were hurt when he failed to indicate that former Fifth Circuit Chief Judge Tuttle, after saying he had confidence in Carswell and would testify in his behalf, had told Carswell he would no longer testify. Carswell's problem was compounded when the Justice Department failed to arrange a meeting between the nominee and three dubious senators.

In the 1986 Rehnquist hearings, senators faced a problem of access to both medical records and documents from the nominee's prior government service that they wished to examine. Some senators thought the former necessary because of Rehnquist's problems with medication to ease back pain, which at one time led to slurred speech at a Court session; the problem perhaps resulted from a doctor's overprescription, not the justice's misuse. Rehnquist waived any rights to privacy in Justice Department documents concerning his role with respect to Army surveillance of civilians, but the administration balked, making them available only after protracted efforts by a bipartisan Judiciary Committee majority and after an initial broad request was narrowed to specific subjects. The documents, examined by staff members from both parties and then by senators, were not made public, but apparently did not provide much new information; however, had the administration persisted in its refusal to release them, confirmation might have been delayed.

The Senate has engaged in no more than two days of debate on all except the most controversial nominations; it used five days each on Fortas (to be Chief Justice) and Rehnquist (both initially and then to be Chief Justice) and seven days on Haynsworth. Until recently the Senate seldom even bothered with roll calls on the nominations, and Senate votes are often unanimous (Scalia, 98-0) or nearly so. Few recent votes in favor of confirmation have been close; 69-33 on Rehnquist to be Chief Justice was the closest, following the 68-26 vote on his initial confirmation. However, opposition has increased recently. Since 1949, eight confirmed nominees have received 10 or more "No" votes. Opposition has occurred even when senators were nominated; Hugo Black and Sherman Minton (a Truman appointee) each received 16 negative votes. In only four twentieth-century confirmed nominations did the negative votes approach one-half the positive vote: Mahlon Pitney (50-26), Brandeis (47-22), and Charles Evans Hughes to be Chief Justice (52-26), all earlier in this century, and Rehnquist to be Chief Justice. Rejections, however, have been relatively close: Parker, 41-39, Haynsworth, 55-45, and Carswell, 51-45.

In addition to those already mentioned, factors that may well affect the outcome of Senate consideration of a nominee include the Senate's partisan and ideological composition and the time during a president's term when the nomination occurs. Senators' liberalism is one element with a strong effect on their votes to confirm, with political considerations underlying votes in 14 instances from Brandeis through Rehnquist's initial confirmation in which at least 10 percent of the Senate's votes were negative. In each of these instances, senators favoring confirmation differed from their generally more cohesive Senate opposition on salient policy issues. In more than three-fourths of the confirmation votes, more than half of those opposing the nomination were clustered at either the most conservative or most liberal end of the political continuum with respect to the policy area at issue, although the ideology of the nominees' supporters was at the opposite extreme in only five cases. Thus "it is primarily dissatisfaction with the predicted policy behavior of the nominee which is the main motive force behind a vote against confirmation,"[70] true as well of the vote on Rehnquist to be Chief Justice. The Democrats' thorough examination of the Scalia and Rehnquist Chief Justice nominations was a message to President Reagan that his nominees to other vacancies should also be of high quality because they would get similar scrutiny, not a free ride. The conflict over some Reagan lower court nominees, like Manion or Sessions, is also related to the Supreme Court nomination process. The thoroughness with which Democrats began to examine such nominees was an indication that they would give comparable, if not in fact more thorough, consideration to Supreme Court nominations, and illustrates that nominations to the Supreme Court are not independent events, but are affected by prior events, also affecting what comes after them.

Timing is another important element. Nominees have been confirmed roughly 90 percent of the time during the president's first three years in office, but less than two-thirds of later nominations have been successful. However, when there is a partisan difference between Senate and president (Nixon's situation and Reagan's after the 1986 elections), the president has had a success rate of roughly two-thirds, but the rate falls to a devastatingly low 27 *percent* (four of 15) in the last year of the president's term. Independent of this matter of timing, the president's success rate is over 90 percent when his party controls the Senate, but only 42 percent when his party is in the minority.[71]

The president cannot control when a vacancy occurs. Warren Harding got four quick vacancies, filling them with Taft, George Sutherland (his campaign manager), Pierce Butler, and Edward Sanford. Nixon was able to fill the chief justiceship immediately and another position a year later, followed by two more shortly thereafter. Others have not been so fortunate. Jimmy Carter, who never had a vacancy to fill, was the first president not to be able to make a nomination to the Supreme Court, but he was not the only one not to be able to do so during his first term. That was FDR's problem. Although FDR, in the course of his three-plus terms, eventually got to name more Supreme Court justices than any other president, the first vacancy, that of Willis VanDevanter, did not come until Roosevelt's Court-packing plan was under heavy fire—and that resignation helped undermine the plan.

President Reagan was not able to control the timing of the vacancy caused by Justice Stewart's departure, which was a surprise because Stewart was one of only four justices under 70, and Justice Powell's retirement in 1987 was also a surprise. However, because the Stewart vacancy came very early in his term, President Reagan benefited from an early administration "honeymoon effect" and could make good on his campaign promise to name a woman to the Supreme

Court. When the Powell retirement came, however, it was late in Reagan's second term and the political environment was quite different.

Despite the problems just noted, the president may in the short run be able to affect the timing of a nomination. For example, immediately after the grueling fight over Haynsworth, the Senate, as suggested by one senator, was prepared to confirm anyone who had not raped a small child, in public, recently. Thus Nixon's delay in sending the Carswell nomination to the Senate misfired, as it allowed the liberals to regain their strength and to discover much negative evidence about Carswell.

Rehnquist's initial nomination, on the other hand, was helped by timing, coming as it did at the end of a session when the necessity of completing normal end-of-session business meant less time for consideration of the nomination, when the Senate was tired from the fight over Earl Butz's nomination to be Secretary of Agriculture, and after substantial effort had been devoted to attacking some anticipated nominations. As this suggests, opposition to a nomination may have a carryover effect. Hoover's nomination of John Parker, which occurred late in Hoover's term, was affected by the earlier controversy over Hughes' nomination to be Chief Justice. Liberal opposition to Warren Burger's appointment as Chief Justice was still simmering when Haynsworth was nominated. That displeasure served to reinforce the deeper liberal and Democratic unhappiness both over the Republicans' having deprived them of the Chief Justiceship when they had blocked the Fortas nomination and over the Nixon administration's not-well-concealed role in helping drive Fortas from the Court. Similarly, when President Ford had to nominate a replacement for Justice Douglas, Ford's earlier unsuccessful attempt as House minority leader to impeach Douglas was in people's minds, and Ford might have had considerable difficulty had he named a conservative rather than the moderate Stevens.

There is some reason to believe that President Reagan, knowing that it would be difficult to achieve the confirmation of a new Chief Justice late in his own second term and concerned that the Democrats might gain control of the Senate in 1986, attempted successfully to bring about Chief Justice Burger's retirement. It was generally believed that the Chief Justice would stay in office through September 1987, his eightieth birthday and the bicentennial of the Constitution, so his June 1986 announcement of his departure was something of a surprise. Although he said he was departing to devote his full attention to the Commission on the Bicentennial of the Constitution, one of his favorite projects, which he could no longer manage *and* devote full time to his work at the Court, the Bicentennial project may simply have been a cover for his real reason. That he appeared to obtain some action on other projects in which he was interested, such as the State Justice Institute (to fund research on state courts), may suggest that there was some negotiation with the administration; it is also possible that Burger, with a strong background in Republican politics, would have responded favorably to a Republican president's appeal that the vacancy be created prompt-ly. One reason it would be quite difficult for Reagan to obtain confirmation of a nominee at the end of his term, particularly with a Democratic Senate majority, illustrates how actions at one point affect actions at a later point. Republicans stalled Fortas' nomination to be Chief Justice because they sensed victory in the 1968 presidential election; that would provide a precedent for Democrats to do precisely the same thing, particularly if a nomination came within several months of the 1988 election—or perhaps even earlier.

Chief Justice Burger's decision to resign seems, in hindsight, to have been a wise one in its timing. Not only did the Democrats capture the Senate, but "Irangate" occurred, further weakening the president and encouraging the Democrats—who would have asserted themselves in any event—to assert them-selves even more. A nomination to the Chief Justiceship would have had much rougher sledding under these conditions than it did when Burger chose to leave the position. If President Reagan sought to obtain Chief Justice Burger's retire-ment, it appears that the unwillingness of Justices Blackmun to step down may have resulted from the Justice Department's strong ideological stance in key cases, also a possible explanation why Justice Powell did not step down sooner. This illustrates that judges are often able to control the president's opportunity to appoint successors.

Another element of the timing of nominations is the president's use of recess appointments to the Supreme Court, such as Eisenhower's appointments of Warren, Brennan, and Stewart. However, this device is likely to produce negative Senate reaction, such as delay in confirming the nominations. Yet there are pressures on the president to fill a vacancy on the Court that arises when the Senate is not in session. To wait to make the appointment until the Senate returns might mean injustice to those with pending cases, which might have to be delayed or reargued. Although the Court's senior justice could serve as de facto Chief Justice, a vacancy in the Chief Justice's position is particularly serious. Coupled with the fact that *Brown v. Board of Education* had already been set for reargument when Chief Justice Vinson died, this probably explains the recess appointment of Earl Warren.

Despite the occasional need to make them, recess appointments cause problems for the president, the Senate, and the Court itself. If the Senate were to convene in special session to consider only the recess nomination, more atten-tion would be focused on a single nomination than it deserved and the Senate's power would increase in relation to the president's. Yet the Senate finds it cannot get necessary information from an already sitting nominee because ethically he cannot respond to questions which touch on cases under consideration by the Court. There is also the possibility that an appointee concerned about Senate reaction to his or her votes might "pull punches" or cases in which the nominee is to write the Court's opinions might be "held" until after confirmation. (Two important opinions by Justice Brennan were not announced until nine weeks after his confirmation.) Even when a nominee is not a sitting justice, senators may have difficulty getting detailed answers to questions bearing on specific issues. That was evident in the hearings on the Scalia nomination, in which the nominee refused to go beyond generalities, leaving some senators rather frustrated but at a loss about how to prompt anything more precise.

Although often the president does no more—and need do no more—than announce the nomination, not only his timing but also his stance toward the nomination may affect the outcome, particularly if opposition arises. Both Woodrow Wilson's support for Brandeis and Eisenhower's support for Earl Warren (a public statement and a letter to the Judiciary Committee) had positive effects, and President Reagan's radio attack on Rehnquist's critics may have been of some help. President Hoover's calling in several Republican senators for discussions to gain support for the Parker nomination was, however, unsuccessful, and Lyndon Johnson's support of Abe Fortas' nomination to be Chief Justice backfired because Fortas was already under attack as a crony of Johnson. President Nixon failed to help the Haynsworth nomination with his initial heavy pressure, a special news conference repudiating anti-Haynsworth charges in detail, and a statement that senators should not take a nominee's philosophy into account; Republican senators did not like Nixon's "arm twisting." Nixon's attempt to maintain a "low profile" for the Carswell nomination was not effective, and he overreacted, even claiming, in a letter to Senator (later Attorney General) William Saxbe (R-Ohio), that he had a right to appoint whom he wanted.

> What is centrally at issue in this nomination is the constitutional responsibility of the President to appoint members of the Court—and whether this responsibility can be frustrated by those who wish to substitute their own philosophy or their own subjective judgment for that of the one person entrusted by the Constitution with the power of appointment. The question arises whether I, as President of the United States, shall be accorded the same right of choice in naming Supreme Court Justices which has been freely accorded to my predecessors of both parties.[72]

Challenging the Senate, as the president did in this statement, is particularly unwise politically. Nonetheless, the question remains whether the burden is on the president, and the president's nominee, to demonstrate that the nominee should be confirmed, or is on the Senate opponents of the nominee to show that the person nominated should not have been chosen. That issue was raised during the Rehnquist chief justiceship hearings, and is quite likely to be raised again.[73]

A Note on the Bork Nomination

On June 26, 1987, the last day of the Court's 1986 Term, Justice Lewis Powell announced his resignation. On July 1, President Reagan nominated Judge Robert H. Bork of the U.S. Court of Appeals for the District of Columbia—the same court from which Justice Scalia had moved to the Supreme Court. Bork, a former Yale law professor, not only had judicial experience but had served as solicitor general. In that position, he had carried out President Nixon's order to fire Special Prosecutor Archibald Cox during the Watergate investigation, after the attorney general and deputy attorney general had refused to do so and had left office.

President Reagan said he was making the nomination because of Bork's belief in "judicial restraint." Although the president did not point to specific issue positions, the nomination was particularly important to him because he had not been able to achieve his social agenda in Congress. Bork's prior positions immediately led civil rights, women's rights, and liberal groups to oppose the nomination, with opponents attempting to portray the nominee as ultraconservative, while the administration painted a picture of him as moderate. The opponents, having anticipated that Bork might be the next nominee, were prepared with materials to use in their campaign of opposition.

The argument over the nomination quickly turned to whether the Senate should reject Bork because of his ideology and whether it was legitimate for the Senate to refuse to confirm someone who might shift the Court's balance. The president and Republican leaders argued that the only issue was the nominee's qualifications and that "politics" should be kept out of the process. This position was, however, disingenuous because the administration itself took ideology into account both in its lower court nominations and in the Bork nomination itself and because Senator Thurmond (R-S.C.), the ranking Republican on the Senate Judiciary Committee, had opposed Justice Fortas' nomination to be Chief Justice in 1969 specifically because of the Warren Court's liberal rulings.

Judiciary Committee hearings, beginning in mid-September, occupied 11 days, with five days of testimony by Bork. The hearings led to a negative shift in public opinion. On October 6, after the Court began its 1987 Term, the committee voted 9-5 to give the nomination a negative recommendation. Bork, even after a clear Senate majority opposed him, refused to withdraw. After three days of Senate debate, the final vote was 58-42 against Bork. The subsequent nomination of Judge Douglas Ginsberg, also of the District of Columbia Circuit, lasted barely a week before it was withdrawn after revelations about marijuana use and possible conflict-of-interest.

Notes

1. *United States v. Woodley*, 751 F.2d 1008 (9th Cir. 1985).

2. *Atkins v. United States*, 556 F.2d 1028 (Ct. Cl. 1977), cert. denied, 434 U. S. 1009 (1978).

3. *Duplantier v. United States*, 606 F.2d 654 (5th Cir. 1979) and 608 F.2d 1373 (5th Cir. 1980), cert. denied, 449 U.S. 1076 (1981).

4. Data from surveys by *National Law Journal*: May 28, 1979, June 2, 1980, July 6, 1981; also *New York Times*, May 18, 1982.

5. *Chandler v. Judicial Council of the Tenth Circuit*, 398 U.S. 74 (1970). For a thorough treatment of the entire Chandler matter, particularly the underlying conflict between Judge Chandler and his fellow judges, see Joseph C. Goulden, *The Benchwarmers: The Private World of the Powerful Federal Judges* (New York: Ballantine Books, 1974), pp. 234–84.

6. Richard Ellis, "The Impeachment of Samuel Chase," *American Political Trials*, ed. Michal R. Belknap (Westport, Conn.: Greenwood Press, 1981), pp. 57–78.

7. Rayman L. Solomon, "The Politics of Appointment and the Federal Courts' Role in Regulating America: U.S. Courts of Appeals Judgeships from T.R. to F.D.R.," *American Bar Foundation Research Journal* 1984 (Spring): 285–344.

8. "Q. & A. With the Attorney General," *ABA Journal* 71 (July 1985): 46.

9. William Overend, "Judges Need No 'Litmus Test,' 9th Circuit Told," *Los Angeles Times*, July 3, 1985, pp. 1,16.

10. Sheldon Goldman, "Reaganizing the Judiciary: The First Term Appointments," *Judicature* 68 (April–May 1985): 314 n.1.

11. Harold W. Chase, *Federal Judges: The Appointing Process* (Minneapolis: University of Minnesota Press, 1972), pp. 36–37.

12. For a description of procedure, see Elliot E. Slotnick, "The U.S. Circuit Judge Nominating Commission," *Law & Policy Quarterly* 1 (October 1979): 465–96, on which I have drawn; Slotnick, "Federal Appellate Judge Selection During the Carter Administration: Recruitment Changes and Unanswered Questions," *Justice System Journal* 6 (Fall 1981): 293–304; Larry Berkson, "The U. S. Circuit Judge Nominating Commission: The Candidates' Perspective," *Judicature* 62 (May 1979): 466–82; and Larry C. Berkson and Susan B. Carbon, *The United States Circuit Judge Nominating Commission: Its Members, Procedures and Candidates* (Chicago: American Judicature Society, 1980).

13. Elliot E. Slotnick, "What Panelists Are Saying About the Circuit Judge Nominating Commission," *Judicature* 62 (February 1979): 322.

14. Ibid.

15. Ibid., p. 323.

16. Slotnick, "Reforms in Judicial Selection: Will They Affect the Senate's Role?" *Judicature* 64 (September 1980): 119.

17. See Alan Neff, "Breaking with Tradition," *Judicature* 64 (December–January 1981): 256–78; and Neff, *The United States District Judge Nominating Commissions: Their Members, Procedures and Candidates* (Chicago: American Judicature Society, 1981): and Slotnick, "Reforms in Judicial Selection," *Judicature* 64 (August 1980): 60–73 and (September 1980): 114–31.

18. See Adlai E. Stevenson, "'Reform' and Judicial Selection," *American Bar Association Journal* 64 (November 1978): 1683–85.

19. Neff, "Breaking with Tradition," pp. 265–66.

20. Slotnick, "Reforms in Judicial Selection," p. 67.

21. Neff, "Breaking with Tradition," p. 275.

22. Slotnick, "Reforms in Judicial Selection," p. 116. See also Sheldon Goldman, "Should There Be Affirmative Action for the Judiciary?" *Judicature* 62 (May 1979): 488–94.

23. W. Gary Fowler, "Judicial Selection Under Reagan and Carter: A Comparison of Their Initial Recommendation Procedures," *Judicature* 67 (December–January 1984): 265–83.

24. Slotnick, "Reforms in Judicial Selection," pp. 69–70.

25. Chase, *Federal Judges*, pp. 130–31, 135.

26. "Q. & A. With the New Attorney General," *American Bar Association Journal* 65 (October 1979): 1502. See also Elliot E. Slotnick, "The ABA Standing Committee on Federal Judiciary: A Contemporary Assessment," *Judicature* 66 (March 1983): 348–62 and (April 1983): 385–93.

27. See Elaine Martin, "Women on the Federal Bench: A Comparative Profile," *Judicature* 65 (December–January 1982): 309.

28.   Goldman, "Reaganizing the Judiciary," p. 316.

29.   David O. Stewart, "The President's Lawyer," *ABA Journal* 72 (April 1, 1986): 61. See also Goldman, "Reaganizing the Judiciary."

30.   Goldman, "Reaganizing the Judiciary," pp. 322, 326; Sheldon Goldman, "Reagan's Second Term Judicial Appointments: The Battle at Midway," *Judicature* 70 (April–May 1987): 327.

31.   S. Sidney Ulmer, "Are Social Background Models Time-Bound?" *American Political Science Review* 80 (September 1986): 957–68.

32.   See three articles by Sheldon Goldman: "Voting Behavior on the United States Courts of Appeals, 1961–1964," *American Political Science Review* 60 (June 1966): 374–83; "Conflict and Consensus in the United States Courts of Appeals," *Wisconsin Law Review* 1968: 461–82; and "Conflict in the U.S. Courts of Appeals, 1965–1971: A Quantitative Analysis," *University of Cincinnati Law Review* 42 (1973): 635–58.

33.   C. K. Rowland and Robert A. Carp, "A Longitudinal Study of Party Effects on Federal District Court Policy Propensities,"*American Journal of Political Science* 24 (May 1980): 300. See also Robert A. Carp and C. K. Rowland, *Policymaking and Politics in the Federal District Courts* (Knoxville: University of Tennessee Press, 1983).

34.   See Jon Gottschall, "Carter's Judicial Appointments: The Influence of Affirmative Action and Merit Selection on Voting on the U.S. Courts of Appeals," *Judicature* 67 (October 1983): 164–73, and "Reagan's Appointments to the U.S. Courts of Appeals: The Continuation of a Judicial Revolution," *Judicature* 70 (June–July 1986): 48–54.

35.   Craig R. Ducat and Robert L. Dudley, "Federal Judges and Presidential Power: Truman to Reagan," paper presented to Midwest Political Science Association, 1986.

36.   Kermit L. Hall, "The Children of the Cabins: The Lower Federal Judiciary, Modernization, and the Political Culture, 1789–1899," *Northwestern University Law Review* 75 (October 1980): 436. See also Hall, *The Politics of Justice: Lower Federal Judicial Selection and the Second Party System, 1829–1861* (Lincoln: University of Nebraska Press, 1979).

37.   Kermit L. Hall, "Hacks and Derelicts Revisited: American Territorial Judiciary, 1789–1959," *Western Historical Quarterly* 12 (July 1981): 279, 284.

38.   J. Woodford Howard, Jr., *Courts of Appeals in the Federal Judicial System*, p. 113.

39.   The data here and some that appear subsequently are drawn from Sheldon Goldman, "Characteristics of Eisenhower and Kennedy Appointees to the Lower Federal Courts," *Western Political Quarterly* 18 (1965): 755–62; and Goldman, "Judicial Backgrounds, Recruitment and the Party Variable: The Case of the Johnson and Nixon Appointees to the United States District and Appeals Courts," *Arizona State Law Journal* 1974: 211–22.

40.   Solomon, "The Politics of Appointment."

41.   Elliot E. Slotnick, "The Paths to the Federal Bench: Gender, Race and Judicial Recruitment Variation," *Judicature* 67 (March 1984): 384.

42.   *McClure v. Carter*, 513 F.Supp. 265 (D.Idaho 1981), aff'd sub nom. *McClure v. Reagan*, 454 U.S. 1025 (1981).

43.   Goldman, "Reaganizing the Judiciary," p. 323; Goldman, "Reagan's Second Term," pp. 330, 334.

44.   Goldman, "Reaganizing the Judiciary," pp. 321-22.

45.   Gottschall, "Carter's Judicial Appointments."

46.   Martin, "Women on the Federal Bench," pp. 310, 312; and Slotnick, "The Paths to the Federal Bench," pp. 375–76.

47.   Slotnick, "The Paths to the Federal Bench," p. 387.

48.   For the data, see Elaine Martin, "Women in the Federal Judiciary," paper presented to Midwest Political Science Association, 1986.

49.   Gottschall, "Carter's Judicial Appointments."

50.   Robert Scigliano, *The Supreme Court and the Presidency* (New York: Free Press, 1971), p. 105.

51.   John R. Schmidhauser, "Judicial Behavior and the Sectional Crisis of 1837–1860," *Journal of Politics* 34 (November 1971): 615–40.

52.   Stuart Nagel, "Comparing Elected and Appointed Judicial Systems," Sage Professional Papers #04-001 (Beverly Hills, Calif.: Sage, 1973), p. 25.

53.   John R. Schmidhauser, *The Supreme Court: Its Politics, Personalities and Procedures* (New York: Holt, Rinehart and Winston, 1961), pp. 31–32.

54.   John R. Schmidhauser, "Stare Decisis, Dissent and the Background of the Justices," *University of Toronto Law Review* 14 (May 1962): 194–212.

55.   Scigliano, *The Supreme Court*, p. 146. His full treatment of the subject is on pp. 125–28.

56.   Edward V. Heck and Steven A. Shull, "Policy Preferences of Justices and Presidents: The Case of Civil Rights," *Law & Policy Quarterly* 4 (July 1982): 333.

57.   Robert Harrison, "The Breakup of the Roosevelt Supreme Court: The Contribution of History and Biography," *Law and History Review* 2 (Fall 1984): 165–221.

58.   Beverly Blair Cook, "Justice Sandra Day O'Connor and the Uses of Federalism as a Decisional Principle," paper presented to American Political Science Association, 1986, pp. 4–5, 9a.

59.   Charles M. Lamb, "The Making of a Chief Justice: Warren Burger on Criminal Procedure, 1957–1969," *Cornell Law Review* 60 (June 1975): 756, 786. See also Lamb, "Exploring the Conservatism of Federal Appeals Court Judges," *Indiana Law Journal* 51 (Winter 1976): 257–79.

60.   This examination draws on Joel B. Grossman and Stephen L. Wasby, "Haynsworth and Parker: History Does Live Again," *South Carolina Law Review* 23 (1971): 345–59; and Grossman and Wasby, "The Senate and Supreme Court Nominations: Some Reflections," *Duke Law Journal* (August 1972): 557–91.

61.   See Robert Shogan, *A Question of Judgment: The Fortas Case and the Struggle for the Supreme Court* (Indianapolis: Bobbs-Merrill, 1975).

62.   For a correction and addition to the study by Grossman and Wasby based on correspondence with Judge Haynsworth, see Wasby, *Continuity and Change: From the Warren Court to the Burger Court* (Pacific Palisades, Calif.: Goodyear, 1976), pp. 27–28, note.

63.   Donald R. Songer, "The Relevance of Policy Values for the Confirmation of Supreme Court Nominees," *Law & Society Review* 13 (Summer 1979): 939.

64.   Sandra D. O'Connor, "Trends in the Relationship Between the Federal and State Courts from the Perspective of a State Court Judge," *William & Mary Law Review* 22 (Summer 1981): 801–15.

65.   See Walter F. Murphy, "In His Own Image: Mr. Chief Justice Taft and Supreme Court Appointments," *Supreme Court Review 1961*, ed. Philip Kurland (Chicago: University of Chicago Press, 1961), pp. 159–93.

66.   Bernard Schwartz, *Super Chief: Earl Warren and His Supreme Court—A Judicial Biography* (New York: Oxford University Press, 1983), pp. 428–29.

67.   Henry J. Abraham and Bruce Allen Murphy, "The Influence of Sitting and Retired Justices on Presidential Supreme Court Nominations," *Hastings Constitutional Law Quarterly* 3 (Winter 1976): 37–63.

68.   Bruce Allen Murphy, *The Brandeis/Frankfurter Connection* (New York: Oxford University Press, 1982), p. 320.

69.   This is based on Grossman and Wasby, "The Senate and Supreme Court Nominations," updated.

70.   Songer, "The Relevance of Policy Values," pp. 935–36.

71.   See Scigliano, *The Supreme Court*, pp. 146–47; updated.

72.   Richard M. Nixon to William Saxbe, March 31, 1970, *Congressional Record* 116 (1970): 10158.

73.   For a recent examination of the nomination and confirmation process, see Laurence Tribe, *God Save This Honorable Court* (New York: Random House, 1985).

4   Lawyers, Interest Groups, and Appeals

PLAYING A CRUCIAL ROLE in the judicial process are people who initiate cases and particularly their attorneys, who present the cases in court. In any examination of the Supreme Court, lawyers—individual attorneys in private practice, government lawyers, and interest group lawyers—are particularly important because of their role in deciding what cases to appeal. Not all types of cases are appealed in the same proportions, and during an appeal lawyers may shift the focus of a case from issues that were central in the trial to other issues. Although individuals may be able to present their own cases effectively in local courts, the assistance of lawyers is essential when cases are complex or when cases reach the higher levels of the judicial system. Because the Supreme Court accepts only cases involving issues of considerable public significance, the role of lawyers is especially important in helping shape those outcomes, which will affect many people in addition to the lawyers' clients. Moreover, although some corporations or wealthy individuals can afford the lengthy process of litigation and appeals, taking a case to the Supreme Court requires most litigants to obtain financial support, at times provided by interest groups.

Those interest groups participating in the judicial process and other well-organized actors are also involved in cases before the Supreme Court because of their stake in long-run outcomes extending beyond the particular facts of individual cases. The government is another party appearing regularly before the courts in general and the Supreme Court in particular. The government acts not only as a prosecutor and defender of its own policies, but also as another major actor trying to affect the Court's shaping of policies in cases in which the government itself is not a party. In this chapter, after some general comments about relations between lawyers and judges, we look first at federal government attorneys—the United States Attorneys, the Attorney General of the United States, and the Solicitor General—and then turn to a more extended examination of the role of private attorneys and interest groups in litigation.

Lawyers, Cases, and the Court

Relations between bench and bar take a variety of forms in and out of court. Lawyers and judges interact not only in formal ways in the courtroom—ways that, because of their frequency, may become regularized—but in a variety of ways differing in their formality outside the courtroom. When lawyers become judges, they may withdraw somewhat from frequent contact with former lawyer colleagues, even when they remain in the same city, but not all such ties are severed. Judges continue to participate in bar association activities, both nationally and at the state and local levels. Those activities include not only social functions but also work on committees that make policy recommendations. Judges also have contacts with the lawyers who serve on advisory committees of both the Judicial Conference of the United States and circuit councils. Lawyer representatives are regularly in attendance at the annual circuit judicial conferences, providing the lawyers an opportunity to criticize judges' work.

Lawyers' involvement in cases is, of course, crucial to the course of the judicial process and its outcomes. The importance of lawyers at all stages of litigation, from initiation to final appeal, cannot be underestimated, even though judges may have the final say in a case. Obviously lawyers help determine the cases that will be brought initially and that form the universe from which appeals may be drawn. Decisions to initiate cases are often the result of implicit interaction between lawyers and judges. On the basis of the precedents established by judges' rulings, lawyers may try to discourage clients from pursuing litigation they are sure to lose. Yet where the law is not clear or fully developed, a lawyer wishing to solve a client's problem may bring to the courts questions the judges have not previously considered. Judges may encourage lawyers to bring cases by making hints or suggestions that particular legal issues have not been raised. On the other hand, by showing firmness in disposing of a matter, they make clear that the court wishes to hear no more litigation on that subject.

Moreover, the general policy orientation of a court affects the cases lawyers bring to court and pursue on appeal. With the departure of Earl Warren and his replacement by Warren Burger, for example, one heard civil liberties lawyers talk about taking fewer cases to the Supreme Court; this view was strengthened as the full dimensions of Burger Court doctrine emerged. Yet despite their negative perceptions of Supreme Court rulings, liberal lawyers continued to bring cases— because clients pressed them to do so, because they believed they might achieve victory even if they estimated their chances of doing so to be slim, because they feared that other lawyers would bring a case raising their issue before they had a chance to do so, and because, out of momentum, they were accustomed to doing so. On the other hand, conservative lawyers, both those representing public interest law firms and government lawyers who saw the Court as more open to their claims, were more likely to appeal cases to the Supreme Court.

In our supposedly adversary system of justice, courts are expected to make their decisions on the basis of material submitted by the parties. This serves to underscore the importance of lawyers' actions in presenting their cases. Reliance on party-submitted material is greatest with respect to factual matters at the trial, which are doubly important because the trial record serves as the basis for appeals. Thus lawyers' actions at one stage of litigation affect later actions and may even foreclose them. At the appellate level, the court's decision is also supposed to be based on material submitted by lawyers: the trial record, briefs, and arguments made in the appellate court. Thus to a greater or lesser degree lawyers' positions place constraints on the decisions judges can reach. If both lawyers in a case press the same position or at least focus directly on the same narrow issue, the judges' freedom of action may be decreased. At other times, however, those constraints are not tight, particularly when lawyers plead multiple claims, press procedural and substantive questions simultaneously, or argue broad grounds about which they are personally indifferent. The constraints are further lessened when interested individuals or (more likely) groups file briefs as an *amicus curiae* ("friend of the court") to urge legal positions related to the issues in the case but often somewhat different from those stressed by the direct litigants.

Judges can increase their freedom of action by expanding or contracting issues ("issue fluidity": see pages 203-4), by relying more on material submitted by an *amicus* rather than by focusing exclusively on the parties' arguments, or by developing additional information through research they and their law clerks conduct. Judges' development of information has been criticized for not being consonant with a pure version of the adversary system and because the litigants don't have an opportunity to evaluate material serving as a partial basis for judges' decisions.[1] However, such use of additional material may be necessary if courts, and particularly the Supreme Court, are to issue decisions affecting more than the immediate parties to the case; only in this way might a judge know, for example, of a case's broader implications and potential effects.

The Government's Attorneys

United States Attorneys

Particularly crucial for the federal judicial process are United States Attorneys and the Attorney General and Solicitor General of the United States. There was no Department of Justice until 1870, but there have been United States Attorneys, one for each judicial district, and an attorney general, serving as the lawyer to the president, since 1789. U.S. Attorneys are formally appointed by the president and confirmed by the Senate, although district judges have the authority to select "court appointees" to fill temporary vacancies. The realities of the appointment process, however, give substantial roles to senators, through senatorial courtesy, and to the Justice Department, which, in making its choices, takes into account the need to maintain good relations with the bench. The senators' role increases U.S. Attorneys' local orientations. On the other hand, the U.S. Attorneys' national orientation is evident in the fact that they generally submit their resignations when a new president takes office, although there have been some instances in which they have refused to do so, thus forcing their removal by the president.[2] The president may also remove a U.S. Attorney for misbehavior, as occurred in the Northern District of Ohio in 1984 after the incumbent was alleged to have improperly disclosed information about a pending grand jury indictment to someone who notified the grand jury's target.

U.S. Attorney offices vary greatly in size, roughly paralleling the relative size of a district's federal bench; they have ranged from an office that comprises the U.S. Attorney and one assistant to that for the Southern District of New York with well over 100 assistants. In the larger offices, the basic work is carried out by the assistant U.S. attorneys, hired by the U.S. Attorneys, with the latter generally acting as managers, although some seek to set policy and shape agency priorities. Although U.S. Attorney offices have responsibility for enforcement of federal law, that for the District of Columbia is unusual in having responsibility for enforcement not only of federal statutes but also of laws of local applicability; moreover, because of its location, it represents many government agencies when their actions are challenged.

U.S. Attorneys and their assistants are at the center of a set of relations—with the judges in their districts, other government agencies, and the Department of Justice, which in turn has relations with executive branch agencies (see Figure 4.1).

Figure 4.1.   United States Attorneys' Relations

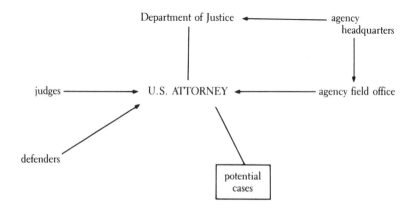

Relations between DOJ (Department of Justice) and the USAs (U.S. Attorneys) vary depending on the district and the incumbent; they also vary over time depending on DOJ efforts at control and the USAs' willingness to resist such control. U.S. Attorneys are under the formal supervision of the attorney general, who can control politically sensitive cases—for example, bribery charges against high government officials—or cases in certain categories such as civil rights and can instruct the U.S. Attorneys about whether or not to try a case. In recent years, the Justice Department has made use of *strike forces* of its attorneys and agents from other government units to go to particular areas of the country to deal with major problems like drugs or organized crime; policies for the strike forces are set by the Justice Department rather than by the U.S. Attorney in the district in which a strike force is working, although there may be cooperation between the two.

In areas of law that the Justice Department considers important, great effort is made to establish priorities for U.S. Attorneys. Overall policy direction is, or at least can be, established by the attorney general and the assistant attorneys general in charge of the department's various subject-matter divisions: Criminal, Civil, Land and Natural Resources, Civil Rights, and Antitrust. In most instances, however, formal supervision is not matched by actual control of their work so that the federal government has "not yet succeeded in establishing complete domination and control over U.S. Attorneys' offices."[3]

U.S. Attorneys have traditionally exercised considerable independence of "headquarters." A few offices, most notably that for the Southern District of New York, have developed significant autonomy—especially symbolic autonomy—because of the high proportion of all federal cases, and particularly of the important federal cases, they handle. Indeed, U.S. Attorneys have considerable autonomy within the federal law enforcement establishment because of their resources, including their standing in the community, access to information that others do not possess, and others' dependence on their work. They have considerable discretion in determining what cases they will bring, resulting in considerable variation from one district to another in the way similar cases are handled.

U.S. Attorneys' activities are affected less by relations with DOJ than by relations with district judges and by interaction with the other federal agencies that initiate cases and on which they may need to rely for information. Because they can refuse to prosecute, U.S. Attorneys and their assistants may be in a superior position in dealing with investigative agencies. However, "many of the cases presented leave little room for the exercise of discretion": good cases cannot be turned down and trivial ones cannot be authorized.[4] Moreover, workload affects decisions about what cases to accept: a heavy caseload may lead an office to decline prosecution of cases that an office with greater resources would have accepted. Judges have particularly significant effects on U.S. Attorneys' offices: they can affect not only case outcomes but also the way in which cases move through the court, and can supervise the assistant USAs, who spend much time in court. However, relations between judge and prosecutor are not unilateral: cases brought by the U.S. Attorney's office are the dominant portion of a district court's caseload and thus affect the conditions of the judge's work and the amount of work the judge has.

Attorney General and the Justice Department

The attorney general has several roles to perform. One is to serve as a member of the Cabinet. Another role is that of chief prosecutor of those alleged to have violated the nation's laws. Still another is as administrative head of the Department of Justice (with 60,000 employees in more than 30 divisions, bureaus—including the Federal Bureau of Investigation—and boards) and of the decentralized collection of U.S. Attorneys and their assistants, although day-to-day administrative coordination is invariably performed by someone else. The attorney general's tasks as administrator may entail resolving friction not only between DOJ and USAs, but also between lawyers in the department's divisions and the political appointees heading those divisions. An example is the continuing conflict between the department's conservative top leadership and the Civil Rights Division's more liberal lawyers.

The Attorney General of the United States, often someone personally close to the president or someone closely involved in his political campaigns, does have special assistants to provide supplementary skills and a deputy attorney general to assist in running the Department of Justice, and specialists are chosen as assistant attorneys general. However, an important question is whether a person chosen to be attorney general on the basis of political party or friendship considerations—such as Robert Kennedy, with little previous legal experience; John Mitchell, a Wall Street bond counsel who was Nixon's attorney general; or Reagan's attorneys general, William French Smith, a corporate attorney, or Edwin Meese, long a close policy adviser to the president—has skills appropriate to being the nation's chief lawyer. There is also a question whether such people can avoid getting into legal trouble related to their close ties to the president, as John Mitchell did, with an independent counsel investigating Edwin Meese for actions as a White House adviser and questions having been raised about his role in the Iran-Contra controversy while he was attorney general. (As one headline put it, "Is Meese Corrupt, Incompetent, or Under Attack by Political Foes?")

Another issue is the attorney general's ideological commitment and closeness of views to the president's policy positions. With the selection of the attorney general and his immediate subordinates in the president's hands, the president would be expected to choose those who would carry out his policies rather than those who would be neutral on such matters. However, it may be difficult for the attorney general—the official supervising government prosecutors—to enforce the law in an even-handed fashion if he continues to play a role in policy making over a wide range of issues, as Attorney General Meese did by presiding over the Domestic Policy Council, a Cabinet group advising the president on domestic and social issues (with a Justice Department staff member coordinating the Council's activities), and particularly if the attorney general seems to be pursuing a particular ideological platform. The Ethics in Government Act provided for independent counsel to prosecute certain cases because of concern that attorneys general would not be appropriately neutral; in a number of cases, judges have ruled that the attorney general failed to follow that law when accusations had been made against senior federal officials, and others have claimed that the attorney general too easily found "credible evidence" warranting appointment of an independent counsel.

Relations between the Department of Justice and other executive branch agencies with respect to litigation are not always easy. The agencies want to control cases they initiate and the Justice Department wishes to maintain a uniform litigation position and to assure that only legally sound positions are pursued, which it claims can be accomplished only if it controls the litigation. At times there are disputes between other agencies, at other times between another agency and DOJ.[5] (There is also conflict *within* the agencies, for example, between general counsel and agency head or simply between factions within the agency.) Conflicts between DOJ and agencies about litigating authority are not new, reaching back to the Justice Department's establishment in 1870. For example, in the New Deal, agency attorneys who had begun to proceed with cases in court found that the Justice Department wished to remove their authority to do so.[6]

Justice Department representation of agencies in court, which puts agencies in the position of being "captive clients," allows the department to control litigation. For example, the Civil Division usually represents administrative agencies in litigation concerning those agencies' regulatory programs. The department has generally pressed hard to increase its litigating authority so that the agencies have had to deal with its "relentless bureaucratic imperialism." For example, in June 1933, the department, by Executive Order, took away control of litigation authority from all existing agencies.[7] There are, however, situations in which agencies, at times as a result of congressional pressure, have had their own litigating authority increased through a "memorandum of understanding" reached with DOJ.[8] In general, when conflicts arise about whether a case should be brought or how it should be argued (that is, the points that should be emphasized), Justice Department officials end up resolving the disputes. During the Carter administration, a Federal Legal Council was created "to facilitate communication and coordination" among agency general counsel and the attorney general.[9]

A crucial role for the attorney general is being the "president's lawyer," a role retained despite the growth of White House staff, which allows the president to obtain legal advice on his immediate responsibilities from his own staff. The position of White House counsel dates only from the Truman administration; as recently as the Nixon administration, the office consisted of only two lawyers,

John Dean and Fred Fielding. Fielding, as President Reagan's White House counsel, had eight to 10 attorneys working for him plus several other professionals assisting on security clearance matters.[10] In the Department of Justice, the work of being the "president's lawyer" is institutionalized in the position of Assistant Attorney General for Legal Counsel, who advises the attorney general in the latter's role as the president's adviser and also provides legal opinions for the heads of executive branch agencies. The advice given is, however, not always followed, particularly on major policy matters where policy and political concerns are likely to dominate.

The attorney general, working with the president and the latter's assistants and at the president's direction, is also chief maker of the nation's legal policy. This role includes making decisions to bring cases or to file briefs to establish particular legal points, such as the Reagan administration's participation in cases as part of its efforts to limit school busing, to restrict "affirmative action" plans for hiring of minorities in public employment, or to restrict the breadth of the exclusionary rule in criminal cases. In trying to develop national policy, the government continues its efforts even after losing in one or more district or appellate courts, not accepting as authoritative a single court of appeals ruling adverse to the government on a particular point of law. Instead the government is willing to relitigate even within the same circuit if some basis can be found for distinguishing later cases from the initial ones. Only when three unanimous courts of appeals decisions have been decided against the government is the government willing to stop litigation on that point of law. This continuous relitigation is part of an effort to create an intercircuit conflict that it is hoped the Supreme Court will accept (see page 212).

The attorney general's role as maker of national legal policy is also visible in changes in the government's litigation position, such as the shift, after the Reagan administration took office, on tax exempt status for private schools that discriminate against racial minorities (from opposition to the tax exemption to support for it) and on a state's obligation to provide education to children of illegal aliens (where the government terminated its support for nongovernmental litigants seeking such educational aid). (The administration lost both cases.) It is also seen in statements made by the attorney general on major policy issues, such as those by Attorneys General Smith and Meese on limitations on federal court jurisdiction, proposed constitutional amendments, "judicial activism," and the need to follow the "original intent" of the Constitution.

Solicitor General

The Solicitor General of the United States is the third-ranking official in the Justice Department. Perhaps best known from appearances before the Supreme Court, the solicitor general, assisted by five deputies and almost 20 assistant solicitors general, plays a crucial part in the executive branch's judicial activity, particularly in the appellate courts. Almost all that activity is in appearances before the courts, but there have been some direct contacts with the justices, for example, when Solicitor General J. Lee Rankin visited Chief Justice Earl Warren to express the Eisenhower administration's concern about the foreign policy implications of a case.[11]

Making up the bulk of the work of the solicitor general's office are decisions whether to appeal cases the government has lost in a district court and whether to seek Supreme Court review of adverse appellate rulings; these actions are closely related to the Justice Department's overall litigation concerns. Such decisions are crucial for federal agencies, as only a few regulatory commissions, such as the National Labor Relations Board (NLRB) have the authority to go to court on their own to seek enforcement of their orders, and only a few, including the Interstate Commerce Commission and Federal Maritime Commission, have statutory authority to appeal their cases without DOJ approval; even for them, absence of the solicitor general's approval is disadvantageous. (Government agency decisions *not* to appeal are seldom reviewed by the solicitor general, much less overturned.) That government agencies need the solicitor general's approval to appeal a case often leaves that official caught in the middle if two agencies take opposing positions, a conflict that may be resolved by allowing one to file its own appeal without his endorsement. The solicitor general must also decide whether to defend the government against appeals from its lower court victories, although this is done routinely; whether to oppose opponents' certiorari petitions; and whether to support or oppose other parties through the filing of *amicus* briefs both in the lower appellate courts and the Supreme Court. In so doing, the solicitor general can be highly selective in choosing precisely the cases in which to press new legal arguments.

Although usually defending the government, the solicitor general may decide that the government should have lost a case it has won, such as a case won because of improper actions like illegal wiretapping. In such instances the solicitor general makes a *confession of error*, that is, tells the justices that the government should lose. Decisions not to appeal government defeats to the Supreme Court may be related to the Court's caseload and the government's general legal policy position, including the desire to restrict the legal effect of the defeat to the district or circuit in which it occurred. In confession of error situations, other factors also come into play. Foremost is the need to protect the department's reputation and thus to increase the chance of winning later cases. Although the department will confess error, at times it chooses instead to narrow the issues in a case. The department, faced with a statute it believes unconstitutional or otherwise improper, may refuse to defend the provision, leaving Congress to provide a lawyer to defend the statute, as happened with the legislative veto case. When the administration adopts this position after the government has won in the lower court, the Supreme Court may have to appoint someone to present one side of the case—which happened with respect to tax exemptions for private schools that discriminate on the basis of race.

The solicitor general's actions carry great weight with the Supreme Court, but at least some justices will not automatically accept a confession of error. When the majority had followed a suggestion by the solicitor general that a case involving promises made to a government witness be returned to the trial court, Justices Rehnquist and Powell and Chief Justice Burger, dissenting, complained that "this Court does not, or at least should not, respond in Pavlovian fashion to confessions of error."[12] Several justices have also criticized the solicitor general for trying to use the Court to remedy U.S. Attorneys' failures to follow Justice Department policy.[13]

Another of the solicitor general's principal functions is to decide when the government will appear as an *amicus curiae* to urge executive branch policies upon the courts in cases to which the government is not a party. The United States and its agencies (when the solicitor general approves), like state and local governments, do not need to seek approval in order to file *amicus curiae* briefs. Because, without the consent of both parties, *amicus* participation comes only upon a petition to the Supreme Court itself, the solicitor general must also decide, in cases in which the government *is* a party, when others will be allowed to appear as *amicus*.

The solicitor general's participation as *amicus* before the Supreme Court and the permission granted to others have varied over time, in part reflecting the Supreme Court's preferences. Thus after the Court seemed in 1949 to want fewer *amicus* participations before the Court, the solicitor general reduced the number of permissions to potential *amici*. Then as the justices seemed to relax their position on *amicus* participation, his consent was given more frequently.[14]

When the government does file an *amicus* brief, it may also ask to appear to present oral argument. Private *amici* are rarely granted such permission, but the Court frequently gives it to the solicitor general—and continued to do so most of the time even after the Court changed its rules in 1980 to eliminate the solicitor general's exemption from the rule that such appearances would be allowed only under "the most extraordinary circumstances"; when the solicitor general does appear in person, it is more likely to win than when it only files a brief. In addition, the Court may *invite* the solicitor general to present the government's position in a case in which the office has not already done so; although such an invitation might suggest that the justices are unsure of the result they should reach, there is lack of support for the hypothesis that the solicitor general would win more frequently when invited to participate than when he does so on his own motion.[15]

There is little question that the Court pays close heed to the solicitor general's arguments—and even to his *not* filing a brief, to which it has given weight although not "dispositive" weight.[16] The solicitor general is far more successful than private litigants in getting the Court to accept the government's petitions for certiorari, doing so at a rate of roughly 70 *percent*; as an *amicus* in support of others' certiorari petitions, the solicitor general is even *more* successful in getting the Court to take cases. [17] When the government is in the Court, either as a party or as an *amicus*, the solicitor general's won-lost record has also been extremely impressive, with far more victories than losses. For example, in sex discrimination cases in the 1971–84 Terms of the Supreme Court, the direction of the solicitor general's brief was highly related to the direction of the Court's result: a liberal brief meant a liberal result in 90 percent of the cases, whereas a conservative brief meant a liberal result only one-third of the time. [18] When "underdogs"—not likely winners in the Burger Court in any event—were supported by the solicitor general, their chance of prevailing was noticeably increased. [19]

One must be careful not to attribute too much influence to the solicitor general. Influence may instead run in the other direction, with the solicitor general responsive to the Court's wishes and policy positions and "guided by the Court's ideological predilections in carrying litigation to the Court." For example, in the 1960s solicitors general authorized appeals in only a low percentage of cases when the government's position was conservative and a much higher percentage when the government's position—like the Court's at the time—was liberal. With changes in the Court's orientation and with the administration and the new Court majority sharing an ideological orientation, as the Reagan administration and the Burger Court did, one would have expected comparable interaction. However, some have suggested that in the Reagan administration the solicitor general's office became increasingly politicized, presenting to the Court positions that reflect directly the administration's conservative ideology without sufficient regard to the Court's position or to more narrowly technical legal considerations. [20] When the office abandons the previous administration's position in controversial cases that are not yet resolved, the charge of partisanship is most likely and the justices are also likely to be unhappy with the change in position.

Solicitor General Charles Fried denied the politicization of the office, but others familiar with it continued to make the allegation, which is also supposed to explain the departure of Rex Lee, Fried's predecessor. Lee, although conservative, may not have adopted explicitly conservative positions readily enough for the president's very conservative supporters, who thought Lee was doing too much to win cases—and thus maintain the office's stature in the Court's eyes—rather than pressing a political agenda. For example, Lee was criticized for not asking the Court to overturn its school prayer ruling when he did argue for a moment of silent prayer in schools. Fried, on the other hand, did ask that the Court's 1973 abortion ruling be overturned and also continued to press the administration's position that there could be no racial preferential hiring and promotion except for specific victims of discrimination, even after all the courts of appeals that considered the position rejected it. His position that voting rights improvements indicated a lack of discrimination against North Carolina blacks prompted a counterbrief from Senate Majority Leader Robert Dole (R-Kansas). (The administration's position lost.) More important, it has been suggested that the change in the solicitor general's posture "has begun to translate into a lack of willingness on the part of the Court to defer to the solicitor general's expertise," because if the solicitor general takes obviously "political" (or "partisan") positions in some cases, the justices cannot be sure the office is not doing so in others.[21] However, Solicitor General Fried did *not* ask the Court to overturn the *Miranda* ruling on interrogations despite Attorney General Meese's attack on that ruling, perhaps both because even the conservative members of the Court seemed to have accepted it and because of Fried's losses when he did directly challenge precedents.

Private Lawyers, Interest Groups, and Litigation

Private Attorneys

Private attorneys, particularly those associated with interest groups, are also crucial to the federal judicial system's operation. Lawyers who bring cases to the Supreme Court have become associated with those cases in several ways. For example, lawyers in Warren Court reapportionment and loyalty-security cases got involved through friendship with potential litigants, while those in civil rights cases had group affiliations.[22] Lawyers also enter cases at various stages of litigation. Despite the importance for appeals of the way issues are raised and presented in the district court and the way the record is shaped there, not all lawyers are in a case "from the beginning." Over 85 percent of those who argued reapportionment and loyalty-security cases in the Supreme Court in the late 1950s and early 1960s were involved from the initial trial onward. By contrast, less than two-thirds of those who argued civil rights cases were involved in the initial trial; the remainder did not become involved until the Supreme Court stage. In criminal justice cases, where most attorneys became involved through court appointment, slightly over two-fifths were involved at the initial trial, another one-third-plus appeared in the case at the first appeal, and the remainder were first involved at the Supreme Court level. Lawyers handling federal criminal appeals are now quite likely to enter cases at the appellate level because the Criminal Justice Act of 1964 provides appointed appellate counsel for those who cannot afford to retain their own attorney. However, lawyers who set out to establish particular doctrinal positions—as by bringing a case in a purposeful challenge to a statute or regulation (a *test case*)—are more and more likely to be involved from the beginning of the case.

Certain lawyers appear much more frequently in the Supreme Court than do others. The "Supreme Court bar" of the Court's early days has dispersed, in part because of the ease of getting to Washington, D.C., to argue a case—a temptation few seem to be able to resist. However, those from the solicitor general's office or representing some major civil rights groups, who appear before the Court regularly, possess experience that serves them well when they argue a case. Because that experience was thought to be lacking among lawyers for state and local governments, a State and Local Legal Center was established in 1983 by the National League of Cities and the Council of State Governments to file briefs and to assist those doing so or arguing before the Court, so that they can make a better presentation. The Justice Department has assisted in this effort by loaning a senior attorney to the National Association of Attorneys General to provide comparable assistance. [23]

It is important to recognize that not all those who have achieved major Supreme Court victories establishing important precedent set out to do so. Attorneys in the major Warren Court criminal procedure cases were often simply trying to win cases for their clients. In that effort, they argued constitutional questions along with everything else they could find to present, thus giving the Court its opportunity to establish the broad rules it announced. By comparison, attorneys who argued sit-in, reapportionment, and loyalty oath cases were far more likely to have had more in mind than to win the case for their client; they were interested in broader goals.

Lawyers do not have identical orientations to the law; those orientations affect their choice of cases and appeals as well as the shape of those cases and appeals. Some lawyers act as the client's agent (or "hired gun") and use the law basically to resolve conflicts. Others, whose view of the social good or public interest may play a greater role in determining the course of litigation, see law and clients' cases more as means for bringing about social change. Lawyers in corporate practice are more likely to be in the former group; those in other types of practice—such as criminal, environmental, consumer, labor and civil rights law, and women attorneys more than men attorneys—are more likely to adhere to the latter view. [24]

The Supreme Court itself helped stimulate an increase in the number of lawyers with a "welfarist" orientation. The Court's ruling in *Gideon v. Wainwright* requiring appointment of counsel for indigents in serious criminal trials, followed and reinforced by establishment of the "War on Poverty" Legal Services Program with its emphasis on "law reform" instead of individual "band-aid" law, helped produce lawyers broadly interested in the problems of the poor. Such lawyers were more likely than others to initiate broad legal challenges, as in the area of welfare policy. Their action reinforced the Warren Court's reach toward broad rules, which in turn further encouraged the lawyers.

Lawyers' differing orientations affect not only the types of cases in which they become involved but also the factors they consider in deciding whether or not to appeal and the relative weights they give those factors. One set of federal appellate lawyers studied generally agreed that the chance of success is quite important, and the timing of a case, an organization's concern, and advice by other attorneys are unimportant factors, but "social welfarists" were more likely than "entrepreneurials" to give the chance of winning greatest weight in deciding whether or not to take a case to the court of appeals, and the "entrepreneurials" gave far less weight to "importance to society" than did the "social welfarists." A greater overall interest in obtaining a forum from which to make issues known led the latter to be more willing to file a petition for certiorari in the Supreme Court when the possibilities of its being granted were low. Women appellate attorneys appeared to want higher "odds" of winning than did the men before they would file a certiorari petition. They were also less likely than men to cite financial reasons, including a client's ability to pay, for appealing and placed more emphasis on strategic concerns than did men.

Interest Groups

Cases are usually brought in the name of individuals. However, in a large proportion of cases, particularly in "public law" cases involving challenges to government actions and in cases brought under new statutes protecting individuals' rights, *interest groups* are associated with the cases in some way. Although many interest groups become involved in the judicial process only infrequently and peripherally, some have become "repeat players," large-volume litigators able to obtain advantages in the choice of courts in which to bring cases, the choice of cases to pursue, and the pace at which they move cases. [25] Interest group participation in the judicial system, although occurring in forms specific to the legal system, serves to reinforce the political character of the judicial process.

The norm is that interest groups should not lobby judges the way they lobby members of Congress or administrative officials; thus direct contact with judges is generally avoided. However, there are occasional violations of the norm. The noted Washington lobbyist Thomas ("Tommy the Cork") Corcoran approached both Justice Black and Justice Brennan on behalf of oil interests in connection with the *El Paso Natural Gas Co.* case. His efforts to discuss the case were firmly and promptly rejected, but nonetheless caused a problem because of concerns that a justice who had been approached should withdraw from the case. [26] The norm also does not prevent many people from writing letters—often critical of particular cases—to the justices. Justice Blackmun, author of the Court's opinion in the 1973 abortion cases, is estimated to have received over 45,000 letters in the 10 years after the decision, most of them unfavorable, with many more since then.

Interest groups involved in litigation include both the "aggressive litigant . . . seeking innovative interpretations of the Constitution" and the "defensive litigant" whose strategy is to convince judges "that prevailing constitutional norms, already favorable to his interests, should be applied." [27] At times, defensive litigants have been at a disadvantage before the Supreme Court. Although effective in invoking precedent and custom before local judges who share their views, at times they have not been prepared to deal effectively with the different—and more nationally oriented—values invoked in the Supreme Court by aggressive litigants seeking social change. An example is provided by the effort to overturn racially restrictive covenants used to prevent the sale of housing to blacks. Defensive litigants were successful in enforcing the covenants in state courts; however, they failed in the Supreme Court (in *Shelley v. Kraemer*, 1948), in part because they were not prepared to defend their position in terms of nationally accepted values and lacked as well an appropriate organizational network for defending their position.[28] The same may be said of those southern attorneys general defending school segregation against the NAACP's attack in *Brown v. Board of Education* and related cases.[29] If "defensive litigants" in those situations are conservatives, now the reverse is true: those defending Warren Court rulings, particularly in the area of criminal procedure, find themselves "defensive litigants" rather than "aggressive" ones.

Beginning with the Warren Court era, many interest groups seeking to produce social change for less advantaged members of society such as racial minorities, women, and the handicapped, or seeking to advance new causes such as environmental protection, played an increasing role in litigation.[30] Labor unions have also long used the courts in pursuit of their goals. However, such groups have no monopoly on interest group participation in the judicial process. A number of groups pursue conservative goals through litigation.[31] For example, Citizens for Decency through Law seeks to limit obscenity; Americans for Effective Law Enforcement attempts to strengthen the hand of police and prosecutor; and the National Right to Work Legal Defense Fund is engaged in limiting unions' authority. Also increasingly involved in litigation have been conservative public interest law firms, including a set of regional units created by the National Legal Center for the Public Interest; these include the Mountain States Legal Foundation, from which James Watt came to the Reagan administration to be Secretary of the Interior. There are also some unaffiliated conservative public interest law firms like the Capital Legal Foundation, which supported General Westmoreland's libel suit against CBS. These are modern-day versions of the dominant social interests favoring the status quo—such as business groups and trade associations—that have long used the legal system to achieve their goals, not only to resolve disputes but also to create rules for their future advantage. In the late nineteenth and early twentieth centuries, they used the courts to attack laws they couldn't defeat in the legislatures, and they were behind the attacks on New Deal legislation during the 1930s, speaking, for example, through the National Lawyers Committee of the American Liberty League.

There has been a noticeable increase in Supreme Court participation by better prepared conservative interest groups starting with the first term of the Burger Court. During the 1969–80 Terms, either a liberal or a conservative interest group or both participated in half the cases decided by the Court. Liberal interest groups were participants, either as direct sponsors of litigation or as *amicus*, in two-fifths of the cases; conservative groups participated at one-half that rate. Thus, although participation by liberal groups predominated, participation by conservative groups was far from insignificant. Moreover, conservative participation increased during the period, although it was more likely to take the form of *amicus* participation than did that of liberal groups. The conservative groups were more likely to be found in cases involving economic regulation, while liberal groups were still more likely to be found in civil liberties cases.[32] It is interesting to note that, despite liberal groups' decreasing win rate in the Supreme Court, "underdogs" *increased* rather than decreased their use of *amicus* participation during the Burger Court, continuing the increases seen during the Warren Court. Where "upperdog" *amicus* filings had far outnumbered "underdog" filings in the Warren Court, with "underdogs" showing a much more rapid increase than "upperdogs," the figures were almost even in the Burger Court.[33]

Types of Participation. Interest group participation is of several different types. Lawyers may be interest group "cooperating attorneys" receiving help in preparing briefs and assistance with expenses; a group may provide the total financing for a case; or a group may provide its own staff lawyers to try a case. Some groups have assisted with the expenses of a trial or an appeal. At times umbrella groups may be established to assist in raising funds, as was done with causes célèbres like the Chicago Seven, Harrisburg, and Wounded Knee trials of the 1960s and early 1970s. Other groups become involved only as *amicus curiae* at the appellate level—an effective way for a group to be involved in precedent-making cases while shepherding scarce resources, although conservative public interest law firms have regularly used the *amicus* device even when they had adequate financing to be more directly involved: they seemed primarily concerned to have the conservative perspective brought before the court so that the liberal view would not be the only one presented.

"Friends of the court" may at first have been thought to serve the court as neutral participants rather than to favor the parties. However, groups usually become involved in a case as *amicus* because they wish to present a position favorable to one side in a case, although they may do so at the stage at which the Court is considering whether to grant review, by arguing either for or against granting review.

Over time, there has been a shift in *amicus* participation from neutrality, actually being a friend of the *court*, to advocacy, being a friend of one of the *parties*.[34] They do not, however, necessarily repeat the principal parties' basic arguments and often either adopt a different perspective or argue positions the principal litigants do not wish to emphasize. Particularly when an *amicus curiae*'s approach to a case differs from the parties' approach, the *amicus*'s role can be quite significant, providing reinforcement for the justices' opinions or even alerting the justices to the importance of certain issues. This may result in a case being considerably transformed in the Supreme Court from what was presented in the lower courts. For example, in *Mapp v. Ohio* (1961) the argument by the parties to the case centered on the issue of convicting someone for "mere possession" of obscene material (that is, without intent to sell) and on the "shocking" nature of the search that led to discovery of the material, but the defendant's attorney had not urged a change in the rule that improperly seized evidence could be used in the trial. The exclusionary issue was raised in the *amicus* brief filed by the American Civil Liberties Union and the Ohio Civil Liberties Union, but it was not central even to their argument.[35] The Supreme Court, clearly eager to reverse its position on the admissibility of improperly seized evidence, reached out to make the admissibility question the central one of the case, and, without reaching the obscenity issue raised by the parties, handed down a landmark ruling excluding illegally seized evidence from state trials.

Amicus participation, particularly before the Supreme Court—it occurs far less in the lower appellate courts—increased substantially starting in the 1960s and was quite likely to be found in civil liberties and civil rights cases, although less so in criminal appeals.[36] The Court has been generous in granting requests to file *amicus* briefs when one or the other of the parties has refused to grant participation, with the Court's "grant" rate running around 85 percent.[37]

Despite the potential importance of *amicus* participation and particularly its symbolic significance for a group wishing to record its position in important litigation, interest groups increasingly have felt that more direct involvement in cases is necessary and that it is best to provide an attorney from the beginning of a case. Groups such as the American Civil Liberties Union, which tended to focus earlier efforts on appellate *amicus* work, now frequently participate in cases from the beginning and often will not become involved in a case unless they can do so. This gives the group a greater opportunity to control the case by shaping the trial record, instead of having to work on appeal with a record created by lawyers for whom the group's interests may not have been central. Control allows a group to concentrate on issues of particular concern and permits it to file multiple cases raising the same or closely related issues in different courts, in turn increasing the likelihood of having a "good" case available for appeal.

From time to time, groups bring lawsuits in their own name. They do so not only to protect their own members, as the NAACP did in protecting against demands for membership lists, but also to assert the group's basic interests. The latter type of involvement is quite likely to be found in environmental litigation, with cases being brought by groups such as the Sierra Club, the Wilderness Society, and the Natural Resources Defense Council. However, in other areas of litigation, interest groups, instead of waiting for potential litigants to come to the group seeking assistance, may seek out litigants who have a case raising issues important to the group and who have a "case or controversy," thus satisfying requirements for access to the courts (see Chapter 5). In such cases, despite the use of the names of individual plaintiffs, the group, not the individual, is bringing the case.

Resources.[38] Resources are a major problem for many litigating interest groups, both conservative—although they have larger financial backing on which to draw—and liberal. The cost of major litigation, particularly when groups are involved from the beginning, is so large that no group can do all that it wants, and must pass up some cases in favor of others. The set of cases constituting *Brown v. Board of Education*, the 1954 school desegregation ruling, cost at least $250,000 (in the preinflation dollars of that time) to bring, with much lawyer time donated. More recently, the Detroit school cases of the mid-1970s—long in the trial court, in the appeals court several times, and twice decided by the Supreme Court—cost the plaintiffs just under $4,000,000; the Dayton school cases, also involving two Supreme Court rulings, resulted in an application for fees and costs for the NAACP and retained counsel of $1,800,000.

On the basis of the frequency with which their names appear in the media, groups trying either to defend or advance the interests of minorities and the otherwise disadvantaged may seem to have adequate resources, but the actual situation is one of quite scarce resources, both absolutely and in relation to goals sought. If cases are long and complex—increasingly true for school desegregation and job discrimination suits and cases challenging conditions in mental institutions and prisons—resources must be stretched. For example, much time is needed to prove a constitutional violation in large northern school districts; additional resources are required to develop remedies; and because of the difficulty of overcoming school board and public resistance to achieve effective desegregation, litigation may have to be pursued for several years. Because there are too many lawsuits to be brought in too many different places, organizations may have to pass up cases because their attorneys are "pinned down in the trenches" somewhere else.

Resources can be stretched by enlisting the assistance of government agencies, at least when those agencies share group goals. Groups may shepherd scarce resources by transmitting individual complaints to those government agencies that have complaint-processing machinery. Indeed, agencies or factions within an agency may not object to being prodded by interest groups to use their resources in a particular way. Such actions serve to bring government pressure on those the interest group would otherwise pursue directly.

Interest groups' in-house legal staffs are not large—perhaps 20 lawyers in most significant liberal groups, and actually much smaller in the conservative public interest law firms. Attorney resources are, however, made considerably greater through use of *cooperating attorneys*. These are lawyers otherwise in private practice who handle cases for the interest group either *pro bono* (for free: *pro bono publico* means "for the public good") or for a fee or honorarium considerably less than their regular hourly rate; the interest group often also assists with expenses. Cooperating attorneys have their own law practices to attend to, and thus often cannot handle long and complex cases, leading to use of staff attorneys. Because cooperating attorneys' priorities may not be identical with the group's, delegating responsibility to them may cause problems and reliance on them leads to organizational decentralization. At times, local attorneys are used for cases in state courts, where they are more familiar with the rules, and national staff attorneys handle federal litigation and any Supreme Court cases. At other times, the relationship is sequential: local attorneys take matters through the lower courts and then "hand them off" to national staff attorneys for appeals.

Such an arrangement may be necessary when a local lawyer does not seek an interest group's assistance until after the trial, requiring the group's staff attorney to begin the group's work with whatever the local attorney has accomplished—or failed to accomplish.

Interest group resources have been increased recently through court awards of attorneys' fees. When a group has supplied an attorney for a lawsuit, has prevailed, and has obtained an award of attorneys' fees, those fees can be plowed back into the organization to finance other litigation. The basic *American rule* has been that the winning party in a lawsuit is *not* entitled to attorneys' fees as part of the costs awarded at the end of the trial. However, the idea that individuals or groups serve as *private attorneys general* to enforce existing laws or constitutional rights—and thus are entitled to attorneys' fees—has been embodied in some statutes, such as the Civil Rights Act of 1964. In 1975, the Supreme Court ruled in the *Alyeska Pipeline* environmental litigation that, because Congress had not specifically provided for them in that type of case, attorneys' fees could not be awarded in cases where the public is said to benefit from pursuit of the lawsuit but where no single individual or small set of individuals may have suffered substantial economic injury. Congress then included attorneys' fees provisions in several substantive statutes and, more important, passed the Civil Rights Attorneys Fees Act allowing the prevailing party in civil rights cases to recover attorneys' fees and the Access to Justice Act allowing recovery of fees from the federal government.[39] The Supreme Court has decided a number of cases dealing with what attorneys' fees are appropriate, and covering such questions as what constituted the "prevailing party" entitled to recover such fees and on what claims recovery could occur (those on which the client prevailed plus others sufficiently intertwined), the basic method of calculating fees (the "lodestar" of hours reasonably expended, multiplied by reasonable hourly rates), and whether the fees could exceed the underlying damages award (the Court said it could).[40]

Because resources are scarce, interest groups' decisions concerning allocation of whatever resources exist are difficult. These include not only decisions about legal issues on which to concentrate but broader decisions about the relative weight to give to litigation, lobbying the legislature and administrative agencies, and developing public opinion. Such resource-allocation decisions are affected by the relative complexity and length of the contemplated lawsuits as well as by availability of cooperating attorneys to try them. Both attorney preferences for certain types of cases and membership concerns may lead to placing new topics on a group's litigation agenda. An example of the effect of membership concerns is civil rights groups' addition of criminal justice issues (police brutality, discrimination in jury selection, and application of the death penalty) to their earlier priorities of education, jobs, and housing.

Strategy.[41] To talk of choices to be made in allocating resources may leave the impression that litigating interest groups have a well-developed litigation strategy. If we define strategy broadly as "overall plans, coordination and direction developed for a major area of litigation, general enough to allow for flexibility and adaptability to changing circumstances,"[42] that may be true in some situations. Some groups define in advance the policy positions to which they will give preference in bringing or defending lawsuits for individuals who seek their aid and may go further in orchestrating an attack on a policy, as the NAACP did with respect to racially restrictive covenants on housing. Yet one of two cases decided by the Supreme Court on this issue was not an "NAACP case" but had been filed by another lawyer. As this indicates, groups are often propelled into a case before a strategy is developed. This also occurred with the sit-in cases, where no strategy existed because lawyers for the "Inc. Fund" (the NAACP Legal Defense and Educational Fund) initially had no idea that so many cases would develop.[43]

Groups can have substantial influence over some cases. Some cases are brought at the trial level with the intent to appeal them to the Supreme Court, but, on the other hand, some are initiated simply to obtain a trial court order and not as a part of a "grand plan." Groups that appear to have a strategy may simply be responding idiosyncratically to cases brought to them or engaging in "an ad hoc search for targets of opportunity."[44] Some groups conducting much litigation remain largely reactive. This was true of the American Civil Liberties Union until relatively recently, when it developed several special litigation projects, such as the rights of women, prisoners, and the mentally ill. Even when a group has a general blueprint, the often unpredictable course of litigation is as influential as any such blueprint. Much litigation, including some cases appealed to the Supreme Court, remains beyond the group's complete control. (This is true also for government agency attorneys trying to bring test cases; like interest groups, those agencies vary in their litigation strategies, and tend to reflect the style of their general counsel.[45])

Why is the existence of interest group strategy in the broad sense problematic? One reason is that groups have a variety of goals they wish to achieve. Some seek to achieve certain outcomes. These might be greater rights for women or minorities, the invalidation of restrictive economic regulations, district judges' detailed rulings on remedies to change public institutions like prisons, or Supreme Court rulings on constitutional principles. Others undertake litigation to achieve leverage for legislation and administrative regulations they want adopted or altered, as Common Cause did in its campaign for election finance laws.

Some interest group litigation goals are short-term because victories are necessary in the short run if the groups are to continue to obtain resources. Thus certain actions must be undertaken for publicity purposes, to show supporters that the organization is alive and well, and to reinforce the group's ideological position. (*Amicus* participation may help in this respect, particularly if the group is short of resources for other types of litigation participation.[46]) Yet attention to short-term concerns may tie up precious resources needed for the longer term and may interfere with development of strategy aimed at achieving long-run goals, which perhaps can be achieved only by a series of cases, each building incrementally on the next but none of them particularly glamorous.

Control of cases is central to group strategy. A resultant question is whether client or group controls a case, particularly when an interest group supplies counsel and when it seeks out litigants. Because resources are scarce, a group is not likely to get involved in a case unless its own interests can be advanced. However, the ethics of the legal profession require that an attorney act in the interest of the client. If the client shares the group's interests, there is no problem, but when interests are not identical, the lawyer may define the client's interests in terms of group interests rather than vice versa. For example, when the client is offered a settlement in a case that might "make new law" if the case were to proceed to trial, the lawyer might be tempted to recommend against acceptance of the settlement instead of "sacrificing" the group's investment in seeking new legal principle. Most groups say that the case is indeed the client's, not the group's, but instances can be found that indicate that the group has settled for a symbolic victory rather than more concrete rewards for the client or that the group has emphasized precedent-setting cases at the expense of actions to enforce the rights won in such cases.[47]

Indeed, groups like the NAACP and ACLU have been accused of *barratry,* more commonly known as ambulance-chasing. This is the stirring up of litigation in which the instigator has no direct interest, usually for a share of the proceeds. The Supreme Court has made clear that a group, as part of its members' right of association, may help protect their constitutional rights through litigation. That groups such as the NAACP and ACLU have not profited financially from the litigation has undoubtedly been a factor in such rulings.[48]

Certain elements of interest group litigation *are* likely to increase separation of client interest from group concerns. Attorneys serving on the staffs of national organizations often have backgrounds and political ideologies different from those of the membership of the groups for which they are working. In addition, professionals such as lawyers often dominate laypersons such as clients. In interest groups such lawyer dominance, which tends to extend beyond the details of litigation to the general setting of policy, is quite likely if the group has a successful litigation record. There is often considerable geographical distance between an organization's staff attorneys (working at headquarters, usually New York City or Washington, D.C.) and the communities in which the group's members/clients are found, and there is often little if any personal contact between the staff attorneys and the clients, with local counsel handling the face-to-face interaction with the client. Contact between lawyer and client is further diminished by use of lawsuits on behalf of large classes of people. Although an organization has to use such *class action suits*—brought in the name of one or more specific plaintiffs on behalf of all those "similarly situated" legally—to stretch scarce resources, those within the plaintiff class who disagree with the dominant class view are quite likely to be submerged.[49]

Environment. Strategy to achieve groups' multiple goals is affected by the environment in which groups must act. In the early 1970s and the 1980s, changes in public opinion, coupled with corollary changes in congressional mood and particularly in the executive branch's posture, produced an atmosphere far less favorable to civil rights interest groups and more favorable to conservative groups than had existed in the 1960s.

Included in a group's environment are not only legislative or administrative receptivity to the group but also existing statutes and regulations. Because, until the mid-1960s, groups representing the politically disfavored were unable to achieve legislation necessary to protect their rights, they regularly turned to the courts; thus, for many years national civil liberties and civil rights policy was made almost entirely in the courts. The passage of the Civil Rights Act of 1964 and the Voting Rights Act of 1965 altered the political environment by requiring group attention not only to maintenance of existing judicial precedent but also to implementation of the statutes through regulations and follow-up litigation.

Supreme Court decisions on both procedural and substantive issues have definitely affected the course of interest group litigation. An example of the effect of procedural rulings is the obstacle that a decision on who may bring lawsuits asserting the rights of disadvantaged individuals (see page 172) posed for attacks on exclusionary zoning by suburbs. However, that ruling did nudge groups toward greater use of state courts, where they received favorable rulings in some states.[50] The Court's decisions on substantive issues also have affected interest groups' litigation strategy, as when NAACP lawyers' efforts received a substantial boost from a ruling that facilitated a new attack on whites-only primary elections.[51] Similarly, the NAACP's shift toward a more direct attack on "separate but equal" facilities came after the Supreme Court ordered desegregation of law schools on the basis of intangible factors, in *Sweatt v. Painter* (1950).

Interest groups turn to the courts not only because they are unable to achieve their goals elsewhere but also because of the *myth of rights*, the idea that litigation can produce statements of rights as well as their implementation.[52] Their belief in this myth is one reason why lawyers return again and again to court even when rights "won" there are not implemented and even when courts like the Supreme Court seem to be less receptive to lawyers' claims.

When they do go to court, the question is which court—state or federal. The answer has varied over time and has depended in large measure on where interest groups believe the judges will be more favorable to their position. In the nineteenth century, business turned to the federal courts for protection while state regulators used state courts. At least since the Warren Court's favorable consideration of civil rights and civil liberties claims, interest groups seeking protection for civil rights have gravitated particularly to the federal courts. One reason why a national interest group might prefer federal over state courts—apart from the question of which provided more favorable rulings—is that federal court litigation is "the surest and fastest route to the Supreme Court" for those seeking constitutional precedent.[53] An organizational factor is that litigating in federal court provides a single legal framework (the federal rules of procedure) that allows staff attorneys to bring cases anywhere in the nation and to coordinate local attorneys' work more effectively. The complexities of the multiplicity of state procedural and substantive legal provisions, which would force staff attorneys to devote scarce time to their mastery, are thus avoided.[54] There are, however, some who argue that the perceived lack of "parity" between federal and state courts in their handling of civil liberties cases is not real, and that courts in at least some states support civil liberties and civil rights claims at least as favorably as the federal courts.[55] Certainly the Burger Court's lessened support for civil liberties claims, as reflected in lower court rulings carrying out the new Supreme Court precedents, might lead an attorney to believe that civil liberties claims stood a greater chance of success in state courts, particularly those using their own constitutions as the basis for decision.

Organizational Factors. Other important intra- and interorganizational factors affect litigation strategy and make the existence and course of planned litigation problematic. One factor is a group's *organizational structure*, such as whether it is membership based, with official policy established by representatives at an annual convention, or is limited to a collection of attorneys and an advisory board and is funded by contributions and foundation grants. There has been an increasing number of the latter, generally referred to as *public interest law firms*, which exist to serve not only liberal causes, such as the National Resources Defense Council or the Mexican-American Legal Defense Fund (MALDEF), but also the conservative ones mentioned earlier.

A group's *longevity* and continuity allow it more strategic flexibility because a group that has been around for some time and is in no danger of collapse can wait out bad times more easily, adjusting the pace of its litigation to changing judicial doctrine. Thus longevity affects a group's ability to control litigation. Longevity can, however, lead to inertia, in which a group continues down tried-and-true paths, unable to adapt to changes in judicial doctrine or political environment. Group inertia or momentum can be reinforced by opponents' resistance to earlier judicial victories and is particularly likely to result from success in the courts: lawyers may feel that "after all, if we've been successful there, we will continue to be." Victorious litigants certainly do not wish to give up, or to be seen as giving up, what they had pressed hard to achieve. Moreover, a group that has developed expertise in presenting cases in court will want to continue to utilize, rather than dissipate, that expertise.

The existence of and *relations with other organizations*, including business groups providing financing (in the case of conservative public interest law firms), are an important part of an interest group's political environment and affect a group's litigation activities. The number of groups litigating in a particular area of the law—thus competing for resources—is part of the interorganizational situation. For example, for a long time the NAACP Legal Defense and Educational Fund (LDF), closely allied with the NAACP, was the dominant if not the sole civil rights litigator, thus having substantial control over litigation when it engaged in planned strategy. Now the NAACP and LDF are separate (indeed, feuding) and there are many, many civil rights litigating units: public interest law firms; private law firms that provide regular fee-for-service lawyering to private clients and also engage in public interest law practice; other private law firms closely affiliated with particular interest groups; individual private attorneys who bring cases, such as employment discrimination cases under Title VII of the 1964 Civil Rights Act, from which they can receive attorneys' fees if they win; and "back-up centers," created through the Legal Services Program, that assist with litigation. A growing "rights consciousness" has also produced more causes—including women, the poor, and the handicapped—for which litigating capacity has developed. The large number of groups in any one of these areas, such as the large number of women's groups, has caused problems of coordinating litigation.

Proliferation of litigating units had led to a loss of control by any single litigator and decreased ability to pursue a concerted strategy. Also important is the presence of groups that, as an ideological matter, do not use litigation and may disdain it. In the 1960s, for example, new civil rights groups, whose style was far more activist and confrontational, felt that the NAACP had not accomplished enough through the courts. The activities of groups such as the Congress of Racial Equality (CORE) and the Southern Christian Leadership Conference (SCLC, the Rev. Martin Luther King, Jr.'s group), caused older groups to shift priorities and resources as well as to pay more attention to membership concerns.

In addition to competition and conflict between groups seeking goals in any policy area, there is considerable cooperation. At times lawyers whose organizations are formally "at war" work together toward common goals—true in the small and cohesive "civil rights bar," in which a convergence of perspectives has developed. At times groups work together explicitly, primarily through exchange of information, which is quite important for control of cases as well as for efficient allocation of resources. Representatives of litigating groups also meet to exchange ideas or even to work out strategy; the three primary plaintiffs' interest group litigants in the church-state area (the American Jewish Congress, American Civil Liberties Union, and Americans United [for Separation of Church and State]) have worked together in this way.[56] On the conservative side, the Heritage Foundation has held monthly luncheons attended by representatives of most conservative litigators. Some groups go even further, perhaps providing auxiliary legal services for other interest groups.[57] Much cooperation is, however, implicit rather than overt. Through awareness of what other groups are doing, groups maintain at least somewhat differentiated central thrusts in which some concentrate on some types of cases while others focus their efforts on other areas. At times, such "comparative advantage" leads to the explicit cross-referral of cases from one organization to another better fitted for the particular task.

Notes

1. Charles M. Lamb, "Judicial Policy-Making and Information Flow to the Supreme Court," *Vanderbilt Law Review* 29 (January 1976): 46–124.

2. On selection of U.S. Attorneys, see James Eisenstein, *Counsel for the United States: U.S. Attorneys in the Political and Legal Systems* (Baltimore: Johns Hopkins University Press, 1978), pp. 35–47. The following paragraphs also draw on Eisenstein's study.

3. Ibid., p. 16.

4. Ibid., p. 156. See also Robert L. Rabin, "Agency Criminal Referrals in the Federal System: An Empirical Study of Prosecutorial Discretion," *Stanford Law Review* 24 (June 1972): 1036–91.

5. See Peter Irons, *Justice at War* (New York: Oxford University Press, 1983), for a story about conflict between DOJ and the War Department.

6. Peter H. Irons, *The New Deal Lawyers* (Princeton, N.J.: Princeton University Press, 1982), pp. 40–41.

7. Ibid., p. 11.

8. See Susan M. Olson, "Comparing Justice and Labor Department Lawyers: Ten Years of Occupational Safety and Health Litigation," *Law & Policy Quarterly* 7 (July 1985): 295, and Olson, "Challenges to the Gatekeeper: The Debate Over Federal Litigating Authority," *Judicature* 68 (August–September 1984): 71–86.

9. Olson, "Comparing Justice and Labor Department Lawyers," p. 290.

10. David O. Stewart, "The President's Lawyer," *ABA Journal* 72 (April 1, 1986): 58–61.

11. Bernard Schwartz, *Super Chief: Earl Warren and His Supreme Court—A Judicial Biography* (New York: Oxford University Press, 1983), p. 248.

12. *DeMarco v. United States*, 415 U.S. 449 (1974).

13. See *Watts v. United States*, 422 U.S. 1032 at 1035–36 (1975) (Chief Justice Burger and Justices White and Rehnquist, dissenting); and *Rinaldi v. United States*, 434 U.S. 22 (1977) (Rehnquist and White).

14. See Robert Scigliano, *The Supreme Court and the Presidency*, pp. 167–68. See also Samuel Krislov, "The Role of the Attorney General as Amicus Curiae," in Luther Huston et al., *Roles of the Attorney General of the United States* (Washington, D.C.: American Enterprise Institute, 1968), pp. 71–104. For a description of the process leading to the Solicitor General's decisions to file or not file amicus briefs in the *DeFunis* and *Bakke* affirmative action cases, see Timothy J. O'Neill, *Bakke & The Politics of Equality: Friends & Foes in the Classroom of Litigation* (Middletown, Conn.: Wesleyan University Press, 1985), pp. 179–91.

15. S. Sidney Ulmer and David Willison, "The Solicitor General of the United States as Amicus Curiae in the U.S. Supreme Court, 1969–1983 Terms," paper presented to American Political Science Association, 1985.

16. See *Container Corporation of America v. Franchise Tax Board*, 463 U.S. 159 at 196 and n. 33 (1983).

17. Scigliano, *The Supreme Court and the Presidency*, p. 176.

18. See Jeffrey A. Segal and Cheryl D. Reedy, "The Supreme Court and Equal Protection: The Role of the Solicitor General," paper presented to American Political Science Association, 1975, p. 11.

19. Ulmer and Willison, "The Solicitor General of the United States," p. 19.

20. Scigliano, *The Supreme Court and the Presidency*, pp. 191–93, for the earlier period; for a comparison of the actions of three solicitors general, see Karen O'Connor, "The Amicus Curiae Role of the United States Solicitor General in Supreme Court Litigation," *Judicature* 66 (December–January 1983): 256–64; and for the Reagan administration, see Lincoln Caplan, "The Tenth Justice," *New Yorker*, April 10, 1987, pp. 29-58, and April 17, 1987, pp. 30-62.

21. Ulmer and Willison, "The Solicitor General of the United States," pp. 16–17.

22. Jonathan Casper, *Lawyers Before the Warren Court: Civil Liberties and Civil Rights, 1957–1966* (Urbana: University of Illinois Press, 1972), tables 4 and 5, pp. 88–89.

23. See Douglas Ross, "Safeguarding Our Federalism: Lessons for the States from the Supreme Court," *Public Administration Review* 45 (Special 1985): 723–31. For recent examination of states' appearance as amicus in the Supreme Court and their relative success, see Thomas R. Morris, "States Before the U.S. Supreme Court: State Attorneys General as *Amicus Curiae*," *Judicature* 70 (February–March 1987): 298–305, and Lee Epstein and Karen O'Connor, "States Before the U.S. Supreme Court: Direct Representation in Cases Involving Criminal Rights, 1969–1984," *Ibid.*: 305–6.

24. Gregory J. Rathjen, "Lawyers and the Appeals Process: An Analysis of the Appellate Lawyer's Beliefs, Attitudes and Values," paper presented to Midwest Political Science Association, 1975; Rathjen, "Lawyers and the Appeals Process: A Profile," *Federal Bar Journal* 34 (Winter 1975): 21–41; Susan Ann Kay, "Sex Differences in the Attitudes of a Future Elite," *Women & Politics* 1 (Fall 1980): 35–48.

25. See Marc Galanter, "Why the 'Haves' Come Out Ahead: Speculations on the Limits of Legal Change," *Law & Society Review* 9 (Fall 1974): 95–160.

26. See Robert Woodward and Scott Armstrong, *The Brethren*, pp. 79–84.

27. Richard C. Cortner, "Strategies and Tactics of Litigants in Constitutional Cases," *Journal of Public Law* 17 (1968): 288.

28. See Clement Vose, *Caucasians Only* (Berkeley: University of California Press, 1959).

29. For the story, see Richard Kluger, *Simple Justice: The History of Brown v. Board of Education and Black America's Struggle for Equality* (New York: Alfred Knopf, 1976).

30. For stories and studies of the work of these groups, see Michael Meltsner, *Cruel and Unusual: The Supreme Court and Capital Punishment* (New York: Oxford University Press, 1973) and Robert Belton, "A Comparative Review of Public and Private Enforcement of Title VII of the Civil Rights Act of 1964," *Vanderbilt Law Review* 31 (May 1978): 905–61, on the work of the NAACP Legal Defense and Educational Fund; Robert Rabin, "Lawyers for Social Change: Perspectives on Public Interest Law," *Stanford Law Review* 28 (January 1976): 207–61, on the NAACP Legal Defense Fund and the American Civil Liberties Union; Frank J. Sorauf, *The Wall of Separation: The Constitutional Politics of Church and State* (Princeton, N.J.: Princeton University Press, 1976); Karen O'Connor, *Women's Organizations' Use of the Courts* (Lexington, Mass.: Lexington Books, 1980), and O'Connor and Lee Epstein, "Beyond Legislative Lobbying: Women's Rights Groups and the Supreme Court," *Judicature* 67 (September 1983): 134–43; and R. Shep Melnick, *Regulation and the Courts: The Case of the Clean Air Act* (Washington, D.C.: The Brookings Institution, 1983); and Susan M. Olson, *Clients and Lawyers: Securing the Rights of Disabled Persons* (Westport, Conn.: Greenwood Press, 1984).

31. Lee Epstein, *Conservatives in Court* (Knoxville, Tenn.: University of Tennessee Press, 1985).

32. Karen O'Connor and Lee Epstein, "The Rise of Conservative Interest Group Litigation," *Journal of Politics* 45 (May 1983): 479–89.

33. Robert C. Bradley and Paul Gardner, "Underdogs, Upperdogs and the Use of the Amicus Brief: Trends and Explanations," *Justice System Journal* 10 (Spring 1985): 78–96.

34. Samuel Krislov, "The Amicus Curiae Brief: From Friendship to Advocacy," *Yale Law Journal* 72 (March 1963): 694–721.

35. Lynn Mather and Barbara Yngvesson, "Language, Audience, and the Transformation of Disputes," *Law & Society Review* 15 (1980–1981): 802–5, and Fred W. Friendly and Martha J. W. Elliott, *The Constitution: That Delicate Balance* (New York: Random House, 1984), pp. 138–39.

36. Karen O'Connor and Lee Epstein, "Amicus Curiae Participation in U.S. Supreme Court Litigation," *Law & Society Review* 16 (1981–1982): 311–20.

37. Bradley and Gardner, "Underdogs, Upperdogs," p. 90.

38. This material and the remainder of this section is based in part on Stephen L. Wasby, "Interest Groups in Court: Race Relations Litigation," *Interest Group Politics*, eds. Allan Cigler and Burdett Loomis (Washington, D.C.: CQ Press, 1983), pp. 251–74.

39. See Karen O'Connor and Lee Epstein, "Bridging the Gap Between Congress and the Supreme Court: Interest Groups and the Erosion of the American Rule Governing Awards of Attorneys Fees," *Western Political Quarterly* 38 (June 1985): 238–49.

40. *Hensley v. Eckerhart*, 461 U.S. 424 (1983); *City of Riverside v. Rivera*, 106 S.Ct. 2686 (1986). See also *Pennsylvania v. Delaware Valley Citizens' Council for Clean Air*, 106 S.Ct. 3088 (1986).

41. In addition to Wasby, "Interest Groups in Court: Race Relations Litigation," see also Wasby, "How Planned Is 'Planned' Litigation?" *American Bar Foundation Research Journal* 1984 (Winter): 83–138; "The Multi-Faceted Elephant: Litigator Perspectives on Planned Litigation for Social Change," *Capital University Law Review* 15 (Winter 1986): 143–89; and "Civil Rights Litigation by Organizations: Constraints and Choices," *Judicature* 68 (April–May 1985): 337–52.

42. Jeanne Hahn, "The NAACP Legal Defense and Educational Fund: Its Judicial Strategy and Tactics," in Stephen L. Wasby, *American Government and Politics* (New York: Scribner's, 1973), p. 396.

43. For an examination of interest group litigation in the field, see Edward V. Heck and Joseph Stewart, Jr., "Ensuring Access to Justice: The Role of Interest Group Lawyers in the 60's Campaign for Civil Rights," *Judicature* 66 (August 1982): 84–95, and Stewart and Heck, "The Day-to-Day Activities of Interest Group Lawyers," *Social Science Quarterly* 64 (March 1983): 173–82.

44. Stuart Scheingold, *The Politics of Rights: Lawyers, Public Policy, and Political Change* (New Haven, Conn.: Yale University Press, 1974), p. 5.

45. See Irons, *The New Deal Lawyers*, pp. 4–5. Irons portrays litigation differences between the Agricultural Adjustment Administration, the National Industrial Recovery Administration, and the National Labor Relations Board.

46. O'Connor, *Women's Organizations*, p. 117.

47. See Stephen C. Halpern, "Assessing the Litigative Role of ACLU Chapters," in *Civil Liberties: Policy and Policy Making*, ed. Stephen L. Wasby (Lexington, Mass.: Lexington Books, 1976), pp. 159–68, for a criticism of group strategy.

48. See *NAACP v. Button*, 371 U.S. 415 (1963), and *In re Primus*, 436 U.S. 412 (1978).

49. See Deborah L. Rhode, "Class Conflicts in Class Actions," *Stanford Law Review* 34 (July 1982): 1183–1261.

50. *Warth v. Seldin*, 422 U.S. 490 (1975). See Michael N. Danielson, *The Politics of Exclusion* (New York: Columbia University Press, 1976), p. 318, and Geoffrey Shields and Sanford Spector, "Opening Up the Suburbs: Notes on a Movement for Social Change," *Yale Review of Law and Social Action* 2 (Summer 1972): 310.

51. Clement E. Vose, *Constitutional Change: Amendment Politics and Supreme Court Litigation Since 1900* (Lexington, Mass.: Lexington Books, 1972), p. 321.

52. Scheingold, *The Politics of Rights*, p. 5.

53. Sorauf, *The Wall of Separation*, p. 111.

54. For the basic arguments about why civil liberties lawyers favor federal courts, see Burt Neuborne, "The Myth of Parity," *Harvard Law Review* 90 (April 1977): 1105–1131, and "Toward Procedural Parity in Constitutional Litigation," *William & Mary Law Review* 22 (Summer 1981): 725–87.

55. For one study, see Robert Solomine and James Walker, "Constitutional Litigation in Federal and State Courts: An Empirical Analysis of Judicial Parity," *Hastings Constitutional Law Quarterly* 10 (1983): 213–53.

56. Sorauf, *Wall of Separation*, p. 82. See also Vose, *Caucasians Only*, pp. 58, 151; Meltsner, *Cruel and Unusual*, pp. 114, 238–39.

57. Heck and Stewart, "Ensuring Access to Justice."

5   Getting into Court

Very few cases filed in federal or state trial courts ever get to the United States Supreme Court, even in the form of a request for review. Most cases that are filed do not proceed to trial. Many are not pursued; a great many civil cases are settled before trial; and most criminal cases, if not dismissed, end with a guilty plea. Of those cases that reach the trial stage, most never proceed further. Of the relatively small proportion taken to the first appellate level, few are pursued beyond that point. State cases that do move further are first appealed through the state court system. The great majority of state cases that the Supreme Court can hear are within its certiorari jurisdiction, allowing the Court to reject the great majority, the same disposition it gives most federal appeals.

In this chapter, we examine both the rules the Supreme Court has developed concerning access to the courts and its doctrines concerning relations between federal and state courts. The Court's requirements on access mean that not everyone can get into court to pursue certain issues; some people with complaints that they wish judges to decide may not be able to satisfy necessary procedural requirements. Others must take care to assure that the rules are satisfied; this may require that issues be shaped in a certain way or that particular plaintiffs be chosen for cases.

Access to the Courts

The formal paths along which cases move are clearly delineated (see Figures 2.1 and 5.1). However, before cases may be moved along those paths, requirements concerning who can have access to the courts and which cases can be brought to court must be satisfied. Congress creates some of these rules in statutes providing *causes of action*, the substantive legal claims that are the basis of lawsuits (see page 173), and provides certain procedural rules, such as those on how appeals should be processed. Beyond those statutory rules, the Supreme Court, through its decisions, sets many rules on access to the federal courts. If the Court is restrictive in those rulings in granting access, major claims may never reach the lower federal courts, much less the Supreme Court itself. Although the Supreme Court cannot tell state courts which cases to hear, it is not bound to accept appeals from state cases when its own access requirements have not been met. The Court has also affected access to the federal courts by developing rules intended to keep cases in the state systems. This is done in an effort to ensure that cases are given complete treatment there before being brought to the federal courts and that once the claims are in the federal court system, review of state court decisions is limited. These include decisions on which set of courts should decide issues that seem subject to decision by both federal and state judges. Among these are rules covering use of habeas corpus petitions in federal courts to challenge state convictions, federal courts' authority to issue declaratory judgments (see below) and injunctions against state laws, and removal (transfer) of cases from state to federal court—rules that affect litigants' ability to challenge the actions of state and local legislators and administrators.

Many rules concerning access to the courts revolve around the stipulation in Article III that courts deal with "cases" or "controversies," a corollary of the idea that courts are legal institutions operating with a specific set of procedures. Although at times rules on access to the courts are dismissed as "narrow technicalities," they are of broad importance and central to the courts' powers in our political system.

> The judicial power shall extend to all cases, in law and equity, arising under the Constitution, the laws of the United States, and treaties made, or which shall be made, under their authority; to all cases affecting ambassadors, other public ministers and consuls; to all cases of admiralty and maritime jurisdiction; to controversies to which the United States shall be a party; to controversies between two or more states; between a state and citizens of another state; between citizens of different states; between citizens of the same state claiming lands under grants of different states; and between a state, or the citizens thereof, and foreign states, citizens or subjects. (Art. III, Sec. 2)

Before deciding a case "on the merits," that is, before turning to substantive issues such as "Did John Jones discriminate against Sally Smith in considering her employment application?", "Did the Giant Corporation attempt to monopolize the business in its field?" or "Did the government prove that the Porn Corporation transported obscene materials in interstate commerce?" a judge must be satisfied that a number of procedural prerequisites have been met. Indeed, the outcomes of cases may be determined by procedural considerations, without the merits being reached.

The procedural prerequisites fall essentially into three interrelated categories: *jurisdiction*, a court's *authority* to hear a case; *standing*, whether the right *person* is bringing a case; and *justiciability*, whether a *case* is appropriate for judges to hear. Justiciability includes the requirements that the parties be adverse to each other and not have manufactured a case to get into court; that the court not be asked for an *advisory opinion*; that the case be both *ripe* (ready for judgment) and not *moot* (the controversy concluded); and that it not entail a *political question* (something to be decided by the other branches). Once the government has imposed restrictions on an individual, it is relatively easy to challenge them. For example, as a defense to a criminal charge, one may question the validity of the law under which the charge has been brought. Thus an individual who has been arrested or indicted by that fact often satisfies requirements to challenge laws on which that action has been based, although the Supreme Court has recently imposed restrictions on who may challenge an allegedly improper search (see page 172). As a result, controversies over access to the courts are most likely to arise when someone wishes to challenge a law and to obtain a *declaratory judgment*, a declaration of legal rights prior to the law's enforcement against that person. The large number of declaratory judgment and injunction actions filed against government officials for violations of civil rights, for improperly institutionalizing the mentally retarded, "double-celling" prisoners, or engaging in police brutality, has produced a substantial increase in cases dealing with questions of access to the courts. During the past two decades, such "1983 actions" (named for 42 U.S.C. §1983 [Section 1983 of Title 42 of the United States Code], the law under which the cases are brought) thus have been at the heart of much Supreme Court activity concerning access to the courts.

> Every person who, under color of any statute, ordinance, regulation, custom, or usage, of any State or Territory, subjects, or causes to be subjected, any citizen of the United States or other person within the jurisdiction thereof to the deprivation of any rights, privileges, or immunities secured by the Constitution and laws shall be liable to the party injured in an action at law, suit in equity, or other proper proceeding for redress. (42 U.S.C. §1983)

The Burger Court, while increasing claimants' access to federal court to proceed against local governments and local officials, restricted access in other ways; state courts' authority was strengthened through restrictions on state prisoners' access to federal courts for review of their convictions and by limits on use of the federal courts to decide issues pending in the state courts. In becoming considerably more restrictive concerning a number of important aspects of access, the justices forced the judicial process toward a more traditional model of our adversary legal system as part of which access rules were initially developed, and toward a more limited role for the courts in our system's separation of powers arrangement, in which they could not intervene almost at will in important policy questions.[1] Parallels between the Court's access doctrines, for example, those excluding the poor and disadvantaged from the benefits of certain constitutional provisions, and its lessened support for civil liberties/civil rights claims were not accidental, and led dissenters to complain that the majority justices, although talking about access considerations, had really based their rulings on their views of the underlying substantive claims.

At times, the justices have treated access rules flexibly to allow them to accept important questions or to reach particular results. The Burger Court majority interpreted the rules on mootness (see pages 175-76) loosely in cases on durational residence requirements for a divorce (where the woman seeking a divorce had already obtained one) and on affirmative action consent decrees (where laid-off workers had been reinstated), reaching a conservative result in those cases (upholding the residence requirement, ruling against layoffs affecting whites negatively); the liberals, dissenting in those cases, took a narrower view of mootness, not surprisingly parallel to *their* result preferences.[2]

As these examples suggest, are the Court's rulings on access, which we are about to discuss in some detail, mostly a cover for the justices' ideology? Before we jump to that conclusion, we should remember that several other elements might underlie access rulings. Judges might want to limit access to facilitate the handling of increasing caseload, an administrative concern; they might limit access because of legal or jurisprudential concerns, a belief in courts' limited role, an aspect of judicial self-restraint; or they might do so for reasons more directly "political"—to "evade certain policy choices and [to] indirectly legitimize preferred policy choices made elsewhere."[3]

For the 1969–75 Terms, none of these possible reasons served to explain access rulings for the Court as a whole, but in varying ways they influenced individual justices, few of whom have been consistent in the direction of their access voting over longer periods. The Court's rulings were, on the one hand, partly "a function of an underlying attitude toward access *per se*," a combination of administrative and legal concerns about proper party and proper forum (court) for cases, and, on the other hand, a function of attitudes about substantive issues ("political" considerations).[4] The access votes of four justices (Powell, Rehnquist, Stewart, White) were predominantly affected by administrative and legal concerns; two, Brennan and Douglas, were affected predominantly by political concerns; and three (Marshall, Blackmun, and Chief Justice Burger) showed no dominance of either set of concerns. Combining these elements, we find that three of the four Nixon appointees (Burger, Rehnquist, and Powell), although with differing motivations, were "willing (and ostensibly anxious) to close access," three (Stewart, Blackmun, and White) leaned toward closing off access, and three (Brennan, Douglas, and Marshall, the Warren Court's liberals) were "generally willing . . . to open access."[5]

Jurisdiction

Jurisdiction is the power of courts to hear a case, that is, their legal authority to do so. Rules of jurisdiction are found either in the Constitution—for example, the Supreme Court's original jurisdiction is stated in Article III—or in statutes, with most detailed matters of jurisdiction being spelled out in the latter. Judges consider matters of jurisdiction so important that they will raise questions of jurisdiction on their own (*sua sponte*) even if the parties have not done so.[6] Yet we must be careful not to assume that the rules on jurisdiction are always clear or that they point in only one direction. "Like other procedural principles, jurisdictional rules may be manipulated to the strategic advantage of private parties and their lawyers"[7]—and to the judges' advantage as well. The rules may be unclear, may be diffuse or "elastic," or may be contradictory (rules, with counterrules, with exceptions), thus giving the user, whether lawyer or judge, much flexibility.[8]

Jurisdiction has a number of components—concerning geography, level of court, subject matter, federalism, the parties to a case, timeliness, and the dollar amount at issue. The first, or horizontal aspect, concerns the question, "Which district court has jurisdiction to hear a particular case?" closely related to *venue*, concerning the proper location for a case when a particular type of court has authority over the particular type of case. The Bill of Rights even specifies venue in criminal trials: "In all criminal prosecutions, the accused shall enjoy the right to a speedy trial, by an impartial jury of the State and district wherein the crime shall have been committed, which district shall have been previously ascertained by law . . ." (Sixth Amendment). A question of jurisdiction is whether the Western District of North Carolina (W.D.N.C.) may hear a Voting Rights Act case or whether it must be heard in the District Court for the District of Columbia (D.D.C.). Another is whether a manufacturer of an allegedly defective car has sufficient "minimum contacts" with a state where it does not directly conduct business that it can be sued there? (No.[9]) Or may a person claiming to have been libeled sue the publisher not where she lives but in another state where the magazine carrying the alleged libel circulated? (Yes.[10]) In some instances, there are alternate locations in which a case can be brought, for example, where the plaintiff resides or at the site of the headquarters of the agency being sued; in others, a court has exclusive jurisdiction, that is, a case can be brought only there, true of the Court of Appeals for the District of Columbia for appeals from some administrative agency rulings.

An instance of subject-matter jurisdiction comes from the struggle, in the federal courts' early years, to work out their jurisdiction. A particular problem was whether there was a common law of crimes, that is, whether federal judges could decide that an offensive act was criminal although it was not so designated in the statutes or could provide punishment where Congress had not designated any. The failure of Congress to specify matters adequately left some judges frustrated. Supreme Court justices were intimately involved in this process, in the course of deciding cases while sitting on circuit. Finally, in 1812 the Supreme Court clearly decided against a federal common law of crimes.[11]

The libel case illustrates another aspect of jurisdiction—timeliness. The plaintiff had sued in the only state where the *statute of limitations* still permitted the suit. The Supreme Court has had to decide numerous cases concerning whether suits are timely. At times the question is what statute of limitations Congress meant to adopt for certain statutory rights it had created, for example, under the antidiscrimination laws (the answer is state statutes of limitations, but then the question becomes, "*Which* state statute of limitations?"). At other times, the question is, "When did the period under the statute of limitations start to run?"—for example, from when a patient realizes a connection between an injury and a doctor's action or whether the patient knows that action may have been medical malpractice.[12]

Another element of jurisdiction is a vertical one—which level of court is appropriate. For example, felonies must be tried in district court, but certain lesser offenses can be tried before magistrates (see pages 49-51). To hear a case, courts must also have jurisdiction of its subject matter, as specified by Article III and, within Article III's limits, congressional statutes. For example, appeals in all patent cases must now go to the Court of Appeals for the Federal Circuit. Courts must also have personal jurisdiction over the individuals who bring the lawsuit and especially those against whom it is brought—a matter of due process.

The federalism aspect of jurisdiction concerns whether a case is properly brought initially in a state or federal court; many cases could be brought in either, indicating that "federal courts have never been primarily tribunals vested with an exclusive special subject matter jurisdiction,"[13] although there are certain crimes triable only in federal court and certain federal statutory claims that have no "match" in state law. One important category of cases that can be brought in either federal or state court are those involving citizens of different states (*diversity of citizenship* cases) (see pages 182-83); they can be brought in federal court, however, only if at least $10,000 is at issue, a statutory requirement. This jurisdictional dollar amount, far less important now than earlier because inflation has eroded its effect, also applied to "federal question" jurisdiction until 1980, when Congress deleted the requirement eliminated earlier in such cases against the federal government and not applicable to cases brought under the civil rights statute (42 U.S.C. §1983). Where the jurisdictional amount blocked access to federal court, cases could still be brought in state court, but Congress felt that the federal courts should be open for rulings on federal law without a dollar threshold having to be satisfied.

Sovereign Immunity.   Under the doctrine of sovereign immunity, a government may not be sued without its consent. The federal courts have had to rule on the extent to which the federal government gave up its immunity in the Federal Tort Claims Act; the *Feres* doctrine, banning suits by members of the armed services for injuries incurred while in the military, has been particularly controversial because of its application to a wide range of situations extending well beyond the battlefield. Far more frequently on the Supreme Court's docket are questions as to whether federal courts may hear lawsuits against states, local governments, and their officials, or whether such suits are barred by the Eleventh Amendment. Ratified in 1798 to overturn an early Supreme Court ruling, that amendment prevents suits against a state by citizens of another state; however, the Court has said it also embodies sovereign immunity so that a state may not be sued by *its own* citizens without the state's consent.[14] In recent years the Court has continued to apply the Eleventh Amendment to bar a variety of claims. Perhaps most important, the amendment is said to bar suits for payments of funds, like welfare benefits, that the state has improperly withheld.[15] The Court has also ruled that a state, by accepting funds under a federal statute, did not waive its immunity, and that the Eleventh Amendment prevents federal judges from ordering state officials to follow state law.[16]

The Court has, however, ruled that congressional action enforcing the Fourteenth Amendment may remove a state's immunity, and has ruled that federal court suits (under 42 U.S.C. §1983) seeking declaratory judgments and injunctions against a state are permissible because they are aimed at *officials* rather than the state itself. The Court has significantly expanded the basis for such lawsuits by saying they could be brought not only when it was claimed that personal *constitutional* rights, such as freedom of speech or the right to associate or property rights, had been violated but also when states were said to violate federal statutes such as the Social Security Act (*Maine v. Thiboutot*, 1981).

Perhaps even more significant was the Court's 1978 *Monell* ruling overturning a 17-year-old decision (*Monroe v. Pape*, 1962) and saying that local governments may be sued for actions implementing official policy statements.[17] This was followed by a decision that local government officers' "good faith" was not a defense to lawsuits against the government itself; however, the Court was unwilling to allow an award of punitive damages when municipalities violated people's rights—for example, by canceling a concert by the rock group Blood, Sweat, and Tears.[18]

The Court has also stripped many state and local officials of at least some of their legal immunity for actions violating people's constitutional rights, thus making them personally liable for damages. The Court took the first step in this direction in *Scheuer v. Rhodes* (1976), a case stemming from the National Guard killings at Kent State University in 1970; the Court ruled that, if state officials violated the U.S. Constitution, their immunity from suit was removed; however, the Court gave high-level officials what amounts to executive immunity by saying that the higher an official's position, the more discretion the official is allowed. The Court then reinforced officials' liability by holding in *Wood v. Strickland* (1975) that superintendents, principals, and school board members would be personally liable if they maliciously or knowingly violated students' rights or did so when they should have known they were doing so.

At the same time, the Court closed off damage suits against those connected with law enforcement and the courts. In addition to granting judges absolute immunity from suit (see page 4), the Court has also granted absolute immunity from civil rights suits to state prosecutors, even when they are claimed to have knowingly used false evidence and to have suppressed material evidence, so they would not have to spend their time defending lawsuits instead of carrying out assigned duties, and to police officers serving as witnesses who supposedly gave false testimony at trials.[19]

Standing

To bring a case, a person must have *standing*, that is, must be a proper party. If no one has standing, the court lacks jurisdiction to hear a case, leaving the possibility that unconstitutional laws will remain on the books because no one can "get at them." Although some rules on standing are found in statutes (see below), most are judge-made, which allows flexibility. As with any judge-made rules on access to the courts, it also allows justices' ideologies to affect those procedural rules.

The basic rule on standing is that the litigant must show real or potential injury to himself or herself or have a personal stake in the outcome; thus a doctor could not challenge anticontraceptive statutes solely on the basis that they would injure his patients.[20] At times, however, the rights of others may be asserted to reinforce one's own claim, particularly where there are obstacles to others' asserting their own rights and where the party in court would assert those rights effectively. Thus a white woman, sued for damages for selling her house to blacks in violation of restrictive covenants, was granted standing to assert blacks' rights to purchase housing; a married man charged with violating a law that prohibited supplying contraceptives to single people but that did not punish the recipients was able to assert their rights; and doctors were allowed to assert the rights of Medicaid patients who might seek abortions in the doctors' suit to recover payment.[21] The Court was not, however, willing to grant standing to a physician who had entered an abortion case as an intervenor seeking to protect the un-born.[22] Standing has also been granted to whites to challenge the exclusion of blacks from juries and to men to challenge the exclusion of women on the basis that all have a right to a jury that is a properly drawn cross-section of the community.[23]

During the late 1960s the Court relaxed the rules on standing, thus permitting more people to sue. For one thing, the Court expanded the scope of those "injured," recognizing in *Sierra Club v. Morton* that injury to "aesthetic and environmental well-being" was among interests that could provide a basis for standing. However, to obtain standing a group would have to do more than state a general interest in the environment; its members would have to be among those injured by environmentally adverse action. Later, when a personal injury claim was added to claims of injury to the environment, the Court was willing to grant standing (*United States v. S.C.R.A.P.*, 1973). The Court has regularly allowed groups to sue on behalf of their own members, doing so most recently when it allowed a labor union to sue on behalf of its members concerning eligibility for certain statutory benefits.[24]

The Court also granted federal taxpayers standing to sue in some instances. Prior to 1968, federal taxpayers alleging that money was being used for an unconstitutional project could not use their taxpayer status to establish standing to sue the government. In 1968 the Court ruled in *Flast v. Cohen*, a case brought to test the 1965 Elementary and Secondary Education Act (ESEA) provisions for assistance to parochial schools, that a federal taxpayer could have standing to sue the government if the challenged program were alleged to violate a specific constitutional prohibition, such as the First Amendment's "establishment of religion" clause. However, in a ruling perhaps indicative of its narrower view of who should be able to raise issues in the courts, the Court refused to grant standing when an organization dedicated to church-state separation challenged a transfer of government property to a religious organization with no payment required, under the clause allowing the government to dispose of property (Art. IV, Sec. 3, cl. 2); there was only a general grievance, said the majority, not any personal injury.[25]

Taxpayer attacks on governmental action on the basis of constitutional provisions more general than the First Amendment's prohibition of establishment of religion have also still not been permitted, because there was little to distinguish taxpayer complaints from general citizen grievances, which are not considered an adequate basis for standing. The Burger Court reinforced this position by refusing to grant standing to a taxpayer trying to force compliance with the Statements and Accounts Clause (Art. I, Sec. 9, cl. 7) of the Constitution because Congress had failed to require the Central Intelligence Agency (CIA) to produce detailed reports of its expenditures; such claims, Justice Powell said, should be brought to Congress, not the courts, with Chief Justice Burger adding that taxpayers could not use federal courts for general grievances. The Court promptly applied this position to deny armed service reserve officers standing when they tried to prevent members of Congress from holding reserve commissions as a violation of the Incompatibility Clause (no executive official should be a member of Congress).[26]

Civil Rights Claims. The Burger Court's restrained view of standing was perhaps clearest in civil rights claims. When both whites and blacks in Cairo, Illinois, the site of serious racial conflict, sued to obtain relief from racially discriminatory judicial bonding and sentencing practices, the Court, in *O'Shea v. Littleton* (1973), denied standing because the plaintiffs had not shown either that they had already been injured or that they could suffer continuing injury from the practices. (Showing that multiple aspects of access doctrine may appear in the same case, the Court's nonintervention was also based on a desire to avoid having the federal judiciary regularly supervise state judges.) Similarly, in a suit against Philadelphia Mayor Frank Rizzo and the police commissioner over improper police practices against minorities and mishandling of complaints (*Rizzo v. Goode*, 1976), the Court said the complainants lacked standing to bring about an overhauling of police disciplinary procedures because their claims rested on what a small, unnamed minority of officers might do in the future and on incidents that *might* happen to others *if* the police procedures were not changed. The extent to which the Court would take this position was made clear when the plaintiff in *City of Los Angeles v. Lyons* (1983), subjected to a police "chokehold" after being stopped for a traffic violation and fearing a recurrence of such police action, was denied standing to enjoin police use of chokeholds because the Court said he did not face a real or immediate threat of recurrence nor had he shown the city authorized routine use of chokeholds.

The Burger Court also demonstrated its law enforcement conservatism in a procedural context when it limited standing to challenge allegedly improper searches. The Warren Court had ruled in the *Alderman* case that suppression of evidence could be urged only by those whose rights were violated by a search, not those against whom evidence is used. The Burger Court built on that by saying that violations of Fourth Amendment search and seizure standards could not be questioned by those who did not own a car that had been searched or its contents or who did not have an expectation of privacy in those parts of the car that were searched (*Rakas v. Illinois*, 1978); that ruling was promptly extended to noncar searches, with the Court overturning a Warren Court ruling in the process.[27] These rulings of course affected use of the exclusionary rule (see pages 379-82), disliked by the Burger Court majority; if fewer people had standing to challenge searches, the exclusionary rule would be applied less often.

In another area of civil rights, the Supreme Court in *Warth v. Seldin* (1975) turned aside all plaintiffs—low- and moderate-income minority residents of a city, a nonprofit corporation trying to alleviate their housing shortage, central city taxpayers, and a homebuilders' association—trying to attack restrictive and exclusionary suburban zoning ordinances: they would have to indicate specifically both how the challenged ordinances would harm them and how judges could protect their rights. (That the majority's position was in part based on the merits can be seen in Justice Powell's comment that "the economics of the housing market," not the ordinances, prevented plaintiffs' move to the suburbs.) Despite this ruling, it proved possible to challenge exclusionary zoning ordinances, at least when a specific rezoning request had been turned down—although the Court then found no intentional racial discrimination.[28]

At times Congress has specified who may or may not bring certain types of cases in the federal courts. For example, in passing the law establishing the National Railroad Passenger Corporation (Amtrak), Congress provided that the attorney general should enforce its provisions; this meant, said the Court, that a railroad passenger group was barred from protesting passenger train discontinuances. The Court similarly limited the ability of trade associations and political action committees (PACs) to invoke Federal Election Campaign Act procedures and restricted the standing of a party national committee to challenge certain election expenditures. An example of expansive interpretation of statutory grants of standing was the Court's ruling that under Congress' open housing legislation, white tenants of an apartment complex have standing to complain about discrimination against blacks.[29]

Closely related to statutory standing issues are those dealing with whether Congress has provided someone a *cause of action* or basis for a lawsuit. Thus the Court has had to decide whether, in the absence of explicit language, Congress intended to allow private citizens to sue to enforce antidiscrimination statutes that provided other remedies; such cases, a result of Congress' failure to make its intent clear, have seriously divided the Court in recent years, as when it ruled that a woman claiming discrimination in medical school admissions practices could sue in federal court under Title IX of the Education Amendments of 1972 (barring sex discrimination in government-funded programs).[30]

The Court also established direct constitutional causes of action for certain civil rights claims, against federal agents for violations of the Fourth Amendment in improper searches; prison officials, for inadequate medical treatment under the Eighth Amendment (cruel and unusual punishment); and members of Congress, for sex discrimination, under the "equal protection" element the Court had earlier written into the Fifth Amendment.[31] The Court was, however, unwilling to give enlisted military personnel such a cause of action for racial discrimination claims because of Congress' structuring of the military justice system.[32]

The Supreme Court decisions on procedures for class action suits (see page 156) require interpretation of federal court rules. Although class actions save time for the courts by avoiding repetitious litigation, the Court has limited their use. The justices have ruled, for example, that a consumer suing a utility could not satisfy the $10,000 jurisdictional requirement for federal diversity-of-citizenship cases by joining his small claim with others' in a class action, and then later ruled in an antipollution case against a paper company that each and every member of the class had to satisfy that $10,000 figure or there could be no class action suit.[33]

Justiciability

Rules on justiciability—the question of cases appropriate for judges to hear—are, like rules on standing, judge-made; they are even more flexible than the rules on standing. The concept of justiciability includes norms against issuing advisory opinions or deciding feigned controversies, moot or unripe cases, or "political questions." There are also cases that fit in none of these categories, as when the Court ruled challenges by Kent State University student government officers to Ohio National Guard riot control rules nonjusticiable because the requested remedy would engage federal judges in constant review of the executive branch, charged with supervising the Guard (*Gilligan v. Morgan,* 1973).

All the categories but that of "political questions" are based on a fundamental rule, settled early in the Court's history, that the Supreme Court will not issue opinions on abstract legal questions but will decide questions of law only when they are presented in the fact context of a particular lawsuit. This basic principle was stated in the course of deciding that the court would not issue advisory opinions, but it extends far beyond that—to other situations where the question would be abstract and the result would be the equivalent of an advisory opinion, such as cases without adverse parties, cases that are not ripe, and cases that are moot. In none of those situations would adequate information be given to the judge: in our adversary system of justice, judges are expected to be passive in the sense of receiving information and legal arguments rather than developing them for the parties. Nor in those situations would the law be given its operative meaning through facts about the law's application. A law might appear to be constitutional "on its face" but be applied in an improper manner, or a law of dubious validity may have been applied—or interpreted by the lower courts—so as to preserve its constitutionality. Judges are likewise reluctant to grant declaratory judgments because prosecution after a violation will bring out fuller sets of facts on the operation of the statute. However, increased use of summary judgments—cases decided on the pleadings—and on motions to dismiss (also on the pleadings) somewhat undercut this idea.

Advisory Opinions. Narrowly defined, an *advisory opinion* is an opinion given by judges to the legislature or executive about a proposed bill or action. Some state high courts do issue such opinions. However, the justices of the U.S. Supreme Court firmly established a rule against the justices giving advisory opinions when President Washington asked the Court for advice on some treaty questions; the justices responded through Chief Justice Jay that they would not do so. Early in the present century, the Court amplified the rule. Congress had passed a law allowing the Cherokee Indians to file suit to test a statute, but in *Muskrat v. United States* the Court said that Congress was seeking a ruling on the law's constitutionality without the presence of a live controversy, therefore in effect asking for an advisory opinion, and the justices would not allow the case to be heard.

Some informal exceptions to the ban on advisory opinions have, however, occurred. In 1822 President Monroe asked several members of the Court about the legality of federal "internal improvements." Justice William Johnson made a general if oblique reply for himself and several other justices, indicating their position that governmental construction of military roads and postroads was constitutional. Certainly Chief Justice Hughes' comment on behalf of the Court about Roosevelt's Court-packing proposal—that the "one Supreme Court" called for by the Constitution could not sit in divisions—could be called an advisory opinion. At other times, individual justices have provided the president with legal advice and have helped draw up legislation, as Justice Frankfurter did for President Roosevelt and Justice Fortas did for President Lyndon Johnson.

In the course of deciding cases, justices also comment on matters on which the Court is not ruling or give suggestions to the other branches about how to deal with problems, making their statements informal advisory opinions. Thus, in striking down a statute regulating a part of the economy, justices have suggested how Congress could deal with the problem by relying on another constitutional clause. More recently, justices have suggested that a statute amending the Voting Rights Act to outlaw at-large municipal elections would be valid and that a statutory revision allowing noncommercial educational broadcasting stations to have affiliates that would editorialize would also pass muster. [34] Because, as the nation's highest tribunal, the Court decides cases intended to be representative of large issues and thus decides more than the particulars of the dispute between the immediate parties, the justices are expected to issue opinions with a reach broader than the facts of the specific case being decided, and thus may make advisory comments. Whenever the Court goes beyond the specific facts of a case to anticipate general questions of policy not yet directly presented to it, it can be said to be issuing an advisory opinion, and some other members of the Court are likely to complain. Justices are more likely to make statements of this sort when they write concurring or dissenting opinions than when they write the "opinion of the Court." When the author of the Court's majority opinion does make comments not necessary for the Court's ruling, the statements are called *obiter dictum* (plural: *dicta*), that is, language beyond the *holding* or basic rule of the case. Although speculation about hypothetical situations not before the Court is clearly *obiter*, often it is difficult to tell what is *obiter* and what is not, and, in later cases, justices may disagree over what was part of a Court's earlier holding and what was *obiter*.

Feigned Controversies. As part of its effort to have the federal courts avoid handing down advisory opinions, the Court insists that litigation not be "made up" simply to obtain a ruling on some matter that the parties would like to see settled, particularly to the detriment of a third party not involved in a case. Thus the parties in a case must be adverse to each other. This rule against feigned controversies is aimed at collusive litigation. It does not mean that the litigants have to be "at each other's throats" but only that their interests be opposed; in short, not all "friendly suits" are barred, but the parties cannot be *too* friendly, or cannot bring a suit to exclude the presentation of their real opponents' views. One of the Court's earliest statements of the rule was in a case, *Lord v. Veazie*, in which a stockholder, claiming ownership of river navigational rights also claimed by someone else, sold some stock based on his own presumed control of the rights. By prearrangement, the stock purchaser, a relative of the seller, sued the seller to determine ownership of the river rights. Both parties obviously wanted the same result, which they were trying to ensure without the third party's involvement. The Supreme Court ruled that no court should hear such a lawsuit. Nonetheless, there have been efforts to get into court with collusive cases from time to time.

An example of the courts *not* throwing out a case as a "feigned controversy" is *Carter v. Carter Coal Co.* (1936), in which the president of a company sued his own company to prevent compliance with the Guffey Bituminous Coal Act. Although both sides had lawyers who made strong arguments in the Supreme Court, the common interest of both parties in getting the law invalidated should have been clear. Moreover, under the then existing rules, the United States—whose statute was at issue—was not a party to the case and was thus at a disadvantage in trying to argue the statute's validity. Because of that situation—in which the Court *did* invalidate the statute, Congress promptly passed legislation that made the United States a party whenever the constitutionality of a federal statute is brought in issue in a case in which the United States is not initially a party. This provision was used in the *Northern Pipeline* bankruptcy case (see pages 51-52) and in an earlier challenge to a union's political expenditures, where the government had not been involved in the lower court but did argue in the Supreme Court after the case was delayed to allow it to do so.[35] States now have the right to become a party to cases in which their laws are being challenged, a parallel to the federal government's right to intervene.

Mootness and Ripeness. Another aspect of the 'case or controversy' requirement is that a case not be moot, that is, that a dispute not be completed or that it not be too late for judges to apply a remedy. The rule has, however, not always been interpreted strictly. Thus when the government made it difficult to challenge its actions either by voluntarily eliminating a questioned rule in the face of a lawsuit while retaining the option of reinstating the rule or by issuing orders of brief duration, each of which would expire before a court challenge could be made, the Court has been willing to hear cases. In the 1960s, changing its basic direction on mootness, the Court made it still easier for courts to decide issues, particularly concerning elections, that were likely to recur. Under traditional mootness rules, challenges to election rules, particularly those excluding candidates, were usually moot before they reached the appellate courts because the election had already taken place. However, because the issue involved in the challenge would recur in a subsequent election, when it might again become moot on appeal, the Supreme Court began to rule on some election cases even after the election had passed.[36]

Prisoners' challenges to their convictions were also made easier when the Court ruled that a prisoner's habeas corpus challenge to a conviction was not mooted by release from prison, because disability resulting from the conviction remained. However, if prisoners were only attacking *sentences* and those sentences expired before a court decided the case, the matter would be moot.[37] The flexible approach demonstrated in those situations was quite evident in the Court's 1973 abortion cases, *Roe v. Wade* and *Doe v. Bolton,* in which Justice

Blackmun, noting that pregnancy was likely to recur, both for the woman challenging antiabortion laws and for other women as well, ruled that, because it was
"capable of repetition yet evading review," it was not subject to traditional rules of
mootness, under which questions related to pregnancy could never be reviewed
on appeal because the pregnancy would be completed. Although mootness has
generally been defined less strictly in recent decades, it can still be applied strictly
when the justices do not wish to deal with an issue. When affirmative action
programs were first challenged in the Court, in the *DeFunis* case, the Court
found the challenge to a law school program moot because the white male who
had brought the case, admitted to the law school while the litigation proceeded,
was about to graduate. Its mootness ruling gave the Court some time to ponder
the issue further before its first ruling on the subject—in the *Bakke* case.

A case also cannot be *premature* or *unripe* if judges are to decide it. Ripeness, like mootness, is related to standing. Someone bringing a case that is not
ripe lacks standing. Similarly, someone without a definite injury lacks standing
because the matter is speculative and thus unripe. For example, because only a
subjective "chill" to First Amendment rights, not actual injury, resulted from
Army surveillance of civilian political activity, the Court—in *Laird v. Tatum*
(1972)—ruled a challenge to that activity not ripe. There are few clear rules
concerning ripeness, the contours of which are established on a case-by-case
basis. For example, the Court held a challenge to anticontraceptive laws not ripe
because, although a prosecutor said he would prosecute those violating the law,
contraceptives were widely available and there had been no such prosecution for
20 years; thus a declaration of people's rights was not necessary, said the majority.
(However, when a doctor opened a birth control clinic, he was arrested, and the
Court then invalidated the law.)[38]

An important element of the rules on ripeness is that a litigant have previously exhausted available administrative and judicial remedies. The administrative ones should be exhausted before one comes to court, so that the administrative agencies' views on the dispute will be known and so that the dispute might
be resolved before ever reaching court; available judicial remedies should be
exhausted before one proceeds to a higher court, to allow the lower courts to play
their proper role in the judicial system, leaving appellate courts free to review
lower court decisions. One must also make full use of state court remedies before
using federal courts to challenge convictions and must avail oneself of appeals
within an administrative body before taking matters to court. For example, the
Court had ruled that challenges to courts-martial cannot be heard by civilian
courts until military courts have completed their review, even where the military's jurisdiction to hold the court-martial is the subject of the challenge.[39] The
exhaustion doctrine in areas such as welfare may exhaust the individual rather
than the remedies and has had a particularly harsh effect on those denied
Conscientious Objector status by their draft boards, where, as a result of statutes

sustained by the Court, review is available only through a challenge to a criminal indictment for refusing induction.

"*Political Questions.*" The most ambiguous part of justiciability is the *political question* doctrine, under which courts will not decide questions the judges think "belong" to the legislative or executive branches under the Constitution's terms or would be more appropriately handled there. The doctrine is closely related to judges' perceptions of "activism" and "restraint" (see pages 283-87); when the Court is unwilling to rule on an issue affecting other branches, a restrained posture, the issue may be labeled a "political question," but when the judges are willing to act, the label is missing.

Over the course of its history, the Court has considered a variety of issues to be "political questions." These include whether a state may rescind its ratification of a constitutional amendment, also at issue with respect to the ERA, and which of two "regimes" in a particular state was the legitimate one—matters that could be dealt with by Congress (in determining the ratification of an amendment or the credentials of members of Congress); whether state constitutions may provide for recall of judges; and whether or not a president should enforce certain laws—something the justices felt should be left to the executive's discretion.[40]

Until the 1960s, the "political question" doctrine had substantial content. However, the Warren Court drastically reduced that content. First, although for many years reapportionment had been thought to be a "political question," in 1962 the Court said in *Baker v. Carr* that complaints about malapportioned legislative districts could be heard by the courts. In 1986, the Court went even further by saying that challenges to partisan gerrymanders—purposeful malapportionment to benefit one political party—were justiciable (*Davis v. Bandemer*). The Court also showed itself willing to interfere in previously undisturbed legislative judgments about the qualifications of their own members. In *Bond v. Floyd*, the Court overturned the Georgia legislature's refusal to seat Julian Bond because of his antiwar statements and in 1968 ruled that Congress should seat Congressman Adam Clayton Powell (D-N.Y.). The ruling in *Powell v. McCormack* came close to rejecting the "political question" doctrine entirely. When President Nixon claimed that the request for the Watergate tapes was nonjusticiable because it was an "in-house" controversy between president and special prosecutor, the Court in *United States v. Nixon* rejected the claim that there was a "political question" and went on to decide the case, just as it did nine years later in overturning the legislative veto.[41]

The political question doctrine is still applied in some situations, almost exclusively involving our relations with foreign nations. The validity of treaties under international law and our recognition of foreign governments are still considered to be "political questions"; thus the courts will not interfere with the executive branch's decisions. The federal courts often used the political question doctrine as the basis for refusing to decide the validity of the Vietnam War under either our own Constitution or international law.[42]

Relations Between Federal and State Courts

Relations between federal and state courts can be smooth or awkward, with much friction. The friction has abated substantially since the early years of the Republic, when there was considerable resistance to judical review of state court rulings (see page 78). Although relations are now less difficult, problems still abound, such as conflicts over federal court interpretation of state law and over review of state criminal convictions; at times, as in the 1986 Texaco-Pennzoil case, conflict stems from federal court rulings, prior to completion of state proceedings, that state courts have not adequately protected certain parties' procedural rights; a federal judge's intervention in the proceedings, by signficantly reducing the appeal bond required by the Texas courts, was seen as an affront to state judges, and the Supreme Court ruled the judge should have abstained from ruling on Texaco's federal court efforts (*Pennzoil Co. v. Texaco*, 1987).

If judicial rulings are the source of much friction between federal and state courts, there are also day-to-day problems of relations between the two levels of courts. One type of problem stems from prosecutors' actions, for example, when federal judges find themselves faced with "penny-ante" drug cases they believe belong in state court. (There can also be cooperation, for example, with state drug cases brought into federal court as federal charges and prosecuted there by state prosecutors deputized as U.S. attorneys, when the state courts are too crowded to handle the increasing number of drug cases promptly.)

In a number of states, administrative and policy matters are handled by *federal-state judicial councils*, most of which were set up after Chief Justice Burger called for them in his 1970 State of the Judiciary message but many of which then became inactive. The councils are primarily mechanisms for exchanges of views, although agreements about how to deal effectively with certain problems may be made. The composition of the councils varies, but usually the chief judge of the federal district court, a resident court of appeals judge, and the state's chief justice are among the members. Questions that have been considered by these councils include habeas corpus petitions, diversity of citizenship litigation, and transfer of jurisdiction. Administrative matters such as overlapping federal and state jury service and the scheduling of conflicting trial schedules for lawyers have also been dealt with, and some councils have worked out joint judicial hearings—with both a federal judge and a state judge present—for certain special cases.[43]

If we return our attention to the Supreme Court's rulings, we find that friction between state courts and the Supreme Court has resulted when the high court's interpretations of the U.S. Constitution's protection of civil liberties have been at variance with state court interpretations. When the Supreme Court rules that the Constitution *permits* but does not require a certain state practice, such as nonunanimous jury verdicts, the states are at liberty to adopt more rigorous standards (by retaining the requirement of a unanimous jury). However, the justices have said that state courts may not require greater protection for civil liberties—by limiting state officials' actions—by interpreting the U.S. Constitution differently from the way the Supreme Court has interpreted it. "A State is free *as a matter of its own law* to impose greater restrictions on police activity than those this Court holds to be necessary under federal constitutional standards. . . . But . . . a State may not impose such greater restrictions *as* a matter of *federal constitutional law* when this Court specifically refrains from imposing them."[44] Such a statement stems from the Supreme Court's views, enunciated in the Little Rock case (see page 79), that not only the Constitution but also the *Supreme Court's interpretation* is the "supreme law of the land."

State courts can both avoid Supreme Court review and establish rules different from those the Supreme Court requires under the U.S. Constitution if they carefully base their rulings solely on their own constitutions (and statutes). Although the Supreme Court seldom used to interfere with state decisions thought to rest on adequate state law grounds, it has become more difficult for state courts to avoid Supreme Court intervention. The justices have insisted that the state courts make a "clear statement" that their decisions rest on state law; otherwise the justices will feel free to treat the state court ruling as based on federal law and thus subject to Supreme Court review.[45] Not surprisingly, such a rule has resulted in the Court's overturning prodefendant state court rulings, despite Justice Stevens' complaint that the Supreme Court's presuming that it has jurisdiction over state court cases "evidences a lack of respect for state courts and will . . . be a recurrent source of friction between the federal and state judiciaries." (He has, however, also complained that state judges do not do enough to rest decisions on state law grounds.[46]

In 1980, the Supreme Court made good on its promise that state courts could establish greater protection for civil liberties under their state constitutions. Although the Supreme Court had said only a few years earlier that leafletting in a privately owned shopping center was not protected by the First Amendment, the California Supreme Court had ruled that it had to be allowed under the California Constitution. Writing for a unanimous court, Justice Rehnquist said that the state court was not prevented from "adopt[ing] in its own Constitution individual liberties more expansive than those conferred by the Federal Constitution."[47] That such a ruling may be made grudgingly is shown by Chief Justice Burger's suggestion in a later case that if state voters don't like state law-based rulings by state judges, they can change that law.[48]

Formal relations between federal and state courts, which the Supreme Court interprets, are depicted in Figure 5.1. The Supreme Court has issued a set of decisions delineating relations between federal and state courts: those concerning habeas corpus and civil rights claims are based on interpretation of federal statutes; others are based on basic conceptions of national court deference to the state judiciary.

Figure 5.1   Relations Between Federal and State Courts

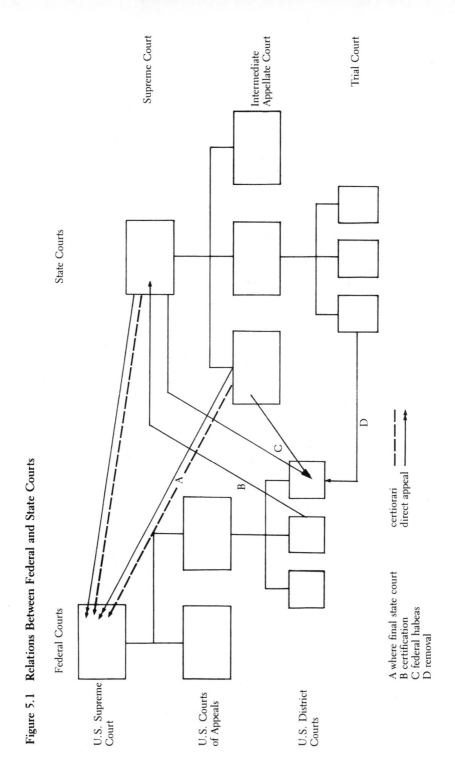

State Courts

Supreme Court

Intermediate
Appellate Court

Trial Court

Federal Courts

U.S. Supreme
Court

U.S. Courts
of Appeals

U.S. District
Courts

A where final state court
B certification
C federal habeas
D removal

certiorari – – –
direct appeal ——▶

Diversity and Removal

Among Supreme Court rulings on federal court-state court relations are those dealing with diversity of citizenship cases and removal, the basic provisions for which are established by statute. *Diversity of citizenship suits* are those between citizens of one state (including corporations) and those of another; they may be brought in federal court if more than $10,000 is involved. Federal courts' application of federal rather than state law in such cases has caused substantial friction within the federal system. In 1842 in *Swift v. Tyson* the Supreme Court ruled that the federal courts could establish their own common law in diversity cases. The Supreme Court did not reverse itself until 1938. In *Erie Railroad Co. v. Tompkins*, the Court declared that its earlier decision was unconstitutional, that there was no federal common law, and that the federal courts should apply the laws of the states in diversity litigation. Despite *Erie*, there is still some use of federal common law in other types of cases, such as labor-management disputes, and there is also the equivalent of a federal common law of procedure because the federal courts have to have a set of rules as to which state's law to apply when different results would occur, but state law now has much greater authority in diversity suits. Although state substantive law is applied, federal procedural rules—particularly those developed under the Rules Enabling Act (see page 75)—supercede conflicting state procedural rules.[49]

Controversy over diversity of citizenship jurisdiction continues, with the Court trying to impose some limits and Congress, responding to pressure from lawyers and judges and a lack of general public concern, not yet having eliminated it. Federal courts' diversity caseload increased by roughly 50 percent from 1960 to 1976. Although it decreased from less than one-third to less than one-fourth of federal civil filings, it remains a significant proportion of federal judges' caseload. Chief Justice Burger, along with the Judicial Conference of the United States, suggested eliminating it altogether to reduce federal court caseload. He argued that state judges are no longer less fair to out-of-state litigants than are federal judges, thus eliminating an earlier rationale for such jurisdiction. Another argument is that federal judges have to take considerable time to ascertain (or guess) the state law to apply and have not helped to develop that law. However, others have argued—and many individual federal judges believe—that diversity cases, which present general legal issues like those often heard in state courts, keep federal judges from becoming narrow specialists and have provided them with a broader perspective.[50] Moreover, there is no state mechanism for handling mass tort litigation that can be consolidated in one federal judicial district; another reason cited for not shifting diversity cases out of the federal courts is that state courts are generally overburdened. Nor, even though the Conference of State Chief Justices argues that federal diversity jurisdiction should be eliminated because it casts intimations of second-class citizenship on the state judiciary, would many state judges like the additional infusion of cases. (Thus, at both federal and state levels, we see judicial leaders' official positions differing from positions of many individual judges "in the trenches.")

Surveys reported in 1980 and 1981, although indicating considerable variation among lawyers from one location to another, show that lawyers remain concerned about local favoritism in state courts but not necessarily about a separate bias against corporations. In their varying relative use of federal and state courts for cases eligible for federal diversity jurisdiction, lawyers pick the court, state *or* federal, that will most expeditiously process their cases. That factor, a preference for the federal rules of procedure, and a concern for judges of high quality (federal courts are given higher ratings) play the largest roles in lawyers' choice of court. [51]

Diversity jurisdiction and *removal* of cases from state to federal court are related because many diversity cases are stated in state courts—where they also can be brought—only to be shifted (removed) to federal court by out-of-state defendants. During the 1960s, removal was attempted in another category of cases—those of civil rights workers in the South who argued that they were being arrested and tried in order to harass them. Their efforts to transfer their cases to federal court failed when the Supreme Court, sensitive to the problem of taking cases away from the state courts, took a narrow view of the federal removal statute. Removal could occur, the Supreme Court said, only when there was a statutorily protected federal right involving racial equality, such as the right to service in a place of public accommodation after passage of the 1964 Civil Rights Act, and a state law or rule prevented the protection of rights in a state trial; an allegation of an unfair trial was an insufficient basis for removal, as errors at trial could be corrected on appeal. [52] The Court has continued to stand by this limited interpretation.

Abstention

Another linkage between federal and state courts derives from federal court interpretation of state law in the course of applying it. Federal judges do not have to decide what state law means when the state law is clear "on its face" or when state courts have provided a clarifying interpretation (or "gloss"). It is considered inappropriate for federal judges to decide what the state law means when it is ambiguous and state courts have not clarified it. *Abstention* is a doctrine that judges have developed to avoid federal court-state court conflict over interpretation of state law. Under this doctrine, federal courts "stay their hand" until state courts have an opportunity to rule on state law questions, because such state court action might allow federal courts to avoid federal questions or might modify those questions so that federal court action would be affected. When the doctrine of abstention was not applicable, "wise judicial administration"—such as avoidance of piecemeal litigation of legal questions—might make it best for a federal court to leave matters to the state courts, particularly when the federal court was several hundred miles from the dispute and state court proceedings had been initiated first. However, federal courts do not invariably abstain from deciding cases when state courts may also be involved in an issue. Justice Brennan has said that abstention was "the exception, not the rule" because federal courts could not abdicate their duty to decide cases unless some important countervailing interest was present.[53]

A specific mechanism for prompt state court interpretation of unanswered state law questions in pending federal cases is for the federal court to *certify* the questions to the state courts, which then provide an answer the federal court applies to the case before it. An increasing number of states have provided for such "downward certification" (different from lower federal courts asking higher federal courts to answer novel legal questions: see page 74). The Supreme Court itself has made use of such a mechanism, for example, remanding a death penalty case to the Georgia Supreme Court for interpretation of that court's opinion.[54] Similarly, the Supreme Court returns cases to state courts for rulings on unanswered questions that might provide an "adequate and independent state ground" to support the state ruling. It also does so when it is unclear whether a state court has used federal law, state law, or both as the basis for a decision, to ascertain whether there were separate state law grounds for the ruling. This is an example of the notion of *comity*—of respect for state courts' ability to decide issues—that the Supreme Court tries to implement.

A closely related matter is the question of whether state court action is "final" so that appeal to the Supreme Court is proper. The Supreme Court does not wish to accept an appeal from a state court in a case in which only some questions have been answered when other proceedings are still pending, because a Supreme Court ruling at that stage may mean interference in state proceedings. On the other hand, not accepting the appeal may mean needless continuation of the trial and thus injury to the appellants if resolution of an issue would terminate the proceedings. On this question of "finality," the Court takes a pragmatic approach despite complaints that the number of exceptions to the finality rule has become larger.

Competing with the preference that state courts decide state law questions is a preference that all claims in a case be heard by either state or federal courts. At times, the preference for having all claims decided in one court may lead to all claims being decided in federal rather than state courts, the reverse of the result produced by abstention. When state matters are raised in federal court along with an adequate federal claim, they may be heard by the federal judge under the doctrine of "pendent jurisdiction." If the federal court then follows normal rules of self-restraint and avoids federal constitutional questions, it may decide the state claim first, thus ironically not resolving the federal questions. Despite the preference for "all claims in one court," the idea is not followed consistently. Eliminating those without $10,000 claims from diversity of citizenship class actions means that the same legal questions may be argued by some plaintiffs in federal court, and by others in state court, with potentially conflicting results. A similar problem can result with prisoners' claims, depending on whether they are embodied in a habeas corpus petition or a civil rights suit. There is no requirement that state remedies be exhausted in civil rights cases, which can thus move directly to federal court, but the exhaustion rule does apply to habeas claims, taking them back to state courts. The same facts may thus be heard simultaneously in federal and state courts, producing duplicative litigation with potentially inconsistent results.[55]

Injunctions Against State Laws

An important issue touching on abstention and comity is whether federal courts should enjoin enforcement of state laws or other action by state officials, or should insist that an individual against whom the state has acted use federal claims as a defense in state court, thus assuring that state courts had the first opportunity to rule on such matters and to apply the Constitution. The Warren Court facilitated obtaining injunctions against improper state action, when, in *Dombrowski v. Pfister* (1965), it allowed an injunction against state prosecution under a broad statute that infringed freedom of speech. When lower federal courts interpreted this ruling broadly, there was a considerable increase in federal court challenges to state laws; these occurred even where state courts, given a chance, might have enforced federal constitutional rights.

Chief Justice Burger felt this practice overused federal courts and denigrated state court authority, and he was clearly determined to put an end to it. The Court's change of position came in 1971 in *Younger v. Harris*. The majority ruled in that case that federal courts were no longer to issue injunctions against already instituted state criminal prosecutions; state court proceedings were to be allowed to continue, except where great and immediate irreparable damage was threatened and that harm could not be prevented by raising the constitutional claims in a later state trial. This rule was to apply, said the Court, even when the challenged statute was clearly unconstitutional. After allowing the plaintiffs in *Steffel v. Thompson* (1974), threatened with prosecution for handing out antiwar leaflets, to obtain a declaration of their rights even when they could not show the irreparable injury necessary for obtaining an injunction, the Court then returned forcefully to the *Younger v. Harris* doctrine and extended it. In *Hicks v. Miranda* (1975), the Court ruled that a federal injunction could not be obtained against a prosecution initiated in a state court *after* the federal challenge had been started—prompting the dissenters' complaint that whether you could get an injunction depended on an improper "race to the courthouse" in which the state could start later and get there first. The *Younger* doctrine was also extended to *civil* proceedings closely related to criminal matters, for example, a state civil nuisance proceeding against a theater showing allegedly obscene movies, and to other matters, both civil and administrative, as well.[56]

If federal court actions against many types of state court actions are barred, state courts also may not prevent the filing of appropriate federal court suits. In 1977 and 1978, the Supreme Court twice had to order a New Mexico judge not to interfere with a litigant's rights to file certain federal cases related to ongoing state litigation concerning obligations under a contract for delivery of uranium in the face of a fivefold price increase. [57]

Federal Habeas Corpus

Filing of habeas corpus petitions in federal court by those challenging state convictions, often many years after state appeals have concluded, is the most controversial present issue concerning relations between federal courts and state courts. Habeas corpus cases are technically civil cases, although they often deal with criminal procedure issues; they provide a clear instance of "diachronic or sequential redundancy" in our dual court system, in which, after one level of courts has decided a case, the parties can turn to the other. [58] (After a federal district court denies a habeas corpus petition, the order denying the petition may be reviewed on appeal only if the district judge who examined the petition, a judge of the court of appeals, or the circuit justice issues a certificate of probable cause, which requires a substantial showing that a federal right has been denied.)

Conflict over habeas corpus is not new, and indeed has been more severe in the past. Prior to the Civil War, there was considerable conflict over the use of habeas corpus in connection with enforcement of the Fugitive Slave Acts. Habeas corpus was sought from state courts to free fugitive slaves rather than have them returned to their owners, and habeas corpus was also sought from state courts when rescuers were arrested by federal officials for violating the Act. Federal officers were held in contempt of state court for enforcing the law, and were released by federal courts on habeas corpus. Federal and state courts were in direct conflict over this matter, central at the time to the future of the Union. [59]

A substantial increase in federal habeas corpus petitions challenging state convictions resulted from Warren Court rulings. The Burger Court reduced use of federal habeas challenges to state convictions. Chief Justice Burger, saying that the lack of finality in criminal cases resulted in considerable extra work for all courts, complained about state prisoners' ability to challenge their convictions for years after the event, and particularly about multiple, successive habeas filings by the same litigant. [60] The Burger Court began to put its views into rulings by deciding that a federal habeas petition could not be filed until the specific claim it contained had been brought before the state courts. The justices then decided that a defendant could not use a federal habeas corpus petition to challenge a grand jury's composition if that issue had not been raised prior to trial, *unless* the petitioner showed "cause" for such an omission *and* actual prejudice to rights from the challenged unconstitutional action. [61] The justices continued to extend this "cause and prejudice" rule concerning state court procedural defaults.

Particularly significant in the Supreme Court's efforts to limit state prisoners' access to federal courts was the rule (*Stone v. Powell,* 1976) that search and seizure claims already reviewed by a state court could not be raised again in federal court. However, the Court was unwilling to extend *Stone v. Powell* to claims that the right to counsel had been improperly denied.[62] The justices also adopted Chief Justice Burger's basic views on successive habeas petitioners, refusing to preclude them outright but defining quite narrowly the standard (the "ends of justice") under which they would be allowed.[63] The Court has also demanded that deference be given to state court judges when it ruled that, in federal habeas proceedings, state courts' factual determinations must be given a "presumption of correctness" and a federal court overruling such determinations must indicate in writing its basis for doing so.[64] We are likely to see more rulings following the Court's path of vesting in state courts greater final authority on criminal procedure matters, with Supreme Court intervention occurring proportionately more on direct review (that is, direct appeal from the state court of last resort) than in collateral proceedings like habeas corpus.

Notes

1. See Antonin Scalia, "The Doctrine of Standing as an Element of the Separation of Powers," *Suffolk Law Review* 4 (1984): 881–89.

2. *Sosna v. Iowa,* 419 U.S. 393 (1975); *Firefighters v. Stotts,* 467 U.S. 561 (1984).

3. Gregory J. Rathjen and Harold J. Spaeth, "Access to the Federal Courts: An Analysis of Burger Court Policy Making," *American Journal of Political Science* 23 (May 1979): 366.

4. Ibid., p. 374.

5. Ibid., p. 380. However, another study shows Burger and Blackmun increasing their support for access claims. Burton Atkins and William Taggart, "Substantive Access Doctrines and Conflict Management in the U.S. Supreme Court: Reflections on Activism and Restraint," in *Supreme Court Activism and Restraint,* eds. Stephen C. Halpern and Charles Lamb (Lexington, Mass.: Lexington Books, 1982), p. 373.

6. See *Marrese v. American Academy of Orthopaedic Surgeons,* 105 S.Ct. 1327 at 1330 (1985).

7. Robert M. Cover, "The Uses of Jurisdictional Redundancy: Interest, Ideology, and Innovation," *William & Mary Law Review* 22 (Summer 1981): 639 n. 1.

8. See Martha Field, "The Uncertain Nature of Federal Jurisdiction," *William & Mary Law Review* 22 (Summer 1981): 686–87.

9. *World-Wide Volkswagen v. Woodson,* 444 U.S. 286 (1980). And see *Asahi Metal Industry Co. v. Superior Court of California,* 107 S.Ct. 1026 (1987), finding no state court jurisdiction over Japanese manufacturer who sold part to Taiwanese manufacturer whose product caused injury in the United States.

10. *Keeton v. Hustler Magazine,* 465 U.S. 770 (1984).

11. *United States v. Hudson and Goodwin,* 7 Cr. 32 (1812). See Kathryn Preyer, "Jurisdiction to Punish: Federal Authority and the Criminal Law," *Law and History Review* 4 (Fall 1986): 223–65, and Robert C. Palmer, "The Federal Common Law of Crime," *Ibid.:* 267–323.

12. The Court said the former, earlier time. *United States v. Kubrick,* 444 U.S. 111 (1979).

13. Cover, "Uses of Jurisdictional Redundancy," p. 640.

14. For a discussion of the application of the Eleventh Amendment to suits against the state, see *Florida Department of State v. Treasure Salvors, Inc.,* 458 U.S. 670 (1982), which produced a badly divided Court.

15. *Edelman v. Jordan*, 415 U.S. 651 (1974); see also *Papasan v. Allain*, 106 S.Ct. 2393 (1986) (trust income for school lands).

16. *Atascadero State Hospital v. Scanlon*, 105 S.Ct. 3142 (1985) and *Pennhurst State School and Hospital v. Halderman*, 465 U.S. 89 (1984), both decided 5-4.

17. The Court has now had to decide what constitutes official policy. See, e.g., *City of Oklahoma City v. Tuttle*, 105 S.Ct. 2427 (1985) (policy of "inadequate training" of police could not be inferred from single incident) and *Pembaur v. City of Cincinnati*, 106 S.Ct. 1291 (1986) (single incident involving instruction from assistant prosecutor can satisfy the test).

18. *Owen v. City of Independence*, 445 U.S. 622 (1980); *City of Newport v. Fact Concerts*, 453 U.S. 247 (1981).

19. *Imbler v. Pachtman*, 424 U.S. 409 (1976); *Briscoe v. Lahue*, 465 U.S. 325 (1983).

20. *Tileston v. Ullman*, 318 U.S. 44 (1984).

21. *Barrows v. Jackson*, 346 U.S. 259 (1953); *Eisenstadt v. Baird*, 405 U.S. 438 (1972); *Singleton v. Wulff*, 428 U.S. 106 (1976).

22. *Diamond v. Charles*, 106 S.Ct. 1697 (1986).

23. *Peters v. Kiff*, 407 U.S. 493 (1972); *Taylor v. Louisiana*, 419 U.S. 522 (1975).

24. *Automobile Workers v. Brock*, 106 S.Ct. 2523 (1986). See also *NAACP v. Button*, 371 U.S. 415 (1963).

25. *Valley Forge Christian College v. Americans United For Separation of Church and State*, 454 U.S. 464 (1982).

26. *United States v. Richardson*, 418 U.S. 166 (1974); *Schlesinger v. Reservists Committee to End the War*, 418 U.S. 208 (1974).

27. *United States v. Salvucci*, 448 U.S. 83 (1980), overturning *Jones v. United States*, 362 U.S. 257 (1960).

28. *Village of Arlington Heights v. Metropolitan Housing Development Corp.*, 429 U.S. 252 (1977). However, the plaintiff did win on remand.

29. *National Railroad Passenger Corp. v. National Association of Railroad Passengers*, 414 U.S. 453 (1974); *Bread Political Action Committee v. Federal Election Commission*, 455 U.S. 577 (1982); *Federal Election Commission v. National Conservative Political Action Committee*, 105 S.Ct. 1459 (1985); *Trafficante v. Metropolitan Life Insurance Co.*, 409 U.S. 205 (1972).

30. *Cannon v. University of Chicago*, 441 U.S. 667 (1979).

31. *Bivens v. Six Unknown Federal Narcotics Agents*, 403 U.S. 388 (1971); *Carlson v. Green*, 446 U.S. 14 (1980); *Davis v. Passman*, 442 U.S. 228 (1979).

32. *Chappell v. Wallace*, 462 U.S. 296 (1983).

33. *Snyder v. Harris*, 394 U.S. 334 (1969); *Zahn v. International Paper Co.*, 414 U.S. 211 (1973).

34. *Rogers v. Lodge*, 458 U.S. 613 at 632 (1982); *Federal Communication Commission v. League of Women Voters of California*, 468 U.S. 364 at 401 (1984).

35. *Machinists v. Street*, 367 U.S. 640 (1971); see Schwartz, *Super Chief*, pp. 371–72.

36. See *Moore v. Ogilvie*, 394 U.S. 814 (1969).

37. *Carafas v. LaVallee*, 391 U.S. 234 (1968) (challenge to conviction); *Lane v. Williams*, 455 U.S. 624 (1982) (sentences).

38. *Poe v. Ullman*, 367 U.S. 497 (1961); *Griswold v. Connecticut*, 381 U.S. 479 (1965).

39. See *Noyd v. Bond*, 395 U.S. 683 (1969); and *Schlesinger v. Councilman*, 420 U.S. 738 (1975).

40. *Coleman v. Miller*, 307 U.S. 433 (1939); *Luther v. Borden*, 7 How. 1 (1849); *Pacific States Telephone and Telegraph Co. v. Oregon*, 223 U.S. 118 (1912); and *Mississippi v. Johnson*, 4 Wall. 475 (1867).

41. *I.N.S. v. Chadha*, 462 U.S. 919 at 941–42 (1984).

42. See Anthony D'Amato and Robert O'Neil, *The Judiciary and Vietnam* (New York: St. Martin's Press, 1972).

43. See John W. Winkle, "Toward Intersystem Harmony: State-Federal Judicial Councils," *Justice System Journal* 6 (Summer 1981): 240–53.

44. *Oregon v. Hass*, 420 U.S. 714 at 719 (1975) (emphasis in original) (Justice Blackmun). For a discussion of doctrinal interchange between the U.S. Supreme Court and state courts, with each drawing on the other's views, see Stanley H. Friedelbaum, "Reactive Responses: The Complementary Role of Federal and State Courts," *Publius* 17 (Winter 1987): 33–50.

45. *Michigan v. Long*, 463 U.S. 1032 (1983).

46. *Delaware v. Van Arsdall*, 106 S.Ct. 1431 at 1442 (1986); *Massachusetts v. Upton*, 466 U.S. 727 at 735 (1984).

47. *PruneYard Shopping Center v. Robins*, 447 U.S. 74 at 82 (1980). The earlier case was *Lloyd Corp. v. Tanner*, 407 U.S. 551 (1972).

48. *Florida v. Casal*, 462 U.S. 637 at 639 (1983).

49. See *Burlington Northern Railroad Co. v. Woods*, 107 S.Ct. 967 (1987).

50. See David L. Shapiro, "Federal Diversity Jurisdiction: A Survey and a Proposal," *Harvard Law Review* 91 (December 1977): 317–55.

51. See Kristin Bumiller, "Choice of Forum in Diversity Cases: Analysis of a Survey and Implications for Reform," *Law & Society Review* 15 (1980–1981): 749–74; and Jolanta Perlstein, "Lawyers' Strategies and Diversity Jurisdiction," *Law & Policy Quarterly* 3 (July 1981): 321–40.

52. *Georgia v. Rachel*, 383 U.S. 780 (1966); *City of Greenwood v. Peacock*, 383 U.S. 808 (1966).

53. See *Colorado River Water Conservation District v. United States*, 424 U.S. 800 at 815–17 (1976).

54. *Zant v. Stephens*, 456 U.S. 410 (1982).

55. *Preiser v. Rodriguez*, 411 U.S. 475 (1973).

56. *Huffman v. Pursue*, 420 U.S. 592 (1975); *Trainor v. Hernandez*, 431 U.S. 434 (1977); *Ohio Civil Rights Commission v. Dayton Christian Schools*, 106 S.Ct. 2718 (1986).

57. *General Atomic Co. v. Felter*, 434 U.S. 12 (1977) and 436 U.S. 493 (1978).

58. Cover, "Uses of Jurisdictional Redundancy," p. 648.

59. See *Ableman v. Booth*, 21 How. 506 (1859), where the Taney Court overturned a Wisconsin Supreme Court ruling holding the Fugitive Slave Act unconstitutional two years after *Dred Scott*, and the earlier *Prigg v. Pennsylvania*, 16 Pet. 539 (1842), a ruling under the pre-1850 Fugitive Slave Act. See Robert Cover, *Justice Accused* (New Haven, Conn.: Yale University Press, 1975), particularly pp. 175–91.

60. See one of his attacks on state prisoners' excessive use of federal habeas corpus, *Spalding v. Aiken*, 460 U.S. 1093 (1983). For a rejoinder, see *Witt v. Wainwright*, 105 S.Ct. 1415 at 1418–19 (1985) (Justice Marshall).

61. *Picard v. Connor*, 404 U.S. 270 (1971); *Francis v. Henderson*, 425 U.S. 536 (1976). The Court did rule that claims of racial discrimination in state grand jury selection *could* be challenged through federal habeas even if the subsequent trial jury had not been improperly constituted. *Rose v. Mitchell*, 443 U.S. 545 (1979).

62. *Kimmelman v. Morrison*, 106 S.Ct. 2574 (1986).

63. *Kuhlmann v. Wilson*, 106 S.Ct. 2616 (1986).

64. *Sumner v. Mata*, 449 U.S. 539 (1981) and 455 U.S. 491 (1982).

6 The Supreme Court: Its Docket and Screening Decisions

LAWYERS' AND GROUPS' DECISIONS to take cases to the Supreme Court, decisions made within the confines of rules on access to the courts, provide the basic pool from which the Supreme Court, using certain regular procedures, takes its cases. By "skimming off" most cases at early stages and disposing of some others through brief orders (summary dispositions), the Court can concentrate on those it considers worthy of full treatment.

All this is part of *docket management*, which provides the Court with opportunities to engage in strategic actions. Selectivity is crucial to the Court's work—not only administratively but also politically: "It helps to keep the Court abreast of new trends in litigation, and it helps to maintain the Court's flexibility in responding to change."[1] Deciding which cases to accept and which to reject is crucial if the justices are to have cases with the best factual settings for rulings they may be predisposed to make and if they are not to have to hand down the wrong decision at the wrong time.

In this chapter, we look first at the cases brought to the Court, that is, the size and content of its docket, and then at the ways in which the justices skim off most of the cases. We turn in the next chapter to the Court's "full dress treatment" of the remaining cases.

The Court's Business

Docket Size

Some claim that the Supreme Court is overloaded with cases. That claim was made repeatedly from the 1970s on, although made earlier as well. To examine that claim, we need to examine the Court's caseload—the number of cases filed—before turning to the question of whether that is an *over*load requiring a remedy—that is, more necessary work than the Court can do, or a burden in which the number of filings exceeds a level with which the justices can reasonably cope. An increased number of filings—even a substantial increase—does not necessarily mean that the Court is overworked, particularly if many of those cases are relatively simple or do not raise important issues of law. Such a judgment depends on what we expect the Court to do with cases brought to it, such as deciding important cases. The fact that the parties, who will have already had at least one appellate review, would like the Court to hear their case does not mean the case is of sufficient importance beyond their own immediate concerns to justify the justices' devoting their time to it.

The idea of "overload" has both subjective and objective components. The subjective ones are the justices' own views of the conditions under which they are working; objective ones might be, for example, increased time from filing to decision, or observers' judgments, based on some agreed-upon standard, of the quality of the Court's output, although many of the standards are themselves subjective. One can agree that Supreme Court justices work hard without necessarily agreeing that they are *over*worked, because the caseload may be manageable, particularly with the management tool the Judges Bill of 1925 gave the Court in making most of its cases subject to the Court's own decision as to whether it should hear them. Through it, the justices can manage the Court's docket and keep the cases to which it gives full (plenary) treatment at a reasonable level for them, regardless of the number of filings. Put differently, we look first at load and then at the question of *over*load.

A variety of factors in combination affect the number of cases *filed* in the Supreme Court. Some are external to the Court. They include "political, economic, and social forces," which may have a general, perhaps thin, effect on several areas of the Court's docket rather than a focused effect on one area; social problems that are transformed into legal issues, as when concerns about women's position in society led to the women's movement and to sexual discrimination cases; and external events, including some external to the United States, like the Arab oil embargo, which ultimately produced cases concerning federal regulations' preemptive effect on state law.[2] They also include Congress' enactment of new legislation and its creation of new federal judgeships and people's propensity to initiate cases and to appeal them, affected in part by their perceptions of the Court's caseload. Others are internal to the Court: the Court's own actions affect its caseload. The justices' willingness to rule on a topic increases the number of cases filed, just as consistent refusal to review cases on a particular subject results in review being sought in fewer such cases. Similarly, adoption of certain doctrinal rules serves to make clear to potential litigants that it will not be fruitful to bring certain types of cases. If, while deciding cases, the justices make statements indicating the Court would welcome cases raising questions not presently before the Court, lawyers are likely to try to bring those questions to the Court for resolution. If, as critics suggest, the justices feel compelled to take more cases instead of allowing lower courts to resolve them, if they operate from an apparent presumption that only *they* can decide certain cases, an increase in filings is likely.

References to the Supreme Court's *docket* are really references to its dockets. Until 1970, there were three: the Original Docket, for the few original jurisdiction cases; the Appellate Docket, containing certiorari petitions or jurisdictional statements (for appeals) in *paid* cases, that is, where the petitions or statements have been printed; and the Miscellaneous Docket, containing the unpaid or *in forma pauperis* (i.f.p.) cases from those, often prisoners, who cannot afford the regular fees. The Appellate and Miscellaneous Dockets are now combined in the Appellate Docket, but paid and i.f.p. cases can still be distinguished because different numbering systems are used for each. (There are also separate dockets for special motions, for applications for stays of lower court proceedings, and for disbarment of lawyers who are members of the Supreme Court bar.)

Someone qualifying for *in forma pauperis* status has the requirement of a printed submission and the payment of filing fees waived. Starting in 1983, the Court began to question whether some people asserting that they qualified for i.f.p. status in fact did so, by giving them several weeks to produce additional documentation or, in the alternative, pay the docketing fees. Several justices objected, saying that if the Court was going to reject the petition for review in any event, which they said was true of the petitions in question, it was simply making more work for itself for it would now have to examine a resubmitted petition again.[3]

With over 4,000 cases filed each year in the Supreme Court, we tend to forget the Court's small early caseload. From 1790 to 1801, the Court's appellate jurisdiction was invoked in only 87 cases, of which 80 were federal cases (36 diversity of citizenship cases, 35 admiralty cases, and 9 civil cases brought by the government).[4] In the earliest years, workload was largely a matter of circuit duty, not the Court's own small docket. As late as the Civil War years (1862–66), the Court still was not handing down many decisions: 240 cases were decided in that period. However, paralleling an increase in federal district court caseload, the Court's output grew to 1,125 for the 1886–90 period. This post-Civil War docket growth resulted largely from statutory changes, including provision for removal of cases to the federal courts and addition to "federal question" jurisdiction. The passage of the act establishing the courts of appeals in 1891 produced an immediate drop in Supreme Court filings—from over 600 in 1890 to 275 in 1892—and the number of petitions for review continued to decline at the rate of 2 percent during the century's last decade.[5]

Despite a rate of increase in filings of roughly 2 to 3 percent for the first half of the twentieth century, as recently as the early 1940s fewer than 1,000 cases were filed annually. The number of filings fluctuated between 1,000 and 1,500 from 1944–54, and then began rather steady increased growth, reflecting an increased annual rate of filings of 5 percent-plus starting at about midcentury. The result was that the Court was dealing in 1971 with three-and-one-half times as many cases as 20 years earlier and roughly seven to eight times the number it had confronted in 1925, when it received full certiorari authority. Despite a slight, uneven decline after 1973, filings again increased, reaching over 4,400 in the 1981 Term,[6] but dropping slightly the following year and staying relatively stable since then. (See Table 6.1.) Roughly half the increase in filings in the 1970s was in unpaid cases, primarily prisoner petitions, which increased in part because of the 1964 Criminal Justice Act provision for appointed counsel for indigent federal criminal defendants. New federal statutes containing new causes of action also contributed to the larger "pool" of cases from which lawyers sought review in the Supreme Court, as did the Court's rulings recognizing new substantive rights.

In evaluating this picture, one should keep several things in mind. One is that the *rate* of increase decreased after 1968, but the larger base meant that absolute increases in filings were substantial. Another is that the increases of the decade ending in 1972, with filings growing from 2,200 to over 3,600, did not continue, with the 1983 Term figure only 16 percent over that for the 1971 Term; had the earlier rate continued, there would have been almost 6,100 cases filed in the 1981 Term instead of the actual 4,400 plus.[7] A third is the possibility that there are cases not being filed because people feel that the probability of obtaining a decision on the merits was not worth the expense or, particularly, the delay. In short, a feeling that the Court has been inundated by filings or is "overloaded" (see below) may lead to the existence of a *hidden docket*. However, given the relative ease of filing cases *in forma pauperis* if one is poor or the existence of many "noncertworthy" petitions now being filed, it may be unlikely that there are many other cases not being brought to the Court that would be plausible candidates for review.

Table 6.1 Supreme Court Filings (rounded)

1955	1,600	1967	3,100	1980	4,200
1956	1,800	1969	3,400	1981	4,400
1960	1,900	1971	3,600	1983	4,200
1961	2,200	1973	3,900	1986	4,300
1965	2,800				

Source: Gerhard Casper and Richard A. Posner, *The Workload of the Supreme Court*, p. 3; updated.

Has the Supreme Court been able to keep pace with the filings? The Court is current with its work in the sense that, except for a few cases set for reargument the next term, all cases argued within a term are disposed of during that same term; in this sense, the Court has no backlog. By the late 1970s, the Court was carrying over for argument roughly the same number of cases as had been on the argument calendar at term's beginning. However, the Court continued to accept more cases for argument without similarly increasing the number of cases argued so that the argument calendar filled up earlier each year—by Christmas recess in the 1981 Term. However, in the 1982 Term, the Court significantly reduced the number of cases accepted for hearing (179 as against 201 in the 1981 Term), and reduced the figure even more—to around 150—the following term. The Court under Chief Justice Burger generally handed down 140 to 150 decisions a year (covering roughly 180 cases, some of which are consolidated in a single decision), up from an average of 115 per term during the 1950s and 1960s. In addition, numerous summary rulings are issued—some 15 to 20 with opinions per term, plus 15 or so summary affirmances with one- or two-line orders, 80 to 90 dismissals of appeals that are rulings on the merits and an additional 40 to 90 rulings in which review is granted and the case is returned to the lower court for further consideration on the basis of intervening Supreme Court rulings.

Although cases are carried over from one term to the next, in most recent years the Court has disposed of roughly as many cases as have been filed, thus not leaving a growing backlog. Although going into Warren Burger's tenure there had been an increase in the carryover, after his first few terms the Court actually disposed of more cases than were filed, particularly in the 1974–76 Terms; this reduced the number of cases not acted upon during the term (carryover + cases docketed - dispositions). The cases remaining at term's end numbered in the high 800s into the early 1980s.[8]

The time the Court has taken to deal with cases, at least with its initial screening decisions, has been fairly steady. Screening decisions are generally made within three months of a case's being filed—except when the filing comes late in the term, in which case no decision is reached until October. Except for the October "bulge," screening decisions issue relatively steadily during the term. Cases accepted for review may remain in the system for extended periods of time, but that depends in part on whether they come from the federal or state courts (longer if from federal court), are appeals rather than certiorari cases (longer for appeals), and whether amicus briefs are filed (longer if they are).[9]

Overload. Is the Court, as some justices and some observers claim, overloaded? High, even increasing caseload, does not necessarily mean *overload*, for increases in supporting staff, such as law clerks, have enabled the Court to cope with higher caseload and, as just noted, the Court has not increased dramatically the number of cases to which it gives plenary (full) treatment each term. Like the bumblebee the physicists said could not fly, the Court continues to function—effectively—even when complaints about caseload might lead one to believe that was not possible. "Overload" complaints were made even when docket size was much smaller, for example, before the courts of appeals were established and again before certiorari jurisdiction was provided. However, in those earlier days, the justices did have to decide all cases—and the Court's ability to delete easier cases means the justices are left with more difficult ones to decide, so that, even if numbers remained the same, workload would increase.

The "overload" argument has, however, been renewed with particular force in the last two decades, and concerns have been raised about the effect of increased caseload on the *quality* of the Court's work. Certainly claims that the Court does not have time for adequate deliberation, or, on the other hand, adequate time to devote to screening cases for review, should be given serious attention. Justice Rehnquist has argued that for the Court to be current in its docket is insufficient: "It is essential that it have the necessary time for careful deliberation and reasoned decision of the very important types of cases which are the staple of its business."[10] However, it has been argued, "History provides little support for the assertion that a smaller docket leads to wiser adjudications or more illuminating opinions," and decisions handed down only after long consideration—like the School Desegregation Cases of 1954 and 1955 and the abortion rulings of 1973—were much criticized not only for their results but also for lack of craftsmanship;[11] with more time, the justices might write more, adding to the "noise" in the system.

In the last few years, more justices have spoken out about workload—even if they do not support a remedy, or any particular remedy, for it. New members of the Court have been more likely to complain about overwork, and to utter such complaints less as they got accustomed to the pattern of work. Justice Douglas said that "no Justice of this court need work more than four days a week to carry his burden," which he claimed was "comfortable" even when he was hospitalized, and he argued that the Court was "if anything, underworked, not overworked."[12] Other justices have agreed with him, needling their colleagues for complaining about overwork when they insisted on taking cases of little importance and did not show sufficient respect for decisions of either the U.S. courts of appeals or the state courts. The justices cannot resist taking cases that will allow them to reach particular results; for the present Court, this is particularly true where the lower court has decided in favor of a defendant in a criminal case. Despite the effect of their ideological proclivities on their choice of cases, the justices find that there are some matters they almost *have* to take, at least eventually if not immediately when they are first presented. Included would be such matters as certain church-state issues, cases that follow up their 1973 abortion ruling, death penalty procedures, and, if it reaches them, the challenge to the constitutionality of the "independent counsel" (special prosecutor) provisions.

The Court's creating more work for itself is a situation that has existed over the years. The justices, if they really wanted to reduce workload, could find reasons *not* to take cases, but they seem to reach in the other direction. Thus the way the Court has limited the "adequate state ground" doctrine (see page 180) allows the Court to take more, not fewer, cases. In earlier years, the Court interpreted federal question jurisdiction in a way that added to its docket, and it was true years ago as it is now that despite the justices' complaints of overwork, "a few important cases decided differently would have had the effect of discouraging much litigation."[13] As Casper and Posner observe, "A frequently overlooked point is the extent to which the Supreme Court itself controls the demand for its services through its power to recognize a new, or extinguish a recognized, federal statutory or constitutional right by interpreting or reinterpreting a federal statute or constitutional provision."[14] Individual justices also make more work for themselves by writing concurring and dissenting opinions—written in addition to their regular "opinions for the Court," not instead of them.

If the Court has in some ways made more work for itself, the justices have also done some things to reduce their workload—just as they did in pressing for the Judges Bill of 1925, which gave them their present discretionary jurisdiction. The justices were at the forefront of the move to eliminate direct appeals from three-judge district courts (see pages 47-48), and have pressed for elimination of remaining mandatory jurisdiction. However, removing diversity of citizenship cases from federal jurisdiction (see pages 182-83), which they also favor, would assist the lower federal courts but have very little effect on the Supreme Court's own burden. In areas of the law where the justices perceive a significant increase in filings, they have acted to limit them, for example, by seeking to limit use of federal habeas corpus by state prisoners. The caseload argument may well be a neutral-sounding excuse for the justices' value positions—particularly as it is the conservative members of the Court who have used the argument when civil liberties claims are turned aside.

Chief Justice Burger suggested that prospective appellants get approval from the courts before they could appeal their cases, and he led moves within the Court to penalize those bringing "frivolous" appeals. In 1983, acting under its Rule 49.2, which permits an award of "appropriate damages" to the appellee when appellant's case is "frivolous," the Court made such an award (of $500) in a case.[15] In 1985, Burger renewed his call for more such action "in egregious cases" in order to "discourage many of the patently meritless applications that are filed here each year," but he was met with a rejoinder from four justices that the time necessary to determine which of the meritless petitions warranted sanctions "would be a time-consuming and unrewarding task."[16]

Since the concern about overload was revived in the 1970s by Chief Justice Burger and the Commission on the Federal Court Appellate System (the Hruska Commission), it has had a specific focus—whether the nation has sufficient judicial capacity to decide cases of national importance and whether the Supreme Court can provide that capacity without assistance from a new court, the National Court of Appeals (see pages 62-63). The claim is that issues requiring a uniform national position, such as interpretations of frequently used statutes, are going undecided, and that intercircuit conflict, conflicts in position between the U.S. courts of appeals, are not resolved promptly. (This is a particular concern of

Justice Byron White, who notes what he feels are intercircuit conflicts when he dissents from the Court's denial of review.) The Commission pressed this view, saying that the absence of adequate capacity for the declaration of national law led to lack of Supreme Court review for cases that 20 years earlier would certainly have been accepted. The Commission also felt that unresolved intercircuit conflict led to repetitive litigation, further increasing filings in the Supreme Court; absent adequate decisional capacity, the Supreme Court would be forced to take cases "otherwise not worthy of its resources" because it was the only court capable of resolving conflicts between the circuits.[17] Yet even with a lower caseload, the Supreme Court has not always handed down many decisions in any particular area of the law and, more important, the area in which it has handed down most decisions—Fourth Amendment search and seizure law—has remained one of considerable confusion, not clarity.[18]

Even if there were consensus on instances of intercircuit conflict, not all need immediate resolution by the Supreme Court. Left alone, some disappear: a trend develops and the "minority position" dissolves. Not resolving a conflict immediately also allows "percolation": lower courts' differing positions provide the Supreme Court with a variety of views on a subject on which the justices can draw when they consider the issue. However, some conflicts may be "intolerable" and should be resolved promptly, for example, "when litigants are able to exploit conflicts affirmatively through forum shopping, or when the planning of primary behavior is thwarted by the absence of a nationally binding rule."[19]

A major difficulty in evaluating claims about overload is that we have lacked a systematic examination of cases to which the Court has granted review. However, such a study was recently undertaken at New York University Law School. Cases were divided into three categories: (1) the priority docket, cases that it was imperative for the Court to hear; (2) the discretionary docket, cases the justices need not hear but could reasonably review; and (3) improvident grants, where the criteria for the first two categories are absent. Specified criteria for the categories were based on clearly stated assumptions about the Supreme Court's roles (see pages 30-36), particularly the notion that the Court should function as a manager of the judicial system, delegating responsibilities to subordinates and presuming their decisions valid. In particular, much weight was given to "percolation" of issues in the lower courts rather than having the Court accept conflicts as soon as they developed.

Close analysis of the Court's 1982 Term showed that almost half (48%) of the cases to which review was granted belonged on the priority docket; included were intolerable conflicts, conflicts with Supreme Court precedents, and resolution of important federalism issues and interbranch disputes. Somewhat more than one-fourth (28%) were located on the discretionary docket; included were cases presenting opportunities to develop federal law. Another one-fourth (24%) were found to be improvident grants. Thus "a significant portion of the Court's present capacity is misused, and might be devoted more productively to other types of cases"[20]; had the Court *not* heard these cases, it most certainly would not have been overworked.

Docket Content

The content of the Court's docket is at least as significant as its size. Over time that content has shifted toward cases raising constitutional questions. In the nineteenth century and extending into the twentieth century, the Supreme Court was primarily a private law court. Cases with constitutional questions began to increase in the 1930s, when matters of due process constituted the greatest portion; other constitutional cases then involved the Commerce Clause, impairment of contract, and full faith and credit. Prior to 1960, nonconstitutional holdings made up two-thirds to three-fourths of the Court's rulings. However, as a result of the Warren Court, constitutional cases constituted one-half to two-thirds of the Court's full-opinion decisions. Cases based on the Bill of Rights were only 5 percent of the constitutional cases in the 1930s, but by the late 1950s they made up over one-third of the cases filed, and *half* in the late 1960s. Much of these changes can be explained by the increase in state criminal cases, almost 100 percent of which entailed constitutional questions.[21]

The Burger Court was expected to give less attention to constitutional problems and more attention to matters of statutory interpretation, in part by shifting from civil liberties cases to commercial or regulatory litigation. At first, there was a shift toward economic issues, with a concomitant decrease in criminal and habeas corpus cases and an increase in private civil actions accepted,[22] but after a few terms, it became clear that the Burger Court, instead of "deconstitutionalizing" its working docket, was going to be largely a constitutional court, and, in particular, to be a *civil rights court*. Cases with constitutional individual rights issues, just over one-fourth of the plenary docket in the 1959 Term, displaced other types of cases on the docket during the 1960s so that by the 1970s they became the plenary docket's largest single component—over two-fifths, and even higher if one adds cases with procedural issues affecting individual rights and those with individual rights as secondary issues.

Criminal procedure cases provided a stable level of business for the Court in the 1970s and 1980s, with a variety of issues making up that business. The predominant issue was search-and-seizure, even after the Court seemed to cut off federal court habeas review of such issues, but there was also significant attention to double jeopardy (particularly in the 1974–77 Terms, when the Court decided more cases than in the preceding 15 terms); right to counsel; self-incrimination; and cruel and unusual punishment—specifically, aspects of the death penalty. Most federal criminal defendants seeking the Court's review came to the Court as indigents, although there were also numerous "paid" petitions seeking review of federal criminal convictions; somewhat more state criminal defendants seeking review of their cases were "paid" than was true of federal defendants, but most of the state cases were also "unpaid." As time progressed, the Court took a substantially greater portion of its criminal cases from state courts—nearly half by the late 1970s—but it was interested in cases brought by state *prosecutors* challenging prodefendant rulings.[23]

The Court's continuing attention to criminal procedure cases, although the Warren Court and Burger Court did so for different reasons (one to protect defendants' rights, the other to limit those rights), raises the question of whether the Supreme Court has an *agenda* and, if so, how it proceeds to implement it. Certainly the Court does not announce an agenda in the way a president or governor or legislative leader would announce it; instead, the agenda is implicit, to be inferred by observers. Changes in the number of criminal procedure cases decided did not, over a 40-year period including the early Burger Court, appear to have reflected changes in the incidence of crime, media coverage of crime, or public concern about crime or changes in that concern, despite all the attention given to "law and order" starting with the late 1960s. What did make a difference were the controlling justices' differing ideologies and changes in chief justices, with the Court significantly more likely to increase the number of criminal justice decisions when liberals controlled the Court than when conservatives did.[24]

If justices have an agenda that they are able to carry out, we must recognize that, while the Court's "agenda-building has purposive elements," it also "varies by policy area," and, at least equally as important, there are constraints on its implementation. For example, independent of the justices' values, the Court needs to take some cases to correct lower court error or to clarify rules. And, because "demands for Court activity are responses to earlier decisions," it takes some time before justices' desires to deal with a particular area of law are reflected in the cases brought to the Court to which review can be granted.[25]

In addition to criminal procedure and free expression cases, equal protection cases and cases on access to the courts have accounted for most of the recent growth in the civil rights component of the Court's plenary docket. The freedom of expression area illustrates that subjects prominent for a while then fade from view as the Court clarifies the law so that it need not take new cases until a new aspect of the problem appears. This was true of a question like access to the ballot by minor political parties and independent candidates. It was also true of obscenity, where there were 20 decisions in the 1959–76 Terms but only three rulings in the seven subsequent terms; the more recent cases dealt with methods for controlling obscenity, not defining it, which had been the earlier focus.

Equal protection cases involving racial discrimination issues increased several-fold from 1959 through the mid-1970s but then declined, remaining as only a small part of the plenary docket. There were, however, few school desegregation cases, with more attention to other aspects of racial discrimination. Although reapportionment received less attention in the 1970s than earlier, there were new areas of equal protection litigation to which the Court gave attention in the 1970s and 1980s: illegitimacy, the rights of aliens, and gender discrimination.[26]

(By contrast to its willingness to deal with women's rights issues, the Court has been unwilling to deal with the concerns of homosexuals and lesbians, and when it did do so in 1986, in *Bowers v. Hardwick*, was resoundingly negative.)

Dominance by constitutional individual rights cases did not mean exclusion of other types of cases from the plenary docket. Cases involving separation of powers, in which the Court performs its role as umpire among the three branches, and federalism, where it serves as umpire among the levels of government, although a smaller proportion of the docket, were present in significant numbers. After the late Warren Court's decrease in interest in federalism issues, interest revived—with a focus on such matters as federal preemption of state powers and whether states had exceeded their authority, especially in matters of interstate commerce. [27]

Cases involving interpretation of federal statutes, earlier accounting for at least 40 percent of the Court's plenary docket, after the 1967 Term took up less than 30 percent of the docket and the subject matter shifted considerably, showing the effect on the Court's docket of laws Congress enacts. New statutes, on environmental protection, occupational health and safety, securities regulation, pension plans, and employment discrimination, along with Freedom of Information Act (FOIA) cases, came to the fore, and older aspects of labor law received less attention in the business regulation area, antitrust provided the largest segment of cases, and there was an obvious decline in Interstate Commerce Commission cases—one "fallout" from deregulation. [28] Among "federal specialties," Federal Employer Liability Act (FELA) cases, once a staple of the Court's business, and admiralty cases were almost totally gone from the docket. Such changes indicate the Court's ability to respond to the need for interpretation of new statutes but also illustrate the "episodic nature of the Court's intervention," which "stands out even more strongly in the realm of statutory law" than elsewhere. [29]

This broad picture of docket content and trends should not obscure the rich variety of particular issues the Court explores in any single term. Although in 1973 there were five antitrust and four welfare rights decisions, and in 1976 there were 10 double jeopardy cases, rarely are there more than one or two cases per term on any single issue, and multiple cases on only a few broad topics such as employment discrimination or search and seizure. This results from the Court's seldom deciding more than 150 cases with full opinion and its attempt to develop law on the many topics on which people have sought its guidance and direction. The range of legal concerns with which the Court deals is illustrated by a partial listing of issues decided during the October 1985 Term:

- scope of bank regulation
- regulation of natural gas sales
- effect of bankruptcy on environmental obligations
- imposition of liability for withdrawal from pension plans

- antitrust implications of rent control laws
- taxability of "unrelated business income"
- state control of liquor prices
- adequacy of notice for farm loans
- state taxes on aviation fuel
- compliance with whaling agreements

The list also includes a wide range of civil liberties matters:

- prosecution by two states as double jeopardy
- dismissal from university for academic reasons
- zoning for adult theaters
- required inserts in utility bills
- liability for shooting of prisoner during riot
- police failure to notify defendant of availability of counsel
- wearing yarmulke on military duty
- probable cause to seize obscene material
- racial use of peremptory challenges of jurors
- aerial view searches
- layoffs under affirmative action plans
- "Baby Doe" regulations
- execution of mentally ill prisoner
- application of Rehabilitation Act to commercial airlines
- open preliminary hearings
- partisan gerrymandering
- ban on advertising of gambling

"Skimming Off": Case Selection

Before reaching those cases to which it will give full (plenary) treatment, the Supreme Court "skims off" many other cases, by denying review and otherwise deciding cases summarily. The decisions denying review and summarily disposing of cases are generally of low visibility. Moreover, reasons underlying them are often well hidden. The sheer numbers of such decisions and the variety of factors potentially playing a part in any particular Court action further mask their meaning but do not decrease their extreme importance, which stems from the fact that such decisions account for the bulk of the Court's actions, far exceeding in number the Court's formal statements of policy. For the Court to make a decision not to hear a case may be as important—not only for the litigants but also for the (unaware) public—as for it to decide particular controversial questions explicitly. The patterns of the Court's actions, reinforced by statements by some of the justices, provide strong evidence that the Court's actions denying review have clear policy implications.

The Court's means for managing its docket have varied. At times the Court has sought additional statutory authority to reduce the proportion of cases it must decide, as when it obtained its discretionary jurisdiction in the 1925 Judges Bill. The Court has also taken its appeals jurisdiction, theoretically mandatory, and made it discretionary in fact. Also, many appeals have been disposed of summarily, a recognition of the Court's flexibility. As early as a hundred years ago, the Court allowed appeals (formerly writs of error) to be affirmed on motion without argument when the appeal appeared to be frivolous or to have been undertaken for purposes of delay.

The important shift toward de facto discretionary treatment of appeals came in 1928, when the Court requested submission of a *jurisdictional statement* stating why the Court should take the case, later extended to indicating why the question was "substantial." For the Court to take an appeal from a state court, the case must contain a "substantial" *federal* question; appeals from federal courts must also raise "substantial" questions. A large proportion of appeals do not meet these standards as the Court has applied them, with many cases dismissed "for want of a substantial federal question" and slightly fewer dismissed for want of jurisdiction; the Court often then treats the latter as certiorari petitions and also denies certiorari. Although dismissal for lack of jurisdiction is not a ruling on the merits, dismissal for want of a substantial federal question is more than a rejection of review. Such a dismissal is formally considered to be a decision on the merits because of the requirement that appeals be decided. The Court has reminded lawyers and judges that in such cases "a federal constitutional issue was properly presented, it was within our appellate jurisdiction . . . and we had no discretion to refuse adjudication of the case on its merits. . . . We were not obligated to grant the case plenary consideration; and we did not; but we were required to deal with its merits."[30]

The Supreme Court expects lower courts to be bound by such rulings, just as it expects them to be bound by full opinion decisions. This causes several problems. Because the Supreme Court has not described the facts and issues covered by lower court rulings in such cases, or explained the basis for its dismissals beyond the "want of a substantial federal question" language, lower court judges are faced with a tedious task in comparing cases they have under consideration with previous Supreme Court summary actions, and then often have a difficult time deciding what the justices intended, for example, *why* they felt no "substantial federal question" was presented. According to Justice Brennan, making such dismissals rulings on the merits also deprives the Supreme Court of lower courts' thinking on complex legal problems: being bound by the dismissals, those courts are expected only to *apply* them, not to explore further the issues in them.

In picking and choosing from among the cases that people wish the Court to consider, the justices rule on about half of those that fall in the appeals category, handling most with summary rulings, and select for further action a small proportion of those brought on certiorari—a proportion that has decreased from

17.5 percent in 1941 to 11.1 percent 10 years later, to 7.4 percent in 1961, and to below 5 percent since 1971 as the number of certiorari filings has increased while the number of decisions by the Court has remained relatively stable.

In managing its docket, the Court must reduce the number of cases to a reasonable amount, but in doing so it does not pick cases at random or through some previously adopted formula. For one thing, there are some cases that the justices find quite difficult to ignore. Included are challenges to major new federal statutes such as the public accommodations section of the 1964 Civil Rights Act and the 1965 Voting Rights Act and instances of extreme resistance to the Court's rulings, such as the Little Rock school desegregation situation, when the Court not only departed from its pattern of not reviewing cases in that area but also held a special session to hear the case. These cases also show that other units of government—Congress, the president, and state officials—have definite effects on the Court's agenda. The justices must, however, take care not to concentrate their efforts disproportionately in one or only a few areas of case law, for that constrains its ability to take up other issues. The Court must also be concerned with the timing of its decisions in relation to external events such as Congress' consideration of legislation and to its own major rulings, which the justices do not wish to undercut. When the court enters a policy area but hesitates to follow through—true with school desegregation after *Brown v. Board of Education*—disobedience to its will may be encouraged. Accepting cases allows the Court to prevent departure from its policy to or indicate that aspects of certain issues have not been settled; rejecting cases allows the Court to show that certain questions are settled, that it does not wish to comment further on the issues.

Despite constraints of these types, the Court does have considerable flexibility in case selection. The wide variety of issues that people want the justices to hear does allow the Court to avoid certain fields completely, at least in the short run, and its pattern of accepting cases for review varies from one policy area to another. In some areas the Court accepts virtually all cases, as it did with sit-in cases in the early 1960s, but in others it may take very few, as it did in school desegregation after *Brown*. Docket management also involves selecting cases of desired breadth or narrowness, weeding out cases with peripheral issues and altering issues presented by the parties. When lawyers seeking review present several questions of varying breadth, the Court can limit its grant of review to one or more of the questions presented. The more issues raised in the request, the more likely the Court is to limit those for which review is granted. The Court may instead choose cases that focus directly on a broad issue "to establish a broad precedent applicable to cases percolating in the lower courts or being readied for the 'launching pad'" and thus to "head off large numbers of cases" coming to Court.[31] The Court can reach the same goal by adding issues to cases—by asking lawyers to address questions not raised in their petitions for review. If offered only a small number of cases in a particular issue area, the Court can use this ability to increase the number of issues to provide complexity otherwise provided by a larger number (and wider range) of cases. Such issue modification is more likely to occur in cases brought to the Court on certiorari than on appeal, because it fits better with the discretionary character of certiorari.

Summary Dispositions

The decision to grant review is linked to the decision on how to process a case. Most cases accepted for review proceed to plenary consideration—full briefing, oral argument, and a full opinion signed by the author. However, some (see page 194) are given summary treatment, being decided solely on the basis of the certiorari or appeals papers, with only a one- or two-line statement issued to explain how the case is being decided. Summary treatment may, however, result in a full but usually unsigned *per curiam* ("by the Court") opinion. First used only to indicate cases with "indisputably clear" substantive law, *per curiam* rulings were later also used for orders in original jurisdiction cases, dismissals of appeals for want of a substantial federal question, and obviously moot cases. There are, however, some *per curiam* dispositions that announce substantive law. This was a relatively uncommon event until the mid-1960s, as the Court generally did not write opinions in cases to which plenary treatment (full briefing and oral argument) had not been given, but it was not uncommon thereafter, particularly with the Burger Court.[32]

Use of a *per curiam* ruling rather than a signed opinion may indicate that a case is considered routine or noncontroversial or may be used to signal that the outcome is obvious and should receive prompt compliance, as in the 1969 ruling ending "all deliberate speed" in school desegregation (*Alexander v. Holmes County*). However, the Court does sometimes use *per curiam* opinions in argued cases when it is very badly divided; there the opinion is limited to policy on which the justices can agree, and each justice or group of justices separately spells out their reasoning.)

Another type of summary disposition is the Court's sending a case back to the lower courts so it can be reconsidered on the basis of a Supreme Court ruling rendered after the lower court first decided the case.[33] Here the Court grants certiorari, vacates the lower court ruling, and remands for "reconsideration in light of" a specified recently decided case. These GVR (granted/vacated/remanded) rulings, which replace the Warren Court practice of using summary reversals to dispose of cases affected by a new and controlling Supreme Court decision, are largely a Burger Court phenomenon: there were 289 in the 1975–79 Terms and 69 in the 1982 Term alone. The implication of the GVR order is that something is wrong in the lower court's ruling; the Court's denying review of some questioned lower court decisions held pending the decision in another case with the same issue, while using a GVR disposition for others, would tend to suggest approval of the former.

All the types of summary dispositions used by the Court have been criticized for providing insufficient guidance to lower court judges and lawyers. Summary decisions without opinion lead people to try to figure out what the Court meant in its brief order with its citation of one or two cases. With a summary affirmance, one cannot tell whether the Court has merely affirmed the lower court's result or adopted its reasoning. The lack of an opinion in summary reversals can leave the lower court in the dark about whether it has applied the wrong law or applied the proper law erroneously. Compounding the difficulties summary rulings produce is that the Court has indicated that they are not to be given the same precedential weight as the Court's full opinions.

When the Court, facing a case involving novel legal issues or significantly changing or extending the law, decides it with an opinion announcing new law but without full briefing and oral argument on the basis of only the certiorari or appeals papers, there are quite likely to be complaints from some of the justices. Such complaints were made when the Court, without full briefing and argument, sustained a 40-year prison term for possession of marijuana against a cruel and unusual punishment claim,[34] and when, in the *Snepp* case, the justices ordered a former Central Intelligence Agency employee to disgorge the profits from his book because he breached his duty to submit material for prepublication review. Recently, dissenters have claimed that the Court's use of such decisions is "one-sided," favoring prosecutors as the Court reverses prodefendant lower court rulings but not proprosecution rulings.[35]

Despite these protests, summary dispositions do provide the justices an additional option for cases to which the Court does not have time for full-dress treatment but on which they wish to act. Summary dispositions also allow the Court to "clean up" a large number of cases in a particular policy area. They may also be used to make clear to lower court judges that their rulings need to be reexamined and cases disposed of more completely in the lower courts. Summary actions may also preserve freedom of action for the justices by providing a result, and thus perhaps an implicit message, without the constraints that full development of doctrinal reasons would impose. However, a summary action's visibility may be too low for the ruling to have its intended effect, particularly when resistance to the Court's policy exists. Thus the Court's mid-1960s attempt to communicate through *per curiam* rulings that desegregation should take place more rapidly was generally ignored, requiring more explicit rulings in 1968 and 1969.

Certiorari: The Process of Choice

The power to grant or deny certiorari is fully discretionary. Yet the Court's choice of cases is not random. This leads one to question whether the Court is a passive body waiting until someone brings a "case or controversy" for decision. A discretionary jurisdiction court like the Supreme Court *is* active. The ability to pick and choose cases makes it like a fisherman of cases: the Court can't place fish in the stream, that is, it cannot create a lawsuit where none exists, but it may stimulate others to stock the stream when the Court's pattern of granting review or the justices' statements prompt litigation to resolve previously undecided or currently unsettled issues. Particularly when those fishing (the justices) change, there may also be changes in those who stock the streams; for example, the change in membership from the Warren Court to the Burger Court led to a partial shift from defendants seeking to suppress evidence or to reverse convictions to prosecutors seeking to have judges' suppression of evidence reversed. In short, the Court's activity may increase the level of nutrients for certain types of fish more than for others, while for other types of cases the Court may provide "acid rain," killing off—or at least reducing—certain types of fish, although it may take considerable time before the Court's actions have an effect.

By *custom*, certiorari is granted by a vote of at least four justices, the "rule of four" that is also applicable to decisions to "note probable jurisdiction" in an appeal. An important norm is that once the "rule of four" has been satisfied, the justices who opposed review, if they comprise a five-judge majority, should *not* turn around and vote to dismiss the case, and *all* should participate in deciding it on the merits. Yet this norm can be violated. Justice Frankfurter did that in Federal Employer Liability Act (FELA) cases; because he thought the Court should not review those cases, he refused to participate in deciding them. If all the justices followed Justice Frankfurter's practice, the Rule of Four would be a Rule of Five, suggested by Justice Stevens as an alternative to adoption of other major changes to deal with the Court's caseload; he said that in between 23 and 30 percent of cases in the 1979–81 Terms, there were only four votes for certiorari; according to Justice Brennan, either the minimum four votes or five votes are cast to hear a case in well over half the Court's screening decisions, with relatively few of the Court's decisions to grant review unanimous (only 9 percent in the 1972 Term).[36]

Despite Justice Frankfurter, adherence to the "rule of four" is generally routine, but controversy can still develop over it. For example, Justice Rehnquist recently complained that the Court violated it by not considering an issue raised in a certiorari petition in a case that the Court decided on other grounds,[37] suggesting that the continued vitality of the Rule of Four is fragile. We can also see this in the context of the Court's policy to "hold" the review decision in some cases until after the Court has decided another pending case with the same issue. A decision to "hold" also requires four votes, but Justice Brennan complained in 1986 that a five-justice majority was subverting that rule by refusing to continue a stay of execution in a death penalty case until the Court had ruled on the certiorari petition in the case.[38]

There are some instances in which four justices, having satisfied the "rule of four" so that a case can be reviewed, do not insist that the Court hear the case. For example, four justices who regularly voted to grant certiorari in obscenity cases, an area in which the Burger Court's majority was firm, said they would not insist the cases be heard because they knew the other five justices would constitute a regular majority on the merits. Justice Stevens has now suggested that such an alignment is a sufficient reason for the four to vote to deny certiorari, rather than going through the motions of a separate statement.[39]

The process by which the decision is made to grant or deny certiorari ends in a vote at a conference of the justices, but for the most part, it is the result of nine individual decisions; indeed, we can talk about nine separate certiorari processes rather than one process.[40] In the earliest years of certiorari review, under the 1891 Act, each justice received the printed record and briefs, and each justice prepared a memo or note about his views, with each petition discussed by each justice at conference. With relatively few petitions, that was possible, and the Court even gave consideration to having oral argument on the petition.

As the number of certiorari petitions increased, detailed conference consideration of each petition was not possible. However, some justices prepare an outline of issues in the petitions and distribute the outlines prior to the Friday conference, and at times there is also an assignment of memo writing, occasionally to two justices, prior to consideration of the petitions. The absence, until relatively recently, of rapid, reliable photocopying machines meant that there would be only one copy of the petitions from most indigents, the *in forma pauperis* or "unpaid" petitions. The Chief Justice, whose task was to prepare a *dead list* of cases that were not to be discussed at conference—and were automatically denied review—unless such consideration was requested by another justice, had particular responsibility for the unpaid petitions, as part of his task of making the conference presentation of most cases. Now, however, with effective copying machines, each justice receives a copy of all certiorari petitions.

The Chief Justice, whose role is still quite significant, now prepares a *discuss list* (to which all capital punishment cases are automatically added); cases not on that list are not discussed and are denied review unless another justice specifically requests it, and the requesting justice makes the conference presentation if such a case is an "unpaid" one. Thus over time there has been a shift from discussion of every case to discussion of every case not on the dead list, to discussion of a case only if it is on the discuss list. Although the factors accounting for a case's being special-listed are not "easily identifiable," cases on the special list during the tenure of Justice Harold Burton (1947–58) seemed to be those where the certiorari petitions (and law clerks' summaries) contained one or more characteristics that served as "demerits" but "no countervailing considerations in favor of review."[41]

There has also been a shift from all justices doing their own screening of all the petitions—with the assistance of law clerks—to use of a "cert. pool." In this arrangement, initiated by Justice Powell and originally joined by Justices Blackmun, Rehnquist, White, and Chief Justice Burger (and more recently by Justice O'Connor when she replaced Justice Stewart), the certiorari petitions are randomly assigned to the combined clerks from the participating justices' offices; a clerk prepares a memo that is then circulated to all the pool justices (and about which non-pool justices' clerks sometimes inquire).

In the offices of the non-pool justices, clerks also prepare memos on cert. petitions, but those memos tend to be less formal than the pool memos. Justice Stevens has his clerks do memos only on cases he considers "certworthy," and Justice Brennan, although he may ask a clerk to do some research before he makes a decision, reads all the cert. petitions himself once the term begins. This is possible, because a justice with experience in dealing with cert. petitions can reduce a large pile of them to a much more manageable pile in short order; after paying greater attention to the reduced pile, the pile can be reduced still further, for consideration at the conference. No matter how much substance clerks contribute to opinions or to suggestions that a case be accepted for review, it is the *justices*, not the clerks, who are definitely in charge, as Justice Rehnquist (once Justice Robert Jackson's clerk) stated. He did assert, however, that the clerks' political orientations were more liberal than the justices' and affected the cases the clerks recommended the Court take for review.[42]

Although the justices (or a majority of them) cooperate in preparation for the ultimate cert. decision, there is relatively little bargaining or vote-trading in the review-granting/denying process. Largely because of the press of time, there is relatively little communication between the justices' chambers about granting review in particular cases before the justices gather at conference, and most of the justices come prepared to vote in most cases. However, there are times when justices seek additional votes for review by circulating a draft dissent from a denial of review; such drafts pick up votes in perhaps 10 to 30 cases per term. There are also times when a justice, not feeling strongly about a case but willing to have it reviewed, will have marked a petition "Join 3"—that is, if three other members of the Court wish the case reviewed, the "Join 3" justice will vote to grant certiorari. (This is, however, not a "courtesy vote" when the potential fourth vote is indifferent, but a somewhat weak proreview position.)

Once having granted certiorari in a case, the justices can change their minds; in such situations, they dispose of the writ by dismissing it as "improvidently granted" (DIG). They do so when developments affecting the legal posture of a case occur after certiorari is granted, or when briefs or oral argument present a picture different from the one gained from the certiorari petition, which presents less information. Frequent use of the DIG "escape" disposition provokes criticism, and specific instances of its use are also criticized. One occurred when the Court, immediately after *Brown v. Board of Education*, after hearing oral argument in a case involving discrimination by a cemetery association, dividing evenly, and receiving a request for rehearing, dismissed certiorari to avoid deciding the case.[43]

There is also concern within the Court that the DIG disposition will be used to undercut the "Rule of Four." Thus Justice Brennan argued that a justice who had voted *not* to grant review should not vote to dismiss the case until and unless all four justices who had favored review agreed in that disposition, but Justice Stevens thought the Rule of Four was satisfied as long as one justice originally favoring certiorari was in the majority voting to dismiss. Later he argued that, while the Court should usually decide a case on the merits once four justices had voted to grant certiorari, there was "*always* an important intervening development that may be decisive in leading a majority to DIG a case—the Court's consideration of the case after full briefing and argument, which might cast new light on it."[44]

Reasons for Granting. The granting of certiorari is discretionary but not random. The Court need not give any reasons in granting, denying, or dismissing review, and seldom does so. Chief Justice Warren claimed that "the standards by which the justices decide to grant or deny review are highly personalized and necessarily discretionary. . . . Those standards cannot be captured in any rule or guidelines that would be meaningful."[45] However, there has also been talk of "*informed* discretion" or "*informed* arbitrariness." References to justices' ability to determine *certworthiness* (a case's significance for review) suggest that even if a large degree of "feel" or educated intuition remains in the process, there are regular criteria on which there is concensus. However, because litigants or potential litigants "differ in their capacity to deduce probable review criteria from the pattern of grants and denials and the Court's meager guidelines on review criteria," those with considerable experience and expertise in the process of seeking review ("repeat players") "tend to benefit from the obscurity of standards for review," while those who are inexperienced lack that advantage.[46]

The court only occasionally says much about why specific cases have been accepted for review. Seldom is the Court's statement more than "We accepted this case in order [to answer the question presented]." At times the importance of the case is noted or a comment is made about the "substantial" or "novel" question presented. Beyond these usual noncommunicative reasons, the need to resolve a conflict between the circuits is the principal reason frequently mentioned. There are, however, times when the Court does tell us more. For example, in a case involving prompt access under the Freedom of Information Act to the Federal Reserve System's monetary policy directives, the Court granted review "on the strength of the Committee's representations that the ruling could seriously interfere with the implementation of national monetary policy." And cases on Indians' treaty fishing rights were accepted to allow the Court to "interpret [an] important treaty provision and thereby to resolve . . . conflict between the state and federal courts . . . and to remove any doubts about the federal court's power to enforce its orders."[47]

In its Rule 17 (formerly Rule 19), the Court has set forth an official statement of some factors it will *consider* in deciding whether to grant certiorari. Rule 17 stresses legal considerations, and thus is incomplete. In addition to the matters raised there, the presence of an "adequate and independent" state ground (see page 180) has also always been understood to bar Supreme Court review or, if it were discovered after review had been granted, to serve as a basis for dismissing certiorari. Where it is unclear whether a state court has based its ruling on state or federal law, the Court can defer acting on a certiorari petition until a certificate is obtained from the state court explaining its action (see page 184) or the Court can grant the petition and vacate the lower court ruling and remand it for such clarification. However, the Court's ruling in *Michigan v. Long* (1983) that state courts must make a clear statement they are relying on state law means the justices will be likely to rule directly on the petition without use of those options.

CONSIDERATIONS GOVERNING REVIEW ON CERTIORARI

1. A review on writ of certiorari is not a matter of right, but of judicial discretion, and will be granted only when there are special and important reasons therefor. The following, while neither controlling nor fully measuring the Court's discretion, indicate the character of reasons that will be considered.

(a) When a federal court of appeals has rendered a decision in conflict with the decision of another federal court of appeals on the same matter; or has decided a federal question in a way in conflict with a state court of last resort; or has so far departed from the accepted and usual course of judicial proceedings, or so far sanctioned such a departure by a lower court, as to call for an exercise of this Court's power of supervision.

(b) When a state court of last resort has decided a federal question in a way in conflict with the decision of another state court of last resort or of a federal court of appeals.

(c) When a state court or a federal court of appeals has decided an important question of federal law which has not been, but should be, settled by this Court, or has decided a federal question in a way in conflict with applicable decisions of this Court.

(Rule 17, adopted June 30, 1980)

Another element to which the Court will not now give particular weight, but that was earlier mentioned in Rule 19 as a consideration, was the situation in which U.S. courts of appeals had "decided an important state or territorial question in a way in conflict with applicable state or territorial law." As that situation would arise only in diversity of citizenship cases, the change perhaps reflected the Court's lessened interest in such jurisdiction.

Beyond Rule 17, individual justices, in off-the-court statements, have indicated what the Court looks for in considering petitions for review. Chief Justice Vinson once said that the Court does not grant certiorari merely to correct errors of the lower courts, but instead uses the writ to deal with cases with broader effects, "questions whose resolution will have immediate importance far beyond the particular facts and parties involved." And Justice Harlan stated from the bench that "the certiorari jurisdiction was not conferred upon this Court 'merely to give the defeated party in the . . . Court of Appeals another hearing,' . . . or 'for the benefit of the particular litigants,' . . . but to decide issues, 'the settlement of which is of importance to the public as distinguished from . . . the parties.'"[48] More recently, Justice Stevens said he did not "believe that error is a sufficient justification for the exercise of this Court's discretionary jurisdiction," because the Court was "much too busy to correct every error that is called to our attention in the thousands of certiorari petitions that are filed each year."[49] That political—and strategic—considerations in the broadest sense are behind the Court's review-granting choices is also clear from Chief Justice Warren's statement that certiorari jurisdiction was "designed by Congress for a very special purpose . . . not only to achieve control of its docket but also to establish our national priorities in constitutional and legal matters."[50]

The Court's actions may also perhaps be explained by the presence of certain *cues* or characteristics of cases. Some of these cues are relatively fixed (an "index"), while others ("signals") are manipulable (not fixed)—like intercircuit conflicts (not fixed because people disagree about whether there is a conflict).[51] The source of a case and the party seeking review are two index items relevant to whether the Court grants review. As to the former, federal appeals are more likely to be accepted than state appeals, but the proportions of state and federal certiorari petitions accepted are more nearly alike.

The party seeking review has regularly been related to the Court's decision to grant review. In 1947–58, certiorari was granted in 49.1 percent of cases in which the only cue was that the federal government favored review, while the Court accepted only 5.8 percent of cases in which all other parties sought review—the same as when no cue appeared.[52] When the U.S. government sought review, at least one justice was likely to vote for review in most cases—impressive in view of the fact that most denials were unanimous.[53] An example of the continuing presence of the government-as-party cue comes in the observation that "in most areas of business regulation, the Court's voice is seldom heard except when the Solicitor General persuades the Justices that an erroneous ruling in the court below threatens an important government program."[54] (See pages 145-46.) Particularly important has been the presence of government prosecutors seeking review. In the 1983 Term, for example, federal prosecutors were granted review in almost every case in which they sought it, compared to a very small fraction of requests brought by defendants being granted.[55]

With respect to subject matter cues, one study showed that presence of an economic issue alone did little to improve chances of review being granted. However, a civil rights or civil liberties issue had significant, positive effects when it was the only cue present, and later analysis showed a high correlation between presence of a civil liberties or civil rights petitioner and granting of review. However, cases with civil liberties issues were certainly not immune from being "dead-listed," although they met this fate less frequently than cases without cues.[56] Cue analysis has also shown that certiorari was granted in 12.8 percent of cases where the sole cues were disagreement between *judges* in a single court, that is, nonunanimous decisions, or disagreement between *courts*, such as where an appeals court had reversed the trial court. Disagreement *within* a court of appeals may provide a stronger signal to the justices than disagreement *between* levels, although the lack of clear findings on this matter is shown by the conclusion of another study that, overall, "the Supreme Court . . . is not primarily guided by lower court agreement—either intercourt or intracourt—in deciding the cases it will hear or reverse."[57] It is, however, clear that intercircuit conflict—even if some lawyers tend to overestimate its existence—is a "signal" related to the granting of review. A study of the 1947–76 Terms showed that the presence of two types of conflict—of a lower court ruling with Supreme Court precedent, and of lower court rulings with each other—both were related positively to the Court's granting of review, with intercircuit conflict actually less of a relevant cue for the Burger Court than it had been for the Warren Court.[58]

There are also times when the justices grant cert. before the court of appeals has ruled on a case. The Court's rules talk of doing so in cases of "imperative public importance" but the justices appear to have done so in other situations as well. Cases falling into the "imperative public importance" category include the Nazi saboteurs case during World War II (*Ex Parte Quirin*), the Steel Seizure Case, the Nixon Tapes Case, and *Dames & Moore* (the Iran hostage case). There are instances in which certiorari before judgment is granted so the Court can join a case to others with the same issue already before the Court; the *Bolling* case from the District of Columbia, decided along with *Brown v. Board of Education*, was one such case. In addition, the Court at times takes some cases on this basis when the case is coming back to the Court a second time or when the parties have erroneously taken a direct appeal from the district court.[59]

What Does Denial Mean? A certiorari denial means formally only that the Court has not accepted the case to decide it, thus leaving the ruling of the lower court undisturbed. As Justice Frankfurter reminded us some years ago, the justices "do not have to, and frequently do not, reach the merits of a case to decide that it is not of sufficient importance to warrant review here." Thus certiorari denial "imports no expression of opinion upon the merits of the case." Such denial "means only that, for one reason or another, which is seldom disclosed, and not infrequently for conflicting reasons, which may have nothing to do with the merits and certainly may have nothing to do with any view of the merits taken by a majority of the Court, there were not four members of the Court who thought the case should be heard." Or, as Justice Jackson observed in the same case, "denial of certiorari . . . creates no precedent and approves no statement of principle entitled to weight in any other case."[60]

These statements about the nonmeaning of certiorari denials are not accepted by many observers of the Court. Some infer consideration of the merits of a case from denials of review. Thus, "when the Court consistently leaves undisturbed decisions at variance with principle, or when it denies certiorari in a notorious case . . . the public may well believe that the Court is implementing an unspoken constitutional judgment."[61] Despite Justice Frankfurter's 1953 ad-monition that "the Bar [was] not to draw strength for lower court opinions from the fact that they were left unreviewed here,"[62] lawyers continue to cite certiorari denials. This further stimulates guesses about the meaning of the denials, al-though such action by lawyers may be no more than their way of indicating that a legal issue is not settled and should therefore be decided, or it may simply be a matter of form (the citation is not complete without noting the cert. denial).

The Court gives reasons as its denial of review even less frequently than when it grants review—indeed, hardly at all. A sample of more than 3,000 denied petitions over 20 years produced fewer than 40 explanations, of which the most common was dismissal on motion of the parties or failure to file timely.[63] In the 1972 and 1973 Terms, 60 percent of the dissenting opinions in certiorari denials stated the need for a national decision to resolve conflicts between lower courts or between the lower courts and the Supreme Court, the presence of statutory questions that needed to be resolved, or "the existence of important questions for decision."[64]

In a way, the Court is better off *not* explaining its denials, at least if it wishes to avoid open disagreement from its own members, as occurred twice in 1978. When the Court indicated in denying review that it appears "that the judgment of the Illinois Supreme Court rests on an adequate state ground," Justice Stevens complained that such statements were "inconsistent with the rule that such denials have no precedential value."[65] And when the Court denied a petition "for failure to file the petition within the time provided" by the relevant statute, Stevens, along with Justices Brennan and Stewart, objected because the lack of precedential value of a certiorari denial meant the notation "serves no useful purpose" and because such explanations are offered only "spasmodic[ally]" and without consistency.[66]

Certiorari denials do, however, have effects. Recognizing this, Chief Justice Warren wrote after his retirement, "Denials can and do have a significant impact on the ordering of constitutional and legal priorities. Many potential and impor-tant developments in the law have been frustrated, at least temporarily, by a denial of certiorari."[67] He did, however, stop short of saying such action was purposeful. More fuel is added to the fire when the justices themselves cite the Court's certiorari denials in concurring or dissenting opinions, at times doing so more than as a matter of form. Justice Blackmun speculated in 1973 that dissents from an earlier certiorari denial were "not without some significance as to [the justices'] and the Court's attitude." This provoked an extended response from Justice Marshall, who said justices may simultaneously agree about an issue's importance and feel the case was not the "appropriate vehicle for determination of that issue." Perhaps too defensively, Marshall even attacked speculation about reasons why certiorari is denied. He said that "the point of our use of a discretion-ary writ is precisely to prohibit that kind of speculation" and asserted, "Reliance on denial of certiorari for *any* proposition impairs the vitality of the discretion we exercise in controlling the cases we hear."[68] This is particularly true if there are different reasons leading individual justices to vote to deny review, as is often the case. As Justice Rehnquist recently observed, "Some Members of the Court may feel that a case is wrongly decided, but lacking in general importance; others may feel that it is of general importance, but rightly decided; for either reason, a vote to deny certiorari is logically dictate[d]."[69]

Justice Jackson, in a significant contribution to the debate, raised questions about certiorari denials' formal meaning. Conceding that "the Court is not quite of one mind on the subject," he continued, "Some say denial means nothing, others say it means nothing much." However, he asserted, "Realistically, the first position is untenable and the second is unintelligible." Jackson felt lawyers could no longer believe denial of review to be meaningless when justices began to file statements dissenting from such denial. Lawyers, said Jackson, "will not readily believe that Justices of this Court are taking the trouble to signal a meaningless division of opinion about a meaningless act." Moreover, he added, "every lower court does attach importance to denials and to presence or absence of dissents from denials."[70]

Despite the absence of time for writing separate opinions and some earlier norms against their use, there has been a substantial increase in the number of dissents from certiorari denials. Although not all dissents deal with the merits of cases, those that do are an indication that review decisions and rulings on the merits are related: "If a denial of certiorari were a purely discretionary act, largely or totally unconcerned with the merits of a particular case, it would be anomalous for Justices to note their dissents."[71] A dissent from a *grant* of certiorari, extremely rare, shows the connection even more clearly; when Chief Justice Burger did this, Justice Blackmun complained that a justice doing so indicates commitment to a result in a case before reviewing most of the materials concerning that case.[72] Justices' ideologies help explain dissents from cert. denials, with the liberals Douglas, Brennan, and Marshall frequently dissenting from denials of review, but justices' proclivity to vote for review also helps explain their behavior. Although some "review prone" justices, like Justice Douglas, have accounted for much of the increase in dissents, others, like Burton and Frankfurter, were "review conservative."[73]

Justice Stevens has recently questioned the validity of dissents from certiorari denials because the strong, perhaps emotional, case the dissenters make can create the impression that the Court, which does not answer the dissenters, "is not managing its discretionary docket in a responsible manner."[74] Without himself going to the merits of the case as the dissenters have often done, Stevens has suggested some possible reasons for denial of review, such as procedural defects, not mentioned in the dissenters' complaints.[75] He also noted that the dissenters' written statements have at times been more persuasive than statements made at the Court's conference and have led other justices to change their votes so that review was granted. However, argued Stevens, such results only justified writing and circulating these memoranda, not publishing them when the dissenters failed to persuade their colleagues.[76] Going further than Stevens, in separate cases Justices Blackmun and Brennan have written statements *in support of* certiorari denials—Blackmun disagreeing with dissenters from the denial and Brennan suggesting alternative procedural resolutions of the problem presented by a case.[77]

Justices exhibit varying degrees of "merits-consciousness," the degree to which they take the merits of a case into account in decisions to grant or deny review.[78] Where the government has won a criminal case in the lower courts, a justice generally favoring criminal defendants (as shown by his votes in full opinion cases) would vote to grant review, while justices who would support the government once the case was accepted would vote not to grant certiorari; when the government was appealing from a ruling excluding evidence in a case, the reverse pattern would occur.

A judge's certiorari votes helped predict the judge's votes on the merits in cases accepted in the 1947–56 Terms. Liberal and conservative voting blocs among the justices could be identified not only from votes on the merits but also at the certiorari stage: a justice who voted with one set of justices in full opinion cases was *un*likely to vote with his remaining colleagues at the review-granting stage.[79] Indeed, on the basis of "paid" cases from selected terms from 1954 through 1975, decisions to grant review can be explained on the basis of whether petitioners are "Upperdogs" or "Underdogs." Although Upperdogs do better than Underdogs in getting their cases accepted, Underdogs' success rate was much higher during the Warren Court (55%) than in the Burger Court (39%), when the justices most clearly differentiated between the two in accepting and rejecting cases.[80] However, judges' attitudes cannot explain the fact that cases most often unanimously denied review have tapped dissimilar ideological matters, such as prisoner petitions and commercial suits by business interests, or the high proportion of unanimous decisions on granting or denying review. Such unanimity is likely the result of shared views about the types of cases to which the Court should devote its attention.

Evidence of judges' strategy in their certiorari votes has also been used to explain certiorari denial in political terms rather than formal-legal ones, for example, to suggest that judges may try to disguise their attitudes from their colleagues or that certiorari votes on particular issues can be explained in terms of the strategies of game theory. Schubert suggested that during 1942–48 in Federal Employers Liability Act cases, a bloc of four justices (Murphy, Rutledge, Black, and Douglas) voted together on certiorari to achieve victory on the merits, parallel to a strategy of never voting for the railroad (the employer) on certiorari but always voting for the worker when the court of appeals had reversed a proworker district court decision, then always voting for the worker on the merits. The four justices had a 92 percent success rate (12 of 13) when they followed that pattern, but only a 73 percent rate (8 of 13) when they voted for workers who had lost in both trial and appeals courts. When the four-justice bloc grew to five, they "won" 13 of 14 cases in the 1956–57 Terms; no justice voted for certiorari in the "lost" case because the appeal was so frivolous.[81]

Justice Burton's docket book showed, however, that members of the "certiorari bloc" showed a lack of consistency, with only votes of nonbloc members favoring workers leading to the Court agreeing to hear some cases, and that some justices voted to grant review with little apparent regard for whether the cases would produce policies they wish the Court to announce. That justices favoring workers on the merits did cast a high proportion of their certiorari votes so as to favor workers does indicate the effect of the justices' ideology, but the other evidence shows limited use of strategy.

Further evidence of the policy implications of certiorari decisions comes from the Court's disposition of cases to which it does grant review. A pattern "too definite to have arisen by sheer happenstance"[82] appears in the Court's reversal of the lower courts in roughly two out of three certiorari cases over the last 30 years. The proportion of reversals in full opinion cases has, with the exception of only a couple of years out of the last 10, hovered around 70 percent, with the proportion higher if *per curiam* rulings are added. Federal court appeals are particularly likely to be reversed in formal opinions, so that the Court could explain the law to the lower federal courts. Such figures seem to indicate clearly a better-than-even chance that the Court approved of lower court decisions to which it did not grant review. Further confirmation comes from Burton's docket book, which indicates that, despite differences between them, justices were more likely to vote to reverse the lower court in cases in which they had voted to grant review than in those in which they did not cast a vote favoring review, and that the Supreme Court reversed the lower court more frequently when five justices (a majority of the full Court) voted to grant review.[83]

Notes

1. Doris M. Provine, *Case Selection in the United States Supreme Court* (Chicago: University of Chicago Press, 1980), pp. 62–63.

2. Arthur D. Hellman, "Case Selection in the Burger Court: A Preliminary Inquiry," *Notre Dame Law Review* 60 (1985): 996, 998.

3. See *Brown v. Herald Co.*, 462 U.S. 928 (1983).

4. Gerhard Casper and Richard A. Posner, *The Workload of the Supreme Court* (Chicago: American Bar Foundation, 1976), pp. 11–12.

5. Ibid., p. 6.

6. See Gerhard Casper and Richard A. Posner, "The Caseload of the Supreme Court: 1975 and 1976 Terms," *The Supreme Court Review 1977*, eds. Philip B. Kurland and Gerhard Casper (Chicago: University of Chicago Press, 1978), pp. 87–98, updating their earlier study.

7. Hellman, "Case Selection in the Burger Court," p. 952.

8. For additional data, see the Statistical Tables in the *Harvard Law Review's* annual (November) issue on the Supreme Court's previous term. See particularly Five Year Tables I and II: 82 (November 1968): 310; 87 (November 1973): 310–11; 92 (November 1978): 336–37; 97 (November 1983): 303–6.

9. These findings are from William McLauchlan, "Managing the Supreme Court's Business, 1971–1983," paper presented to American Political Science Association, 1986; the data are based on paid petitions.

10. William H. Rehnquist, "The Supreme Court: Past and Present," *American Bar Association Journal* 59 (April 1973): 363.

11. Arthur D. Hellman, "The Proposed Intercircuit Tribunal: Do We Need It? Will It Work?." *Hastings Constitutional Law Quarterly* 11 (Spring 1984): 383–84.

12. *Warth v. Seldin*, 422 U.S. 490 at 519 (1975); *Tidewater Oil Co. v. United States*, 409 U.S. 151 at 174-76 (1972).

13. Mary Cornelia Porter, "Politics, Ideology and the Workload of the Supreme Court: Some Historical Perspectives," paper presented to Midwest Political Science Association, 1975, pp. 8, 10.

14. Casper and Posner, *The Workload of the Supreme Court*, p. 31.

15. *Tatum v. Regents of University of Nebraska-Lincoln*, 426 U.S. 1117 (1983).

16. *Talamini v. All-State Insurance Co.*, 105 S.Ct. 1824 at 1825 (Burger), 1827 (Stevens) (1985). See also *Hyde v. Van Wormer*, 106 S.Ct. 403 (1985).

17. Commission on Revision of Federal Court Appellate System, *Structure and Internal Procedures* (Washington, D.C., 1975), pp. 29–31.

18. Hellman, "The Proposed Intercircuit Tribunal," p. 415.

19. Samuel Estreicher and John E. Sexton, "A Managerial Theory of the Supreme Court's Responsibilities: An Empirical Study," *New York University Law Review* 59 (October 1984): 725.

20. Ibid., p. 709. See also Estreicher and Sexton, *Redefining the Supreme Court's Role: A Theory of Managing the Federal Judicial Process* (New Haven, Conn.: Yale University Press, 1986).

21. Glendon Schubert, *The Constitutional Polity* (Boston: Boston University Press, 1970), p. 10.

22. J. Woodford Howard, Jr., "Is the Burger Court a Nixon Court?" *Emory Law Journal* 23 (Summer 1974): 757.

23. Arthur D. Hellman, "The Supreme Court, the National Law, and the Selection of Cases for the Plenary Docket," *University of Pittsburgh Law Review* 44 (Spring 1983): 549.

24. Gregory A. Caldeira, "The United States Supreme Court and Criminal Cases, 1935–1976: Alternative Models of Agenda Building," *British Journal of Political Science* 2 (1981): 457–61, 463.

25. Richard L. Pacelle, Jr., "The Supreme Court Agenda Across Time: Towards a Theory of Agenda-Building," paper presented to Midwest Political Science Association, 1986, p. 20.

26. Arthur D. Hellman, "The Supreme Court and Civil Rights: The Plenary Docket in the 1970s," *Oregon Law Review* 58 (1979): 3–60; Hellman, "Case Selection in the Burger Court," pp. 1004–5.

27. See Hellman, "Case Selection in the Burger Court," p. 973, and Hellman, "The Supreme Court, the National Law," p. 585.

28. For this material, see Arthur D. Hellman, "The Supreme Court and Statutory Law: The Plenary Docket in the 1970's," *University of Pittsburgh Law Review* 40 (Fall 1978): 1–45.

29. Hellman, "The Supreme Court, the National Law," p. 631.

30. *Hicks v. Miranda*, 422 U.S. 332 at 344 (1975), also quoting Justice Brennan, *Ohio ex rel. Eaton v. Price*, 360 U.S. 246 at 247 (1959), to the same effect.

31. S. Sidney Ulmer, "Issue Fluidity in the U.S. Supreme Court: A Conceptual Analysis," in *Supreme Court Activism and Restraint*, eds. Stephen C. Halpern and Charles Lamb (Lexington, Mass: Lexington Books, 1982), p. 339.

32. See Arthur D. Hellman, "Error Correction, Lawmaking, and the Supreme Court's Exercise of Discretionary Review," *University of Pittsburgh Law Review* 44 (Summer 1983): 825–26.

33. Arthur D. Hellman, "'Granted, Vacated, and Remanded'—Shedding Light on a Dark Corner of Supreme Court Practice," *Judicature* 67 (March 1984): 389–401; Hellman, "The Supreme Court's

Second Thoughts: Remands for Reconsideration and Denials of Review in Cases Held for Plenary Decisions," *Hastings Constitutional Law Quarterly* 11 (Fall 1983): 17–20.

34. *Pennsylvania v. Mimms*, 434 U.S. 106 at 115–116 (1977) (Justice Marshall), 117 (Stevens); *Cooper v. Mitchell Brothers' Santa Ana Theater*, 454 U.S. 90 at 95 (1981) (Stevens); *Hutto v. Davis*, 454 U.S. 370 at 387 (1982) (Brennan).

35. See *United States v. Benchimol*, 105 S.Ct. 2103 at 2106 (1985) (Brennan).

36. John Paul Stevens, "The Life Span of a Judge-made Rule," *New York University Law Review* 58 (1983): 17; William Brennan, "The National Court of Appeals: Another Dissent," *University of Chicago Law Review* 40 (1973): 479.

37. *Thigpen v. Roberts*, 468 U.S. 27 at 33 (1984).

38. *Straight v. Wainwright*, 106 S.Ct. 2004 at 2006–7 (1986).

39. *Dyke v. Georgia*, 421 U.S. 952 (1975) (obscenity); *Liles v. Oregon*, 425 U.S. 963 (1976) (Justice Stevens).

40. For much material in this section, I have drawn on two papers by H. W. Perry, Jr., "Indices and Signals in the Certiorari Process," presented to Midwest Political Science Association, 1986, and "Deciding to Decide in the U.S. Supreme Court: Bargaining, Accommodation, and Roses," presented to American Political Science Association, 1986.

41. Provine, *Case Selection*, p. 82.

42. William H. Rehnquist, "Who Writes Decisions of the Supreme Court?" *U.S. News & World Report* (December 13 1957): 74–75, reprinted in *The Courts: A Reader in the Judicial Process*, ed. Robert Scigliano (Boston: Little, Brown, 1962), pp. 166–69.

43. *Rice v. Sioux City Memorial Park Cemetery*, 349 U.S. 70 (1955).

44. *Burrell v. McCray*, 426 U.S. 471 (1976); *New York v. Uplinger*, 407 U.S. 246 at 250 (1984). For an account of *Burrell*, see Robert Woodward and Scott Armstrong, *The Brethren* (New York: Simon and Schuster, 1981), pp. 424–25.

45. "Retired Chief Justice Warren Attacks . . . Freund Study Group's Composition and Proposal," *American Bar Association Journal* 59 (July 1973): 728.

46. Provine, *Case Selection*, p. 4.

47. *Federal Open Market Committee v. Merrill*, 443 U.S. 340 at 344 (1979); *Washington v. Washington State Commercial Passenger Fishing Vessel Association*, 443 U.S. 658 at 675 (1979).

48. Fred M. Vinson, "The Work of the Federal Courts," *Courts, Judges, and Politics*, eds. Walter F. Murphy and C. Herman Pritchett (New York: Random House, 1961), pp. 55–56; *Jones v. Mayer*, 392 U.S. 409 at 478–79 (1968) (Justice Harlan).

49. *Idaho Department of Employment v. Smith*, 434 U.S. 100 at 105–106 (1977).

50. "Retired Chief Justice Warren Attacks . . . ," p. 728.

51. Perry, "Indices and Signals," pp. 16 ff.

52. Joseph Tanenhaus, Marvin Schick, Matthew Muraskin, and Daniel Rosen, "The Supreme Court's Jurisdiction: Cue Theory," *Judicial Decision-Making*, ed. Glendon Schubert (New York: Free Press, 1963), p. 123.

53. Provine, *Case Selection*, p. 32, Table 1.4 and p. 82.

54. Hellman, "The Supreme Court, the National Law," p. 632.

55. Steven Duke and Patrick Malone, "An Overzealous Supreme Court," *Washington Post*, October 21, 1984, p. C5.

56. Tanenhaus et al., "Cue Theory," p. 123; Provine, *Case Selection*, p. 82.

57. J. Woodford Howard, Jr., *Courts of Appeals in the Federal Judicial System*, p. 67; Richard J. Richardson and Kenneth N. Vines, *The Politics of Federal Courts* (Boston: Little, Brown, 1970), p. 153.

58. S. Sidney Ulmer, "The Supreme Court's Certiorari Decisions: Conflict as a Predictive Variable," *American Political Science Review* 78 (December 1984): 908. For an important earlier study, see Ulmer, William Hintze, and Louise Kirklosky, "The Decision to Grant or Deny Certiorari: Further Consideration of Cue Theory," *Law & Society Review* 6 (May 1972): 637–44.

59. See James Lindgren and William P. Marshall, "The Supreme Court's Extraordinary Power to Grant Certiorari Before Judgment in the Court of Appeals," *The Supreme Court Review 1986*, eds. Philip B. Kurland, Gerhard Casper, and Dennis J. Hutchinson (Chicago: University of Chicago Press, 1987), pp. 259–316.

60. *Brown v. Allen*, 344 U.S. 443 at 491–92 (Frankfurter), 543 (Jackson) (1953).

61. David Adamany, "Legitimacy, Realigning Elections, and the Supreme Court," *Wisconsin Law Review* 1973: 801, drawing on Jan Deutsch, "Neutrality, Legitimacy, and the Supreme Court," *Stanford Law Review* 20 (1968): 207.

62. *Brown v. Allen*, at 491.

63. Tanenhaus et al., "Cue Theory," p. 114.

. Commission on Revision, *Structure and Internal Procedures*, pp. 48–49.

65. *Illinois v. Gray*, 435 U.S. 1013 (1978).

66. *County of Sonoma v. Isbell*, 439 U.S. 996 (1978).

67. "Retired Chief Justice Warren Attacks . . . ," p. 728.

68. *United States v. Kras*, 409 U.S. 434 at 443 (Blackmun), 461 (Marshall) (1973).

69. *Huch v. United States*, 439 U.S. 1007 at 1008 (1978).

70. *Brown v. Allen*, at 542–43.

71. Peter Linzer, "The Meaning of Certiorari Denials," *Columbia Law Review* 79 (November 1979): 1255.

72. *Darden v. Wainwright*, 106 S.Ct. 2464 at 2484–85 n. 9 (1986).

73. Provine, *Case Selection*, p. 114.

74. *Chevron USA v. Sheffield*, 105 S.Ct. 2686 at 2686–87 (1985).

75. See *Huffman v. Florida*, 435 U.S. 1014 at 1018–1019 (1978); *Vasquez v. United States*, 454 U.S. 975 at 975–76 (1981).

76. *Singleton v. Commissioner of Internal Revenue*, 439 U.S. 940 at 943–47 (1978).

77. *Kerr-McGee Chemical Corp. v. Illinois*, 459 U.S. 1049 (1982) (Blackmun); *James v. United States*, 459 U.S. 1044 (1982) (Brennan).

78. Provine, *Case Selection*, pp. 110–13.

79. See S. Sidney Ulmer, "Supreme Court Justices as Strict and Not-so-Strict Constructionists: Some Implications," *Law & Society Review* 8 (Fall 1973): 27–28; and Ulmer, "Voting Blocs and 'Access' to the Supreme Court: 1947–1956 Terms," *Jurimetrics Journal* 16 (Fall 1965): 8, 12.

80. S. Sidney Ulmer, "Selecting Cases for Supreme Court Review: Litigant Status in the Warren and Burger Courts," *Courts, Law, and Judicial Processes*, ed. Ulmer (New York: Free Press, 1981), pp. 284–98; see also Ulmer, "Selecting Cases for Supreme Court Review: An Underdog Model," *American Political Science Review* 72 (September 1978): 902–10.

81. Schubert, "The Certiorari Game," in Schubert, *Quantitative Analysis of Judicial Behavior* (Glencoe, Ill.: Free Press, 1959), pp. 210–54.

82. Schubert, *Quantitative Analysis*, p. 66; for his data, see pp. 55–57.

83. Provine, *Case Selection*, p. 127.

7 The Supreme Court: Full-Dress Treatment

IN THIS CHAPTER WE examine the "full-dress" treatment given cases accepted for review. In describing the Court's basic procedures for reaching decisions, particular attention is given to oral argument, the Chief Justice's practices in opinion assignment, and the release of opinions. Then we analyze disagreement within the Court and the alignments of the justices as they decide cases. The Court's power of judicial review and the considerations the justices take into account in reaching their decisions and writing their opinions—matters of precedent, strategy, and activism and self-restraint—are examined in the next chapter.

Procedure in the Court

Although the Supreme Court's annual term begins on the first Monday of October, as it has since the late nineteenth century, in earlier years the Court's sessions were brief. For example, in the early nineteenth century, there were only two sessions of roughly two to three weeks, in February and August; by 1840, there was a continuous January-March session, a period that grew to roughly four months-plus by the post-Civil War period.[1] The Court's term now extends formally until the beginning of the next term; however, the Court's public sessions and the announcement of decisions continue only until the first few days of July, with the justices using the summer to prepare for the next term. The justices hear oral argument from the beginning of the term through late March or early April, although in special situations such as the Nixon Tapes case of 1974 argument can be heard as late as June. The Court has also held special sessions— in 1958 for the Little Rock school desegregation case and in 1972 for the Democratic National Convention delegate challenges. Cases to which the Court grants review early in the term are argued in the same term and are decided within the term; those accepted later in the term are not argued until the following term.

Six justices constitute a quorum for doing business. The Court can thus operate during vacancies, illness, and a justice's withdrawal from a case (recusance). However, when the Court is evenly divided 4-4 or 3-3, the lower court's ruling is affirmed and no opinion is written. In order to avoid such tie votes, the Court has tried to delay deciding controversial cases that might produce such a division until vacancies are filled and there is a full complement of nine justices. When this cannot be avoided, as when illness causes a justice to miss oral argument, cases might be "returned to the calendar" for reargument later in the same term or in the next term. This occurred in the 1984 Term when Justice Powell missed oral argument in 56 cases because of surgery. Some cases were released as 4-4 affirmances and some were set for reargument, with the Court not explaining why it chose one option rather than the other.

A justice's participation in a case solely to create a full Court is not necessarily proper, illustrated by a problem involving Justice Rehnquist that was used against him during the debate on his nomination to be Chief Justice. Shortly before he initially joined the Court, Rehnquist, as assistant attorney general, had testified before Congress on military surveillance of civilian political activity and had commented that a pending case challenging such surveillance was nonjusticiable—the central issue in the case. The lower court had ruled that the case could be heard, and the Supreme Court granted review before Rehnquist began his service on the Court, but did not hear argument until later. Without Rehnquist's participation, the vote would have been 4-4, sustaining the lower court. However, Rehnquist participated and cast the crucial fifth vote to reverse the lower court, thus eliminating the challenge to the government activity (*Laird v. Tatum*, 1972). This prompted the American Civil Liberties Union (ACLU) to petition for a rehearing of the case in which Rehnquist's disqualification was specifically requested. The Court denied the rehearing petition without comment—its usual procedure. Rehnquist, however, wrote a memorandum supporting his participation. He said he had only been the government's attorney, expressing the administration's position, not necessarily his own. He added that someone in government service prior to joining the Court was quite likely to have made statements of opinion on subjects that would arise later in litigation. To have a blank mind on such subjects would, he said, "be evidence of lack of qualification, not lack of bias." The American Bar Association code of judicial ethics showed a clear preference for avoiding even the appearance of impropriety, but Rehnquist stressed a duty to participate, particularly where his vote was necessary to resolve the case.[2] The ACLU again tried to reopen the case in 1986 on the basis of information from government memoranda made available during the process of confirming Rehnquist as Chief Justice. The ACLU claimed that he had not merely served as the administration's spokesperson, as he had said earlier, but had played a role in drafting the surveillance plan. Without comment, the Court refused to rehear the case.[3] In evaluating this situation, one might keep in mind that there have been earlier situations in which justices who had, prior to coming to the Court, participated actively in developing laws, as justices sat to hear cases involving those cases. Justice Jackson is said to have ruled on an immigration issue he had handled as attorney general. As a senator, Justice Black had been an author of the Fair Labor Standards Act (the minimum wage law) and Justice Frankfurter had played an important role in enactment of the Norris-LaGuardia (anti-injunction) law, yet both sat on cases involving the constitutionality or scope of those laws.

Justices usually recuse without explanation or comment because of acquaintance with the parties or their lawyers; financial interest, however small or indirect, usually from ownership of stock; or involvement with a case before the justice began Supreme Court service. For example, Justice White, who had been deputy attorney general before becoming a justice, recused himself from a number of cases involving the U.S. government, as did Justice Thurgood Marshall, who had been solicitor general; Marshall also recused from some NAACP-supported cases because of his long connection with that organization, and did so even many years after he joined the Court. Justices Brennan, Stewart, Stevens, and Scalia, former appellate judges, removed themselves from cases coming from the courts on which they had sat. Financial holdings apparently accounted for the disqualification of Justice Powell, Justice Stewart, and Stewart's successor, Justice O'Connor, in a number of cases. In 1980 the Court amended its rules to require that when corporations file papers with the Court, the papers "include a listing naming all parent companies, subsidiaries (except wholly owned subsidiaries) and affiliates of each such corporation" (Rule 28.1). This was apparently done to facilitate identification of cases in which a justice, a justice's spouse, or other close relatives might have a financial interest, after some apparent embarrassments when justices participated without knowledge of such matters.

Although they no longer ride circuit (see page 44), each Supreme Court justice still has responsibility for one or more circuits for emergencies and other matters that must be dealt with when the Court is not in session or before the full Court can meet to consider them, such as requests to stay executions, often at the last moment. (School board efforts to block busing orders in connection with school desegregation also often have come at the last moment, shortly before the school year was to begin.[4])

A circuit justice can order someone released on bail and can stay lower court orders until the full Court has a chance to act on petitions for review; this is the situation often faced in death penalty cases as more and more Death Row convicts exhaust their appeals and execution warrants are issued. Most stays of execution are requested within days of the scheduled execution date; the Court has increasingly been refusing stays and even lifting lower court stays at the state's request. The majority has complained about "abuse" of the habeas corpus process by the filing of multiple habeas petitions and about the multiple hearings that defendants require before state and federal courts.[5] In some instances, the Court has refused to grant stays to condemned prisoners even when their time to file a certiorari petition had not expired or when they raised an issue the Court was going to consider in cases to which it had granted review.[6] Such actions have prompted Justices Brennan and Marshall to complain about the Court's "indecent desire to rush to judgment in capital cases" and its "unseemly and unjustified eagerness" to allow the prisoner's execution.[7]

Most requests to a circuit justice are passed along to the full Court. Because the action of "the lower court, which has considered the matter at length and close at hand," is presumed to be correct,[8] a circuit justice acting alone does not decide a case on the merits but grants a stay only when the applicant makes a strong showing that the lower court's decision is erroneous and that irreparable injury would occur without the stay; the circuit justice also decides (really predicts) that the other justices would consider the matter sufficiently serious to grant review. Although formal action on a stay request is the circuit justice's alone, occasionally other available justices are consulted, and when the circuit justice considers the matter too important for a single justice's decision, colleagues are consulted, at times by telephone.

The difficulties that can arise when a stay is requested in a controversial matter are illustrated by what occurred during the controversy over the bombing of Cambodia. A district judge had enjoined the bombing and the court of appeals had stayed the injunction. Those seeking to stop the bombing sought to have Justice Thurgood Marshall, the Circuit Justice, set aside the appellate court order, but Marshall said that as a single justice he would exceed his authority if he were to do so because he thought the appellate court had not acted improperly. Then, as sometimes happens when petitioners are unsuccessful with the first justice they contact, the plaintiffs went to Justice Douglas, who did set aside the appeals court stay on the grounds that the case was like any capital punishment case in which one tries to avoid having someone die unnecessarily. Douglas was, however, overruled *the very same day*. Justice Marshall, indicating he had communicated with all other members of the Court, directly stayed the district court injunction.[9]

Oral Argument

Oral argument, the next major step after briefs are filed, was used long before written briefs but is now used to supplement the briefs and other records submitted in a case. The Court's rule that submission of a case solely on the briefs is disfavored, with the Court able to order argument nonetheless (Rule 38.1), shows the importance the Court attaches to oral argument. At one time, argument went on without limits. Then in 1848, the Court imposed a limit of *eight* hours per case (two hours per attorney, two attorneys for each side). A significant further reduction to two hours per side came in 1871, with a further reduction to one and one-half hours per side coming in 1911. However, the Court had limited the parties in some cases deemed less meritorious to 30 minutes per side. During Chief Justice Taft's tenure, the Court reduced the length of argument to one hour per side (in 1925) and also declined to hear the appellee (respondent) if the petitioner's opening argument was not persuasive. Further reduction, to the present one-half hour per side, came with Chief Justice Burger. However, additional time is allowed in exceptional cases or in some cases when the government appears as *amicus* to present argument; consolidation of several cases on the same issue may mean more attention to basic issues common to the cases, which also occurs when two or more cases on the same subject are heard consecutively. The Court now hears argument on Monday through Wednesday, hearing twelve cases during that period; Thursday is left open so the justices can prepare for Friday conference.

Lawyers wishing to argue before the Court are supposed to be members of the bar of the Supreme Court. If a lawyer who wishes to argue a case is not yet admitted to the Supreme Court bar, that lawyer's admission *pro hac vice* (p.h.v.) for that particular case can be moved by another lawyer or the agency employing the lawyer, and such requests are usually granted. Joining the Supreme Court bar—often largely symbolic, as few lawyers really intend to argue cases there—is usually a routine matter. The lawyer must have been a member of the bar in good standing in his or her home state for at least three years, must pay a small fee, and must be recommended by two present members of the Supreme Court bar. The Court used to swear in lawyers in an admissions ceremony at the beginning of its public sessions, but as the number of lawyers seeking admission increased—it is now roughly 7,000 per year—that was discontinued as too time consuming.

Only a few applications to become a member of the Supreme Court bar are rejected each year, and those rejections are generally not made public. However, starting in 1979, Chief Justice Burger filed written dissents to the admission of several lawyers who had received disciplinary sanctions or were under investigation for disciplinary violations in their home states. He felt those lawyers failed to meet the Supreme Court's standard that the "applicant appears . . . to be of good moral and professional character" (Rule 5.1) and were using their admission to the Supreme Court bar to "'launder' their professional records." In 1986, shortly before leaving the Court, Chief Justice Burger concurred in the Court's decision to admit a lawyer whose admission Burger (joined by Justice O'Connor) had severely criticized in 1982; the lawyer, who had felt strongly he had been improperly maligned by the Chief Justice, had resigned from the Supreme Court bar and had applied for readmission to obtain vindication.[10] (When a state disbars a lawyer who is a member of the Supreme Court bar, the Court issues an order leading to the prompt removal of the lawyer from the Supreme Court bar.)

Oral argument, although it may not determine the result in a case, is often quite important in the decision.[11] Justice Harlan stated that there was "no substitute" for this "Socratic method of procedure in getting at the heart of an issue and in finding out where the truth lies," and Justice Brennan said he would be "terribly concerned" were he to be denied the opportunity to participate in oral argument because there had been "many occasions when my judgment of a decision has turned on what happened" there.[12]

The justices' questions at oral argument are particularly important. Lawyers appearing before the Court seldom get to make uninterrupted speeches, and the justices often engage in exchanges with them. Although a lawyer may use notes, the Court has made clear that it does not wish to have a lawyer read from a prepared text (see Rule 38.1). Other aids are generally prohibited, but the Court recently allowed a deaf lawyer—arguing the *Rowley* case concerning the amount of assistance a school district had to supply a deaf child—to use a video display screen from which he could read the justices' questions typed into the system by a stenotypist.

Some justices are more frequent questioners than others, and the Court as a whole usually asks more questions of one side than of the other. For example, in the *Briggs* school desegregation case argued along with *Brown*, John Davis, defending segregation, was interrupted only 11 times, but Thurgood Marshall was interrupted 127 times.[13] The justices not only ask questions; they make statements and suggest positions not raised by the lawyers. In so doing, they often disagree with the lawyers. In the Little Rock school desegregation case, when the state's lawyer tried to gain sympathy for Governor Faubus' position by recalling Chief Justice Warren's service as governor of California, Warren forcefully pointed out that he had as governor abided by rulings of the courts, adding, "I never heard a lawyer say that the statement of a governor as to what was legal or illegal should control the action of any court."[14]

Oral argument performs a variety of functions. Because there is no assurance that the justices have actually read the briefs although it is quite likely that they have done so, it serves to assure the lawyers—and through them their clients—that the Court has actually heard the case. It also helps both lawyers and judges by forcing the lawyers to focus on the arguments they consider most important. Judges' questions quickly lead to a separation of central from collateral issues, a distinction often not discernible from the lawyers' briefs, which are organized point after point in correspondence to the facts and statutes involved in the case, and which often intentionally lack emphasis as the lawyer, never knowing which argument(s) might be persuasive, tries to convince the Court in as many ways as possible.

For the judges, for whom it is probably more important, oral argument not only legitimizes their judicial function but can also be used to obtain support for their positions or to assure them about an outcome toward which they are already inclined. Judges also use oral argument to communicate with their colleagues, asking questions of counsel that are of greater concern to their associates than to themselves and debating each other through those questions. A justice hammering on a particularly difficult point may be trying to persuade colleagues that they will have to resolve that point to decide the case in a certain direction.

Oral argument is basically intended to provide the judges with information. Sometimes they simply want to clarify the lawyers' positions; for example, the differences in rates at which Marshall and Davis were asked questions in the *Briggs* argument can be explained in large part by that need for clarification. However, the particular frequency with which Marshall's 1953 argument attacking the "separate but equal" doctrine was interrupted—53 times in roughly three-quarters of an hour—also resulted from the fact that it was the central part of his case and it derived from his position as the person wishing the Court to adopt a major new position.[15] Oral argument also can provide judges with information to assist them in determining the Court's strategies, that is, how the Court should exercise its broader political role. Questions as to how many people might be affected by a decision and where the Court might be heading if it decided a case a certain way help elicit this type of information.

Conference and After

With the exception of Christmas and Easter recesses and recesses for opinion writing, the justices meet in conference throughout the term. They meet during the last week of September to deal with certiorari petitions that have accumulated over the summer. Although the Court held Saturday conferences when argument time per case was longer, now the justices meet Wednesdays and Fridays when the Court is hearing oral argument. The Wednesday conference is devoted to voting and deliberating on the previous Monday's argued cases, and the Friday conference, which runs from 9:30 to 12:30 and then continues after lunch, disposes of the cases argued the previous Tuesday and Wednesday and certiorari petitions and appeals. At times there may be memoranda exchanged by the justices in advance of the conference at which a case will be considered; a justice may even be assigned to write a memo, with others invited to do so; consensus may develop from this process, which may also serve to identify the justice who will be asked to write the Court's opinion.

In the conference, the Chief Justice makes the initial presentation concerning a case, including his own comments about it. Each justice, the most senior justice first and the most junior last, then comments. Tradition had been to take a formal vote in order of reverse seniority so that the most junior justice would not be influenced by the senior justices' votes, but in most cases a separate vote is not necessary because the justices' votes are clear from their initial statements. The initial conference vote is considered only tentative, allowing justices to change positions before the final vote is taken later. Thus at times what began as the majority becomes the minority, and vice versa.

After the vote, the Chief Justice, if in the majority, assigns the task of writing the Court's opinion. In the past, this was done the day after each conference, but now is done after two weeks of argument and conference. If the Chief Justice is not in the majority, the assignment is made by the most senior justice in the majority. Chief Justice Burger is reported to have tried to control opinion assignment even when not in the majority. Apparently blocked from making this change, Burger is also said to have "passed" his vote at conference until the other justices' alignment was evident, so that he could vote with the majority (even when this did not appear consonant with his conference comments) and thus assign the opinion.[16] Chief Justice Rehnquist, on the other hand, may be more open at conference about his position, thus leaving him in dissent and losing him the opportunity to assign opinions. The justice assigned the opinion circulates drafts to all the other justices for comments, doing so each time changes are made in the opinion. To provide other justices the opportunity to express additional views in a concurring opinion or in a dissent from the majority's views, each justice must see all that every other justice has written. No one assigns the writing of a minority opinion, although dissenters may decide informally among themselves who will write.

Although some justices may engage in joint action in advance of initial conference consideration of a case as they attempt to put together a majority, there is considerable exchange, even caucusing, among the justices between opinion-assignment and completion of the opinion. Negotiation may take place, with a justice "holding out" his vote until the author of the opinion adds, deletes, or modifies language. Thus an opinion issued under one justice's name, for example, Chief Justice Burger's opinion in the Nixon Tapes case, may really be an amalgam of several justices' contributions.[17] There may be threats to file dissenting opinions or separate concurring opinions. Well-stated drafts of such opinions may prompt changes in the language of the proposed opinion of the Court, leading the latter's writer to withdraw the opinion.[18] A persuasive draft dissent may even attract votes and lead to reversal of the Court's original position, with the dissent becoming the opinion of the Court. When the justice writing the opinion for the majority loses a majority, the opinion-writing task is reassigned.[19] The justice assigned to write the Court's opinion, upon reexamining the case materials, may also completely change position, perhaps taking the majority along. The ability of the justice writing the Court's opinion—or a justice writing a separate (concurring or dissenting) opinion—to attract other justices to that opinion is an indication of that justice's influence. When a justice decides not to join the opinion of the Court but instead to write a separate opinion, that is an indication that the writer of the opinion of the Court has failed to exercise influence.

In the give-and-take leading to the final result in a case, personal friendships between justices may affect voting, and in particular cases the opinion author may find cross-pressures developing, with pulls in different directions coming from different friends on the Court. Justices also look to the longer run as well, and *may* vote against conscience in a particular case to attract a colleague's support in later cases. More common have been instances when justices, to obtain eventual support on other matters, have ingratiated themselves to colleagues—by writing positive responses in the margins of circulated draft opinions ("returns"). All such exchanges are not surprising in a multimember "collegial" body that is expected to work together cohesively. However, justices (for example, Justice Douglas) may desire isolation from colleagues or may refuse to seek others' votes (said to be true of Justice Stevens); if a justice objects to others' "prosletyzing," obtaining necessary agreement may be quite difficult.

From initial conference and vote to the ultimate outcome in a case, actual shifts can be significant and the Court's decision making at times is highly contingent. A recent important shift occurred in *Bowers v. Hardwick* (1986), in which the Court upheld Georgia's sodomy statute; apparently because Justice Blackmun's proposed opinion was too strong for Justice Powell, who had initially indicated he would vote to overturn the statute, Powell changed his mind and cast the decisive fifth vote for upholding such laws. An example of the contingent nature of the Court's decision process can be found in *Baker v. Carr* (1962), when the Court ruled reapportionment controversies to be justiciable (see page 178). Justice Stewart, the necessary fifth vote to set aside *Colegrove v. Green* (1946) (reapportionment a political question), did not want to reach the merits of the case, that is, whether Tennessee's reapportionment was valid, but would only rule that courts could hear such cases. Chief Justice Warren assigned the opinion to Justice Brennan with the understanding that, to avoid losing Stewart's vote, Brennan would not go further than that position. Then Justice Clark, originally in the minority, both shifted to the majority and was willing to reach the merits; had he joined the majority earlier, *Baker v. Carr* would have dealt with the merits *and* the Court would have adopted a different standard for reapportionment than the "one person-one vote" standard adopted in *Reynolds v. Sims* (1964).[20]

For selected terms during Justice Harold Burton's tenure, there was no change from 88 percent of the justices' original conference votes to their final votes; in 3 percent of the votes, changes were made from not casting a vote to voting either to affirm or reverse the lower court or from such votes to nonparticipation, while in 9 percent of the votes there was *strong fluidity*, a change from a vote to affirm to a vote to reverse or vice versa. No justices changed their votes in 39 percent of the cases, but in the remaining 61 percent, at least some shift occurred. In four-fifths of those cases, only one or two justices changed their votes. The original minority actually became the ultimate majority in 14 percent of the cases in which there were vote changes. The majority remained intact in the other cases, increasing its size five times as often as it lost size. The picture was much the same during Justice Clark's tenure. If individual votes are examined, strong fluidity took place 10 percent of the time and weak fluidity 3 percent. In one-sixth of the cases with vote changes, a minority became a majority, but most majorities remained majorities and increased in size—68 percent compared to the 24 percent that lost votes.[21]

On the whole, exchanges among the justices in the postconference period produce increased agreement concerning the way the justices view the cases. As changes are more likely to be in the direction of the initial majority, "the movement suggests that postconference activity led to increased similarity of perceptions, which in turn led to greater agreement." The studying and discussing of issues after the conference is what produces the increased similarity of perception. During this period the justices do not change their basic values or their role conceptions—neither of which changes easily—but they can change perceptions. [22]

Opinion Release

The Court's decisions and the justices' opinions are not final or binding until announced by the Court. After that, there are to be no further changes (except in grammar, punctuation, or case-citation) in the opinions because that would deprive other justices of the opportunity to comment on *all* the language in all opinions. Such instances have, however, occurred. Before present-day uniform methods of release of the Court's opinions, Chief Justice Roger Brooke Taney, in the *Dred Scott* case, held back his opinion and added "a considerable amount of material that few if any of the other justices heard or read before its publication,"[23] adding to the friction the case produced. When the Court struck down limitations on pharmacists' advertising of prescription drug prices, Chief Justice Burger changed his concurring opinion between the advance sheets (the initial official released opinion) and the final, bound Court reports. Initially he described pharmacists as "no more render[ing] a true professional service than does a clerk who sells lawbooks." After criticism of this description, the opinion was changed to delete all reference to "true professional service" and to read: "the pharmacist performs largely a packaging rather than a compounding function of former times."[24]

The Court has been particularly careful to assure that its opinions do not become public until they are officially announced, even maintaining is own print shop for the printing of opinions, including drafts. The Court's present word processing system is "integrated with the printing and publishing of final opinions." This word-processing system, access to computerized legal research at the Court, and a computer system for record keeping by the Clerk's office, are significantly advanced from the beginning of Chief Justice Burger's tenure, when the Court lacked even photocopying machines. Such systems are part of the Court's more general pattern of "maintain[ing] its own administrative and research capabilities rather than rely[ing] on the more generally available administrative support office."[25]

The Court's attention to secrecy in the preparation of its opinions stems partly from the public embarrassment suffered by the Court when President Buchanan referred to the soon-to-be-announced *Dred Scott* case in his inaugural address, and partly from fear that people who were able to learn about the Court's intended decisions, particularly those with financial implications, could benefit unfairly from such information. More recently, in the 1978 Term, there were leaks in two cases. One concerned the Chief Justice's authorship of a Nebraska prisoners' rights-parole case; the other, more serious, came when ABC News reported, two days before the Court announced the major libel case of *Herbert v. Lando*, that Justice White had written an opinion for the Court in which the media would suffer a defeat. After the latter incident, the Chief Justice fired a typesetter from his job in the Court's printshop. At the end of the 1985 Term the result the Court reached in the Gramm-Rudman budget case also appears to have leaked.

Justices once read extended portions of their opinions in open court. This practice has been eliminated; justices now read short statements of the facts and issues in a case and what the Court has decided. Until 1965, Monday was the only Decision Day, the day when decisions are announced. In 1965, under Chief Justice Warren, the Court began to use other days as well, to allow greater media coverage of its opinions, and also moved its public sessions from 12:00–4:30 P.M. to a 10:00 A.M. start to help the media meet deadlines. The Court has an information officer, but that person's basic task is only to see that the news media get the opinions, not to explain them or to respond to questions about what the Court or individual justices may have intended. Thus the opinions are released without additional comment—by the justices or other Court personnel. The Burger Court has, however, assisted the press in its task of digesting rulings unassisted by having the Reporter of Decisions prepare a case *syllabus* or head-note, a concise summary of facts, issues, and the Court's holding, for every full opinion case and released when the decision is issued, a change from the earlier practice of not having it prepared until months later for the official reports. (The headnote, not officially part of the opinion of the Court, does not digest any dissenting opinions; only when there are plurality opinions are opinions concurring in the result included.)

The first day of each term, the "first Monday in October," is the day the Court announces the results of the justices' summer labors concerning which cases shall be heard and which denied review, although such decisions are also issued regularly throughout the term. On the first day of the 1985 Term (October 7, 1985), the Court disposed of:

- 1 summary affirmance
- 749 certiorari petitions (21 granted; 8 granted, vacated, and remanded for consideration in light of particular cases; 2 dismissed, and 718 denied)
- 41 appeals (probable jurisdiction noted in 2, 20 dismissed for lack of a substantial federal question and 19 dismissed for lack of jurisdiction—17 of which were then denied as cert. petitions)
- 1 original jurisdiction matter (set for argument)
- 73 miscellaneous matters (including 4 petitions for habeas corpus, 9 for mandamus, and 2 for rehearing; 38 case-related motions (petitions to file amicus

briefs, to retax costs, etc.), 7 petitions to proceed *in forma pauperis*; and 8 disbarment matters.

Use of Monday as the only Decision Day—except when Monday was a legal holiday, with Tuesday used instead—meant that large numbers of important full opinion cases—not to speak of certiorari denials and other orders—were handed down on the same day. This was a particular problem at the end of the term, with the media being deluged with cases. After the Court shifted in 1965 to using non-Mondays as well as Mondays as Decision Days, only one-fourth of the Court's full opinion cases were issued on days other than Mondays in the new practice's first full term, but the Court made only minimal use of non-Monday Decision Days in the remaining three Warren Court terms. Moreover, toward the end of the term, when spreading out cases might have helped out most because most decisions were handed down then, Monday remained the only Decision Day. Thus there were such unusually high outputs as 12 (June 10, 1968), 13 (June 12, 1967), and 14 (May 20, 1968) cases, many announcing significant constitutional doctrine. [26]

Chief Justice Burger's tenure saw non-Monday Decision Days used with increasing frequency, rising to two-thirds of all signed full opinions cases in the 1975 Term, with more than half the Court's signed full opinion cases handed down on non-Monday Decision Days in subsequent terms. During any term, greatest use of non-Monday Decisions Days occurs in the January-March period; once the Court ends hearing argument for the term, in April or May, it is more inclined to release cases on the Monday following the Friday conference and on the Thursday following the Wednesday conference.

As a result of the changes produced by Chief Justice Burger, the Court developed a pattern of handing down cases on several days each week at the end of the term, even overcoming Monday's late-term predominance. The Court thus succeeded in spreading out cases more when the flow was heaviest. There might be more than 20 signed opinions in a week, but no more than five or six were likely to be issued on any one day. Except for such situations as the end of the 1972 Term, with one day of 12 opinions and two each of 14 opinions, eight or nine seemed to be the new upper limit for a single day's output.

Changes in Decision Day practices have not been accompanied by changes in the flow of cases throughout the term. Few opinions can be expected in October, November, and December when oral argument has just begun, but disparities in output between the second three months (January–March) and the last three (April–June) have been considerable. As Table 7.1 indicates, only a small portion of the Court's output appears by the end of December. Less than half the Court's full opinions have been announced by the end of March.

Not only does the Court release most of its output in the last third of the term, but as much as one-third of the Court's entire output for the term is announced in the last six weeks, with more than two-fifths of the opinions appearing in that period in some terms. The end of the 1981 Term was extraordi-

Table 7.1 Opinion Flow—Signed Cases

	Term											
	1975		1976		1977		1978		1979		1980	
October, November, December	6	4.3%	10	7.9%	9	7.0%	11	8.5%	9	6.9%	11	8.9%
January, February, March	41	29.7	36	28.6	33	25.6	34	26.2	40	30.5	36	29.2
April, May, June	91	65.9	80	63.5	87	67.4	85	65.4	82	62.6	76	61.8
TOTAL	138		126		129		130		131		123	

	1981		1982		1983		1984		1985	
October, November, December	11	7.8%	9	5.9%	4	2.6%	5	3.6%	10	7.0%
January, February, March	39	27.7	36	23.7	45	29.8	52	37.4	33	23.2
April, May, June (and July)	91	64.5	107	70.4	107	70.4	82	59.0	99	69.7
TOTAL	141		152		151		139		142	

nary, however, with over two-fifths of the term's output (42%) released in the last *three weeks* of the term and almost one-fifth (18.4%) released in the last week of the term alone. In the 1985 Term, over one-fourth of the term's output appeared in the last two weeks, and just under half in June alone. (*Per curiam* rulings tend to be released relatively evenly across the term's trimesters, because, although a brief opinion must be written in such cases, the decision process for them is much less extended than for full opinion cases.)

Consensus and Dissensus in the Court

Unanimity and Dissent

Lack of unanimity among judges of a multijudge court results from a variety of causes, including intellectual processes of reasoning about past doctrine; differences in judges' values; attitudes about judicial role; personal animosity, such as that between Justice Frankfurter and several other members of the Court, including Chief Justice Warren[27]; and leadership (or lack of it). The desire to have judges put aside personal values and engage in deliberate, logical consideration of cases, so that the result is determined only by the facts of the case and relevant precedents, makes all these reasons except the first somewhat suspect, and helps explain the sharp criticism of a justice whose decisions seem fully controlled by personal attitudes.

Justice Douglas was the target of such criticism, not only for his civil liberties decisions—as predictable in the liberal direction as Justice Rehnquist's have been in the conservative direction—but for his tax rulings as well. Although Douglas prior to 1942 supported the taxpayer less than did the Court as a whole, his support of the taxpayer then became very much higher than the Court's average. In 1943–59 the taxpayer won one-fourth of the time, but Douglas' votes favored the taxpayer in 47 percent of the cases, increasing to 73 percent in the next five years, while the taxpayer was winning only 17 percent of the cases. In 1964–73, Douglas supported the taxpayer in 59 percent of his decisions, well over the taxpayer's 26 percent "win rate."[28]

Even if not in such an extreme fashion, justices' attitudes are important in Supreme Court decision making. Were this not so, shifts in the Court's direction would not stem, as they do in fact, directly from changes in personnel, although other factors soften or reinforce the effects of these changes. It should also be no surprise that justices, not newcomers to major political issues prior to judicial service, do not decide all cases unanimously and that they disagree about the opinions explaining the Court's results. Such disagreement is not necessarily destructive. Conflict within the Supreme Court "makes for alertness, clarifies issues, raises alternative approaches, and tests the intensity of justices' commitments to given positions." It can, however, be destructive if it "becomes highly emotional and antagonistic."[29] We might recall that Justice Holmes once referred to the members of the Court as "nine scorpions in a bottle."

One would expect division on controversial cases. From that perspective, the alignment in a case like *Bakke*, with Justice Powell casting the deciding vote for two different four-vote groups of his colleagues (in a 4–1–4 alignment) should not cause concern, nor should 5–4 rulings on other major issues. What does cause concern, however, is the perceived lack of stability in the Court's decisions and in the fracturing of majority voting groups so that either several concurring opinions appear in addition to the opinion of the Court or, more serious, there is only a plurality opinion rather than an opinion of the Court.

A *plurality* or prevailing opinion is one in which some majority justices join the Court's judgment (its decision or result) but not what would otherwise be the "opinion of the Court," thus leaving fewer than five justices supporting the basic opinion. An example would be a case in which the justices divided 5–4, with three of the majority justices favoring one opinion and the other two concurring only in the result—but not the opinion.

Plurality opinions officially have no binding effect, although they have persuasive value and, as time passes, people may come to treat them as precedent—long true of Justice Frankfurter's plurality opinion in *Colegrove v. Green* that reapportionment was a "political question." Nonetheless, plurality opinions frustrate the lower courts—trying to apply the Supreme Court's doctrine—as well as the other justices. For example, the Court's longtime inability to produce an opinion of the Court in obscenity cases during the 1960s led Justice Tom Clark to say, with some irritation, that his colleagues were "like ancient Gaul . . . split into three parts."[30] The absence of leadership is likely to increase such outcomes.

The Court at times is so badly split that it must resort to a *per curiam* announcement of the basic policy on which the justices agree. Examples are *Furman v. Georgia*, the 1972 death penalty case, and the *Pentagon Papers* case *(New York Times v. United States)*, in both of which each majority justice appended a separate opinion to the brief *per curiam*; *Buckley v. Valeo*, the 1976 campaign finance ruling where five justices dissented from at least some parts of the ruling; the *Norris* pension plan case (1983), where there were different majorities on the constitutional issue and on the remedy; and *Bazemore v. Friday*, a 1986 ruling on racial discrimination, where majorities varied with the particular discrimination issue. (Although there was an opinion for the Court in *Pennzoil v. Texaco* in 1987, and the vote was unanimous, there were six separate opinions.)

Disagreement among the justices does not mean that they *express* that disagreement through dissenting opinions or separate opinions concurring with the majority. The latter opinions, written less often than dissents because they are less useful to later justices and less frequently cited by them, either provide additional thoughts or agree only with the majority *result* but on the basis of different reasoning. Because a justice must write separate opinions in addition to opinions of the Court, they add to a justice's workload and thus limit the frequency with which they are prepared. There are additional constraints as well,[31] some of which are strategic. For example, dissents are said to encourage noncompliance, particularly with controversial rulings like school desegregation. The Court may also be criticized for being divided frequently, just as justices are criticized for writing concurring opinions if doing so results in plurality opinions rather than opinions of the Court. A justice contemplating a dissent must also remember that, apart from the fact that open disagreement may be interpreted as an attack on the Court's integrity, a strong dissenting opinion may make the majority opinion more visible and thus more damaging than would silence. On the other hand, dissents may give the losing side the feeling that someone has listened to their position. Dissents, which also make the majority justices sharpen their reasoning, may allow them to write more forcefully because they do not have to compromise with the dissenting justices.[32]

Individual justices, or groups of justices, nonetheless dissent (or concur separately) to state principled opposition to the majority's doctrine, and to appeal to the dissenter's colleagues and the Court's immediate audience. Dissents may, for example, be written for present lower court judges in the hope that if those judges dislike the Supreme Court majority's position, they will see ways in which to limit it. For example, Justice Brennan, who recently suggested that dissents can serve both as "damage control" to limit the sweep of the majority's position and as "practical guidance" to those wishing to circumvent the majority ruling, himself wrote in a dissent in a criminal procedure case that the Court's rule did not "preclude a contrary resolution of this case based upon the State's separate interpretation of its own constitution."[33] In so speaking to state judges, the dissenters may be more persuasive than the Supreme Court's rulings, which are not binding on matters of state constitutional interpretation.[34]

Dissents may also be speaking to future lawyers and judges. Although many dissenters are defending an outdated status quo (see pages 118-19), dissents are indeed potential majority opinions of the future, and certain "Great Dissenters" such as Holmes and Brandeis are certainly well remembered for their contributions in this regard. Although other factors contribute to the Court's overruling of past decisions, in three-fourths of the Court's overruling actions from 1958 through 1980, justices gave dissents in earlier cases as the basis for overruling those decisions, or based overruling opinions on ideas from the prior dissents.[35]

Judges vary in the extent to which they continue to state a dissent on a particular issue, being more likely to continue so stating in constitutional than in statutory cases. That they stop making the dissenting statement does not, however, mean they have abandoned their initial position; they are more likely to be acquiescing temporarily in the disliked precedent.

Considerations such as the encouragement of noncompliance and the appearance of attacking the Court's integrity also do not prevent dissenters from directly attacking not only the majority's policy positions but also its intelligence and ability—perhaps an extension of friction in the Court's conference meetings, which, according to Justice Blackmun, were "marked by 'impatience' and 'short temper'" in the 1985 Term.[36] At times, the language of the justices' opinions becomes rather testy, raising questions about the "respect" in "I respectfully dissent." In a 1978 case, for example, Justice Brennan accused Justice Rehnquist of writing an opinion that "reaches a result supported by neither policy nor precedent, ignores difficult legal issues, [and] misapprehends the significance of the proceeding below." As if that were not enough, he accused Rehnquist of "ignoring wholesale the analytical framework" of a recent important case, of committing "case-reading errors," and of avoiding discussion of certain important issues.[37]

Rehnquist showed himself able to hand out comparable criticism in his dissent in the 1979 school desegregation cases, where he said of the Court's "lick and a promise" opinions that "perhaps the adjective 'analytical' is out of place, since the Court's opinions furnish only the most superficial methodology."[38] In a more recent criticism of a particular opinion, he said that if it "were to be judged by standards appropriate to Impressionist paintings, it would perhaps receive a high grade, but the same cannot be said if it is to be judged by the standards of a judicial opinion."[39] In a particularly sharp attack in a case involving federal preemption of state regulatory action, Justice Blackmun criticized Justice Sandra O'Connor for a "rhetorical assertion" about federalism that was "demonstrably incorrect" if it were to be taken literally. He then added that "while Justice O'Connor articulates a view of state sovereignty that is almost mystical, she entirely fails to address our central points."[40] Among the sharpest recent statements have been those of Justice Brennan, in part reflecting his minority position on civil liberties issues. Thus, in a case involving the *Miranda* warnings, he wrote that "the Court mischaracterizes our precedents, obfuscates the central issues, and altogether ignores the practical realities of custodial interrogation that have led nearly every lower court to reject its simplistic reasoning" and also criticized the "Court's marble-palace psychoanalysis."[41]

The extent of disagreement within the Court has varied over the years. In the Court's earliest years, each justice wrote an opinion in each case and there was no "opinion of the Court." Chief Justice John Marshall brought an end to these seriatim opinions. Indeed, he wrote most of the Court's opinions, even when he did not agree with the result: from 1801 to 1804, the Court handed down 26 decisions containing opinions, and Marshall wrote for the Court in 24. The "first dissenter"—in the context of unified opinions—was a Jefferson appointee, Justice William Johnson. His dissents not only served to break Marshall's monopoly but led to present practices of opinion-assignment by the Chief Justice, although pressures remained strong to limit the statement of separate views.

Despite year-to-year variation, the level of disagreement within the Court has generally increased over the years; there has been a marked shift from justices acquiescing in all except very major cases to more routine expression of dissent, as expectations of what is appropriate changed. Because most of the Court's cases in the late nineteenth century did not then give rise to controversy, all but a few were decided unanimously. The period of the Taft Court (1921–29) was also one of low dissents, for example, less than one for each six cases in the 1925 Term—leading to the comment that it "may have been the 'Roaring Twenties' in the speakeasies, but it was the 'Boring Twenties' at the Supreme Court."[42]

The shift from mandatory to discretionary review, by eliminating the less controversial cases, produced more disagreement. After 1925, an increase in dissent first appeared in the appeals jurisdiction, from which less important cases had been removed and shifted to the certiorari category. This left the more controversial appeals cases, which would naturally produce more dissent. As winnowing progressed in the certiorari cases as well, dissent later increased there, as did the number of concurring opinions.[43] In short, the cases the Court accepted were disproportionately complex or controversial ("hard" cases), likely to produce dissent, contributing to the long-term trend, extending from well before 1925, of an increase in sharply divided cases (those with 5-4 rulings).[44]

In 1930, only 11 percent of the Court's cases were split decisions. That percentage more than doubled in each of the next two decades. In particular, the time of Harlan Stone's chief judgeship (1941–46), with his ineffective leadership, produced much higher dissent rates, with rates of disagreement between the justices reaching one-third.[45] But Stone alone was not responsible: dissent rates continued to rise after his tenure, reaching 61 percent in 1950, during Fred Vinson's chief judgeship. After Earl Warren became Chief Justice, the figure rose to over three-fourths of the cases in 1957. Only about two-fifths of the Court's full opinion cases in the early 1960s were unanimous. That figure dropped to one-third in the Warren Court's last term, but relatively few of the cases then were decided by close votes. Moreover, most justices' dissent rates were low. In the last Warren Court term (1968), four justices had fewer than 10 dissenting votes each and four cast no "solo" dissents.

The transition to the Burger Court produced an obvious drop in consensus. In Burger's first three terms, the Court achieved unanimity in only roughly one-third of its full opinion cases, falling to one-fourth in the 1972 Term before rising above one-third (to 36%) in the 1975 Term. For the remaining terms of the Burger Court (through the 1985 Term), the proportion of unanimous cases never fell below one-fourth, but it did not rise to one-third until 1981; the proportion then moved higher, exceeding two-fifths in both 1983 and 1984 before dropping sharply (to 28.9%) in Burger's last term. (See Table 7.2.)

The size of majorities may reflect disagreement even more clearly than the proportion of cases that are unanimous. During the 1969 Term, Burger's first, there were wide margins (at least four votes) in 62 percent of the signed cases. The proportion fell to under half the next year, with one-vote margins in over one-fourth of the cases. After 1972, the proportion of cases decided by wide margins returned to over one-half, reaching 70 percent in the 1975 Term and over 60 percent in the 1983 and 1984 Terms, but the proportion of cases decided by one-vote margins remained high—over one-fourth of the cases in 1970, and 20

Table 7.2 Distribution of Votes—Full Opinion Cases

	1981	1982	1983	1984	1985
Unanimous	33.3%	36.1%	42.4%	40.3%	28.9%
8–1	8.5	11.2	8.6	5.6	10.6
7–2	10.6	12.5	8.6	9.4	9.9
Other*	1.4	—	2.6	11.5	.7
"Wide Margins"	53.9	59.9	62.3	66.9	50.0
6–3	20.6	15.8	17.9	17.3	21.8
5–4	22.7	22.4	17.2	11.5	26.1
Other**	2.8	2.0	2.6	4.3	2.1
"Close Votes"	46.1	40.1	37.7	33.1	50.0
Total	141	152	151	139	142

* Includes 7–1, 6–1, 6–2
** Includes 6–2, 5–3, 4–3
Not included: 4–4 votes.

percent or more in 1978 and 1981 through 1982, jumping to over one-fourth in the last Burger term. One factor explaining the high dissent rate is the type of cases the Court decided: cases with constitutional issues were far more likely than those with statutory questions to produce multiple dissents. Thus in the 1981–84 Terms, nearly half of the constitutional decisions had at least three dissenting votes, and only a little more than one-fourth of those cases were unanimous; by contrast, only one-third of the statutory cases had three or four dissenting votes and nearly half were unanimous. Of 250 civil rights cases decided on the merits during that period, there were not even 40 in which all the justices joined in a single opinion, yet there were 70 statutory decisions with all the justices supporting a single opinion. (Likewise, constitutional questions accounted for all but two of 24 cases in which there was only a plurality opinion instead of an opinion of the Court.[46])

Also part of patterns of disagreement is the number of concurring and dissenting opinions. The number of concurring opinions, 40 in the 1962 Term and 67 ten years later, reached a new high of 85 in the 1975 Term. That number was exceeded in four of the next six terms, before dropping into the 60's for three terms (see Table 7.3). The period from 1976 through 1985 produced an average of roughly 120 dissenting opinions per term, although the figure ranged from 101 (1980) to a high of 144 (1985). The relationship between the number of *votes* and the number of *opinions* shows that the justices were more likely to join in other justices' dissenting opinions than in their concurring opinions. A recent examination of justices' joining in each others' concurring and dissenting opinions, as a measure of influence, showed little overall influence of justices on

Table 7.3 Concurring and Dissenting Opinions and Votes—Full Opinion Cases

| | | OPINIONS | | |
	Concur	Per Case	Dissent	Per Case
1981	91	.65	121	.86
1982	65	.43	126	.83
1983	61	.40	106	.70
1984	60	.43	110	.79
1985	75	.53	144	1.01
Average	70.4	.49	121.4	.84

| | | VOTES | | |
	Concur	Per Case	Dissent	Per Case
1981	129	.91	264	1.87
1982	99	.65	272	1.79
1983	94	.62	248	1.64
1984	100	.72	212	1.53
1985	123	.87	289	2.04
Average	109	.75	257	1.78

each other, but in the Burger Court, the liberals mutually influenced each other more whereas during the Warren Court, the nonliberals had shown higher mutual influence.[47]

That there are many dissenting and concurring opinions is, however, only one indication of disagreement within the Court. Professor (now Judge) Frank Easterbrook has suggested that if we look at "whether the Justices who do not join the majority disagree with the Court's rationale," instead of engaging in counting, one sees far less change in conflict within the Court; indeed, "the level of disagreement has been remarkably stable for the last forty years," with "the rate of real disagreement hover[ing] around 20 percent."[48]

Whereas Chief Justice Warren had been an infrequent dissenter, Chief Justice Burger was one of the Court's two most frequent dissenters in his first term. Although his rate of dissent decreased as the Nixon bloc came to control the Court, he continued to dissent frequently, along with Justice Rehnquist, as the liberal justices became the Court's most frequent dissenters. Rehnquist was not either the most frequent dissenter—those "honors" went to Brennan (for dissenting votes) and Stevens (dissenting opinions)—or, as alleged at his 1986 confirmation hearings, the most frequent *lone* dissenter: when both were on the Court together, Stevens dissented solo more than did Rehnquist. The level of dissent within the Burger Court cannot be explained solely by the liberals' dissents or by Justice Douglas' prodigious dissent frequency (57 dissenting votes in the 1971 Term, 15 solo, and 60 the following term).

An important part of the reason for the Court's high level of explicit dis-agreement was that newer members of the Court knew their own minds and did not wait to assert their positions. The suggestions that justices "bide their time" before assuming a position at either the liberal or conservative side of the Court, perhaps staying "in the middle" for several terms before "making their move," and that each waits cautiously to cast his first dissent in a case of substantial importance have not applied to the recent justices. Perhaps as a result of their past judicial and legal experience, they have spoken out in dissenting and con-curring opinions within a short time of reaching the bench. Thus Justice Ste-vens, despite his nonparticipation in roughly one-third of the cases in his first term, dissented in 19 cases; Justice O'Connor promptly joined the Court's conservative bloc.[49]

Variation in the frequency of dissent is an indication of the Court's overall alignment. Thus it should be no surprise that those at the ideological extremities of the Court cast the most dissenting votes, with Brennan, Marshall, Rehnquist, and Chief Justice Burger rivaling each other for the "prize" in this regard. The high rate of dissent for the Chief Justice was perhaps more surprising—and certainly more remarked upon—than Justice Rehnquist's behavior, because of our expectation that a Chief Justice will try to "mass" the Court and will cast fewer dissents as part of that effort.

The size of the Court's majorities may be affected by a tendency, noted by students of small-group decision making, for decisions to be made by *minimum winning coalitions*, that is, the smallest majority necessary. A body threatened from the outside is, however, thought to increase the size of the decision-making coalition. During the period of Justice Burton's Court service, when coalitions at the initial conference vote were smaller than minimum winning, they were likely to become minimum winning by the conclusion of the case, probably because the justices wished an "opinion of the Court." However, when original coalitions were larger than minimum winning, they were unlikely to shrink to minimum-winning size. When justices changed position, size of majority increased far more often than it decreased (see pages 228-29).[50]

In the Warren Court, in nonthreat situations, 31 percent of the *decision coalitions*—justices joining in the vote for the result in a case—and 40 percent of the *opinion coalitions*—justices joining in support of the Court's principal opin-ion—were minimum winning and 17 percent were unanimous. However, under conditions of threat, for example, legislative proposals to limit the Court's juris-diction, only 13 percent of decision coalitions and 23 percent of opinion coali-tions were minimum winning, 44 percent unanimous; the same relations hold if six-justice coalitions are added to combinations of five justices. Furthermore, large coalitions formed under threat conditions were more likely than otherwise to include justices with divergent policy positions, but opinion coalitions smaller than the decision coalitions were more likely than other coalitions to contain ideologically "connected" justices.[51]

Chief Justice: Leadership and Opinion Assignment

The Chief Justice is expected to play a wide variety of roles. In addition to participating in the deciding of cases, writing a share of the Court's opinions, and serving as the Court's presiding officer, he serves as a circuit justice (for the D.C. and Fourth Circuits), and also is court manager, court defender, third branch chieftain, and statesman. Being court manager entails such matters as allocating circuit justice duties, signing certificates of disability for Supreme Court justices should that be necessary, working with the Court's officials—the clerk of court, marshal, reporter of decisions, and librarian—and serving as "building manager" for the Court; it also encompasses being a protocol leader and a major host to foreign dignitaries. Serving as court defender means "press[ing] the Court's case before coordinate branches of the national government" and perhaps "mobiliz-[ing] public opinion" in order to protect the Court's status.[52] The role of "third branch chieftain," one to which Warren Burger gave great attention, concerns administration of the federal judiciary (see pages 64-71). The "statesman" role is extrajudicial: in it the Chief Justice serves on a variety of commissions (as provided by statute) and may accept additional assignments (see pages 291-93).

With respect to the Chief Justice's colleagues, there are three leadership roles that have to be performed within the Court—roles that the Chief Justice may assume but that may be assumed by other justices. These are task or intellectual leadership; social leadership, through which solidarity is produced among the justices and their "emotional needs . . . as individuals" are attended to; and policy leadership, moving the Court toward a particular position over the long term. The Chief Justice may be the Court's social leader (like Taft) or the task leader, although apart from Hughes it does not appear that chief justices have been the task leader. It is possible that the Chief will perform both social *and* task leadership roles, as Hughes did. When the Chief Justice performs neither role (like Stone or Burger), an extremely uncohesive Court results. If the Chief Justice does not perform one of the necessary roles, someone else will; for example, Justice Willis Van Devanter was task leader when Taft was social leader.

Even if the Chief Justice does not perform either role for the Court as a whole, he can perform both roles or neither for a bloc of justices. Chief Justice Burger may have done the former (both roles) for the Nixon appointees during the early years of his tenure, although he did not do so subsequently, and criticisms of Burger as a weak Chief Justice were legion. One must, however, take into account his attention to judicial administration; a Chief Justice devoting much attention to matters outside the Court is less likely to be an in-Court leader than one who invests most of his energies in the Court itself. If the Chief does not lead, others will fill the vacuum, even in (or particularly in) the Court's most crucial cases, as appears to have occurred in developing the opinion in the Nixon Tapes case. Even where the Chief does lead—clearly the case, from most accounts, of Earl Warren, called the "Super Chief"—others may also play a large role. We must be careful not to assume leadership on the part of the person in the "center chair"; even during Earl Warren's tenure, Justice Brennan was a major influence on the Court's doctrinal landmarks, for example, when his dissent in the welfare residency case of *Shapiro v. Thompson* became the majority view and a suggestion he made to Justice Douglas became the right to privacy basis of the *Griswold* contraception case, which led directly to the Court's 1973 abortion rulings. [53]

The Chief Justice's leadership is affected by the degree to which he dissents: a dissenter may exercise *policy* leadership, but exercising leadership over colleagues in the short term is difficult if one is often in dissent. Thus Chief Justice Stone's lack of leadership is reflected in the fact that he dissented in a larger proportion of nonunanimous cases than did any other Chief Justice, and Chief Justice Burger's dissent rate—more than 14 percent for the 1969 through 1980 Terms—helps explain claims that he did not provide strong leadership. The dissent rate when earlier Chief Justices presided was affected by "the attitudes of the justices toward dissent or expressing dissent, the varying complexity of cases being decided, and interpersonal feuding in the Court."[54] If the absence of "conflict cases" indicates more effective leadership, Chief Justice John Marshall (1801–35) has the highest place as a leader: 92.7 percent of the cases during his tenure did not reveal conflict. In the second rank (87–90 percent nonconflict cases) are Chief Justices Salmon P. Chase (1864–73), Morrison R. Waite (1874–88), Edward White (1910–20), and William Howard Taft (1921–29). At the next level (83–85 percent nonconflict cases) are Roger Taney (1836–63), Melville Fuller (1888–1909), and Charles Evans Hughes (1930–41). Far behind are Chief Justices Harlan F. Stone (1941–46) (almost half the cases during his tenure involved conflict), Earl Warren, and Fred Vinson (1946–53) (with almost three-fourths of the cases involving conflict). A problem with this indicator is that the cases facing the Court have varied over time in complexity and controversiality, as have justices' attitudes toward dissent and the level of interpersonal friction in the Court.

Opinion Assignment. The assignment of opinions by the Chief Justice is one of the ways in which he can attempt to exercise his and his colleagues' influence outside the Court—on the Court's multiple audiences, particularly lawyers. There are, however, numerous constraints on the Chief Justice's choice of an opinion writer for the Court. These include his efforts to influence his colleagues through the assignment of opinions and the necessity of distributing the writing workload evenly among all the justices, something not easy to do if some colleagues are frequently in dissent. Justices are expected to be "generalists," that is, to write opinions in all fields of law, but informal specialization appears from time to time—for example, Justice Stephen Field in land law and, apparently, Justice Powell in business cases. Cases may also be assigned to justices because of their past positions, for example, Powell as a former American Bar Association president writing on lawyer advertising and lawyer residence requirements for admission to the bar, and Tom Clark, as former attorney general, writing in criminal procedure cases. The Chief Justice must participate in writing opinions, and he thus retains some cases. It is expected that the Chief Justice will write in some of the Court's "big" cases, but the Court's internal social relations prevent him from keeping all the most important ones.

Danelski has suggested two strategies that the Chief Justice might use in assigning opinions to accommodate some of these pressures:

> RULE 1: Assign the case to the Justice whose views are the closest to the dissenters on the ground that his opinion would take a middle approach upon which both majority and minority could agree.

> RULE 2: Where there are blocs on the Court and a bloc splits, assign the case to a majority member of the dissenters' bloc on the ground that he would take a middle approach upon which both majority and minority could agree and that the minority justices would be more likely to agree with him because of general mutuality of agreement. [55]

Those justices never "closest" to the assigners are usually given unanimous cases or cases in less controversial areas of the law. There are other strategic concerns as well, for example, that of assignment of a case when the Court changes position, where assigning to a prior dissenter may produce too "sharp" an opinion. [56]

In close political cases through 1962, Chief Justice Warren, seeming to follow the strategies suggested by Danelski, "overassigned" cases to justices who joined the majority through votes inconsistent with their usual positions. In the 1962 Term, he also assigned Justice Goldberg, closest to the Court's center of the five reliable liberal votes, six of his 12 opinions in 5-4 rulings. In economic cases, however, Warren assigned opinions to maximize the liberal policy position. [57] When majorities were large, he tended to overassign to those in the midmajority position. Although assigning justices have generally favored justices "closest to them in various issue areas," [58] Warren used those large majorities to help create an opinion of the Court considerably different from his own particular position. The rule of assigning cases to moderate justices was evident in Justice Clark's opinions in cases with liberal results, such as *Mapp v. Ohio* on the exclusionary rule for improperly seized evidence, where his background as attorney general was probably thought to produce a better reception in the law enforcement community than if a justice with a predictably liberal record had written for the Court. As had Chief Justice Vinson before him, Warren underassigned to himself, although toward the end of his tenure, he seemed to keep more of the Court's important cases than he had earlier.

In his first two terms, Chief Justice Burger did not allocate workload evenly, but illness and vacancies may help explain that. Thereafter, the writing of the Court's signed opinions was divided relatively evenly among the justices. [59] Again, exceptions are explained in part by a justice's illness (Powell's 1984 Term surgery) or newness to the Court (O'Connor, 1981 Term), and in part on the basis of ideology: Brennan and Marshall wrote fewer opinions for the Court than the average in several terms, White and Rehnquist somewhat more than the others. The proportion of times the Chief Justice assigned a case to each justice when that justice was available (not in dissent) did vary, with Burger choosing Rehnquist and White a disproportionately high percentage of the times they were available; he chose Brennan a low proportion of the relatively small number of times he was available. Many of Brennan's opinions for the Court (12 of his 15 opinions in the 1981 Term) came from self-assignment when he was senior justice in the majority; this self-assignment was an important source of his power within the Court. Justices Blackmun and Marshall also received a significant portion of their opinion-writing assignments from Brennan.

Certain justices at times write for the Court more frequently in particular situations. For one thing, there appears to be some subject-matter specialization assignment of opinions, but specialists in particular civil liberties and civil rights areas are also the Chief Justice's ideological allies, so that issues specialization can be seen as resulting from assignment based on ideology.[60] Burger definitely used his assignment of opinions to reward Justices White and Stewart, the Court's centrists, and particularly the other Nixon appointees. Although assignment of Rehnquist to write criminal procedure opinions ran counter to the strategy of using mid-Court members, it may have resulted either from the majority coalition's single-mindedness in this policy area or from a feeling that the coalition was sufficiently solid that Rehnquist's positions would not lose votes. (Despite the supposed tradition that a new justice's first opinion comes in a noncontroversial, unanimous case, both Justices Powell and Rehnquist wrote for divided courts in their first opinions; the "tradition" was, however, true for Justices Stevens, O'Connor, and Scalia.)

Table 7.4 shows that some justices write more frequently when the Court is unanimous or nearly so, others when the Court is more seriously divided. Thus, in the last five Burger Court terms (1981-85), more than half of Justice Marshall's opinions for the Court came in unanimous cases, and Justices Blackmun, Rehnquist, Stevens, and the Chief Justice wrote roughly half their opinions for the Court when it was unanimous or there was only one dissenting vote. On the other hand, Justices Powell and White, at the Court's center, wrote roughly half their opinions for the Court when it was seriously divided; so did Justice Brennan, but that resulted from his self-assignment, particularly in 5-4 cases. Chief Justice Burger's self-assignments did not at first come in major cases, but after the first few terms, he began to self-assign in important cases like the *Swann* and Detroit busing cases and the major obscenity case of *Miller v. California*. Although he wrote in fewer "close" cases than some other justices, he did not avoid such cases, for example, taking nine 5-4 rulings in the 1975 Term—in contrast to Chief Justice Warren, who wrote most often in cases with wide vote margins or unanimous votes.

Table 7.4 Assignments, 1981–1985 (combined)—Full Opinion Cases*

	Burger	Blackmun	Powell	Rehnquist	O'Connor	White	Stevens	Marshall	Brennan
Unanimous	43.0%	40.0%	27.7%	39.8%	27.5%	27.1%	43.6%	55.4%	29.0% (19/1)
8–1, 7–1, 6–1	10.1	10.7	12.7 (9/1)	9.7 (8/1)	17.5 (13/1)	5.4	6.4 (4/1)	8.1	8.7 (5/1)
7–2, 6–2	15.2	8.0 (5/1)	10.1 (6/2)	16.1 (14/1)	16.3	14.1	15.3	1.4 (-/1)	10.1 (3/4)
6–3, 5–2	20.3	21.3 (10/6)	17.7	15.1	15.0	22.8 (20/1)	17.9 (13/1)	18.9 (10/4)	17.4 (4/8)
5–4, 5–3, 4–3	11.4	20.0 (4/11)	31.6 (20/5)	19.4 (17/1)	23.8 (16/3)	30.4 (22/6)	16.7 (8/5)	16.2 (4/8)	34.8 (2/22)
Total Assignments	79	75 (57/18)	79 (71/8)	93 (90/3)	80 (76/4)	92 (85/7)	78 (71/7)	74 (61/13)	69 (33/36)

Note: Where two numbers are separated by a slash (9/1), the first number indicates opinions assigned by the Chief Justice; the second indicates those assigned by others when the Chief Justice was in the minority.

*These are inferred assignments, calculated from final vote, not initial vote (data not available). Fluidity might mean assignments have shifted from the original assignment. When the Chief Justice concurred, it is assumed that he assigned and then wrote separately.

245

Over a longer span of Court history, Chief Justices have assigned majority opinions to themselves relatively more often than they have to their colleagues, but they have done so *less* in the post-World War II period. However, in important cases, all Chief Justices have engaged in higher self-assignment. Here, too, there have been differences between justices, with Stone and Warren using their self-assignment prerogative least and Chief Justices Taft and Hughes "pursu[ing] the relatively most advantageous self-assignment policy in important cases."[61] The Chief Justices have also been likely to assign themselves unanimous opinions and to write less frequently for highly divided courts. This is true even in important cases: they are more likely than their colleagues to write for a unanimous Court in important cases and less frequently for a moderately or highly divided Court. This means that, on the whole, the Chief Justice is not put in the position of writing frequently for badly divided courts in a large proportion of major cases.

Judicial Values and Alignments

The votes of Supreme Court justices are patterned, not random. A number of factors help account for the patterned nature of the justices' votes, which have both a short-term component and a long-term one. The short-term component includes the other justices with whom they serve, the presentation of cases, and the decisional environment, plus political and other events of the time. The long-term component includes the justices' pre-Court socialization, which can be a function of the generation in which they were raised; their experience on the Court; their ideology; and their personality.

Attitudes and values are among the central elements in justices' voting. The justices' ideologies or broad preferences as to the proper scope of government and the content of government policy are another. That these elements are central does not, however, mean they are the exclusive causes of justices' voting. The particular fact situations in cases may affect the outcome and recurrent fact situations may allow us to predict the Court's actions. Thus a recent study of the Court's rulings on search and seizure, an area thought to be one of instability and confusion, showed that knowledge of items such as where the search had taken place (e.g., home or business or car), the extent of the search, its prior justification (was there a warrant?), and whether it occurred in connection with an arrest increased substantially one's ability to predict the Court's result, although conservative rulings—by both the Warren and Burger Courts—were easier to predict than liberal ones and the Burger Court's liberal decisions were harder to predict than the Warren Court's. That there was a difference in predisposition toward search issues between the Warren and Burger Courts was clear, but, given the differing predispositions, they treated the factors just discussed in roughly the same way.[62]

Although studied less than attitude or ideology, personality is another major factor that helps explain the pattern of Supreme Court votes, particularly because of its effect on a justice's role conceptions and on interpersonal relations within the Court. An individual's ability or difficulty in assimilating a wide range of often contradictory information and the individual's ability (or inability) to change an initial mindset about a case clearly will affect the processes of communication and negotiation within the Court, and a justice's willingness to admit error (or a change in position) would facilitate development of the law over time.[63] Problems in this regard can be illustrated by Justice Felix Frankfurter, who, "intense, nervous, arrogant, [and] domineering, . . . could not accept serious, sustained opposition in fields he considered his domain of expertise." Thus when he reached the Court, where he could no longer operate as a behind-the-scenes adviser, but was "formally committed to sharing power with strong-willed individuals who had ideas of their own," he "reacted to his opponents with vindictive hostility."[64] His suppressed self-doubts made it difficult for him to work out contradictions in his belief system "between his endorsement of judicial self-restraint," for which he is perhaps best known, "and his belief in the existence of a hierarchy of constitutional values."[65] Not only did he "harden his stands," but he became "preoccupied with the motives of his judicial opponents," attributing impropriety to them; colleagues differing on how to decide cases were not simply fellow professionals with whom one had reasonable disagreements but opponents to be battled as if one were under seige.[66] When he was not trying to ingratiate himself to his colleagues (before he gave them up as lost causes), he was deluging them with suggestions both about cases and about court procedures—something that drove them further away instead of attracting them to his position.[67] To be sure, with Frankfurter or any other justice, personality is not a sufficient explanation, but it is important: "a simple, 'rational' explanation cannot account for [a justice's] personal style on the Court."[68]

Closely related to personality may be biological processes of aging and senescence, which not only cause problems when an older judge becomes ill and is unwilling to leave the Court, true of Justice Douglas after he suffered a serious stroke,[69] but that can also affect an individual's thought processes, for example, leading to rigidity of thinking, and that may help explain increasing conservatism among judges.[70] Such considerations seem particularly relevant in explaining the increasingly conservative voting behavior of Justice Black, who, like Justice Douglas, was most liberal in midcareer. The shift in Black's judicial behavior in civil liberties cases, like that of some other twentieth-century justices, may also have reflected new types of civil liberties cases facing the Court as well as responses to changes in the Court's action. In Black's case, the new types of cases involved not "pure" free speech (speech not connected with action), but "free speech plus," particularly civil rights demonstrations to which he had a strong negative reaction.[71] Also affecting such change is personal learning over time. We have seen justices change their positions—both generally and in particular areas of the law. For example, Justice White recently discussed the change in his position in libel cases from the 1964 ruling in *New York Times v. Sullivan* to the

Gertz case ten years later.[72] A broad change occurred with Chief Justice Warren, whom we remember as a liberal justice but who did not start out firmly planted in the Court's liberal wing, moving there only after two terms in the Court's center.[73] And, more recently, Justice Harry Blackmun, who started his tenure on the Court closely allied with Chief Justice Burger and with a shared conservative view of the world, with considerable deference to government, moved in the 1980s not only to a more liberal voting pattern but to considerable compassion for individuals (other than criminal defendants) negatively affected by government actions or who lacked the resources to contest those actions.

Most studies of the relationship of justices' values or attitudes and their voting have been based only on the justices' recorded votes, supplemented by their papers and, recently, by their docket books, which provide initial conference votes. Materials from a justice's experience prior to Court service have, however, been used to shed light on their values such as morality, tradition, or religion—for such experience could affect the justice's perceptions concerning those values. There was a congruence between the values evident in justices' speeches prior to Supreme Court appointment and the justices' judicial positions reflected in solo dissents but the justices' pre-Court values sometimes caused them internal conflict. For Justice Pierce Butler, these noncongruent values were patriotism and individual freedom. Butler resolved the conflict between them by deciding in favor of patriotism in free speech cases but in favor of individual freedom in criminal procedure cases.[74]

Studies of the justices' voting have been based primarily on their voting interagreement (bloc analysis) and on Guttman scaling. The period used is often that of a *natural court*, that is, a set of nine justices without personnel changes and a period shorter than the broad "Burger Court" or "Warren Court" periods, which included personnel changes. *Guttman scaling*, based on the idea that the case is a stimulus and the judge's vote a response, is used for testing the consistency of attitudes underlying a set of decisions. Scales are sets of cases in which the justices were aligned so that a consistent underlying attitude accounted for their votes. If attitudes do underlie justices' votes in a set of cases, the Guttman scale will indicate a "breakpoint," the case or cases where a justice's votes shift from support for a value to opposition, and a justice whose value or attitude influences his or her voting will vote consistently on either side of the "breakpoint." (However, when two justices vote the same way, it is not clear whether they are treating the same stimulus or perceiving different ones.)[75]

Most bloc analysis studies have been based on the voting interagreement of pairs of justices. The pairs are arranged in a matrix, with blocs identified from sets of high interagreement scores. However, if a bloc is defined as a cohesive group whose members vote together regularly, so that a "bloc" really exists only if Justices Jones, Green, and Brown vote together frequently, and if the three together are frequently found alone, bloc behavior may not be very frequent. If they vote together primarily when they are also voting with others, they do not constitute a bloc. Similarly, the members of several pairs of justices do not constitute a bloc unless all the members of the pairs in the set are in high interagreement. For the 1963–65 Terms, for example, it was difficult to determine the identity of blocs that persisted over time, and identifiable blocs "voted together alone less than half the number of times [they] voted together." Moreover, three- and four-judge dissenting blocs seldom joined in the same *opinion* even when they voted together, making tenuous the idea of "stable, persistent and exclusive . . . blocs, whose members interact substantially as a bloc."[76] Even when two (or more) justices vote conjointly, that does not necessarily mean they share an ideology. Perhaps the best example of this phenomenon is Brandeis and Holmes. Both "believed that the executive and legislature should be given wide latitude in the formulation of social and economic policy," but Brandeis' basic premise was that scientific expertise in government could resolve the problems brought to the government for solution. On the other hand, Holmes was a skeptic and Social Darwinist: the best-fitted would win in the end, so he should not interfere.[77]

Whatever their methods, researchers have regularly discovered blocs in the Supreme Court. For example, in the 1931–35 Terms, the Court that displeased FDR, there was a "Left bloc" of Stone, Cardozo, and Brandeis, and a "Right bloc" of Van Devanter, Butler, Sutherland, and McReynolds. Justice Roberts and Chief Justice Hughes were members of the Right bloc in terms of overall interagreement, although in dissent Roberts was independent and Hughes was marginally affiliated with the Left bloc. In the 1935 Term, however, when the Court shifted to the right, Roberts "was closely aligned with the conservative bloc" in cases where bloc voting occurred and Hughes, who had been slightly left of center, moved slightly right of center.[78]

An examination of judicial voting in terms of game theory was undertaken for this period. Schubert calculated what Hughes and Roberts ("Hughberts," because of their closely-joined voting) would have to have done in the 1936 Term to increase their power, that is, their ability to determine the outcome of the Court's decisions. A "pure" strategy for them would have been to have formed a minimum winning coalition of five with the Left bloc when possible, to join with the Right bloc when the first strategy was not possible, and to join the rest of the Court (Right and Left together) when all agreed, so as not to be isolated. The Hughes/Roberts behavior indeed closely approximated the specified strategy: the two were affiliated with the Left in total interagreement, voting with the Right only when they could not form a majority with the Left.[79]

Part of the "conventional wisdom" concerning the Court's response to FDR's attack was that only Roberts had shifted his position to produce the "switch in time that saved nine." Roberts' own explanation was that he had earlier indicated his change in positions on the validity of minimum wage legislation. However, when a case containing the appropriate challenge did arise, Justice Stone's illness produced a delay in decision of the case, which as a result was not decided until after the Court-packing plan.[80] Schubert's analysis, which led him to conclude that both Roberts *and* Hughes had shifted, contradicts both explanations but is reinforced by a radical shift in bloc dissenting rates from the five previous terms to the 1936 Term. Furthermore, the study covers an entire term of Court, not just a few cases, and reveals patterned rather than idiosyncratic behavior.

Justices' interagreement in the Warren Court and afterward indicates the presence of blocs as well as variance in patterns of interaction within and between those groupings.[81] In the Warren Court's first few years, the Chief Justice and Justice Tom Clark voted together in 95 percent of the cases in which both voted and occupied the Court's "center of gravity" before Warren shifted toward the liberal end of the Court. The later liberal "Warren Court" was still not to materialize, with the Court "splintered into warring factions, with no group able consistently to attact the decisive votes of the centrist judges" in the 1958–62 period.[82]

The 1962–64 Terms, the Warren Court's middle period, produced a liberal bloc of Douglas, the Court's most liberal member, Black, Warren, Brennan and Goldberg—whose arrival had for the first time provided a reliable fifth liberal vote—and a conservative bloc of Clark, Kennedy appointee Byron White, Eisenhower appointee Potter Stewart, and John Marshall Harlan, the Court's most conservative justice.[83] Stewart's center position on the Court is shown by his pairing with liberal bloc member Goldberg as often as with the conservative Harlan. In the 1964 Term, change was revealed: Warren's interagreement with Black, Douglas, and Goldberg decreased, as the liberals, "having achieved full control over the court . . . broke ranks . . . and new alignments emerged."[84]

When Justice Fortas replaced Justice Goldberg, fundamental changes in bloc alignments did not occur, although there was greater fluidity, with the Chief Justice voting more with Justices Clark, White, and Fortas than with Douglas and Black. Black's movement, to a point between the liberal and conservative blocs, meant a liberal majority was not assured, but Justice Marshall's arrival led to an extremely cohesive bloc of Warren, Brennan, Fortas, and Marshall—with Douglas a reliable liberal vote even if not a cohesive bloc member.[85]

The Warren and Fortas departures and Chief Justice Burger's arrival immediately affected voting alignments, but results were to be unpredictable, as alignments never fully solidified in the "Burger Court." There certainly was not a Burger Court in the new Chief Justice's first term, with Burger "most out-of-step with the majority" in civil liberties cases. A clear indication of change was that Justice Black voted with Chief Justice Burger more than with former voting companion Douglas. When Burger acquired Justice Blackmun, the other "Minnesota Twin," they voted together in 90 percent of the 1970 Term's nonunanimous cases and in all but one criminal procedure case. The effect of the other Nixon appointees, Powell and Rehnquist, is an indication of freshman justices' potential role, particularly when "several new justices form a voting bloc"—or when, as in the Warren Court, they "use their votes to strengthen an existing bloc."[86] Once Powell and Rehnquist did join the Court, Burger's highest inter-agreement was with Rehnquist (95 percent of the nonunanimous cases). At the same time, Burger voted with Douglas only 4.2 percent of the time, and Brennan, only 10.9 percent, a polarization extreme for the modern Supreme Court. The two-thirds Douglas-Rehnquist disagreement rate was "a modern Supreme Court record," and seven pairs of justices had disagreement rates above 50 percent.[87]

Typical of the next several terms was the 1972 Term pattern in which Burger, Blackmun, Powell, and Rehnquist were together in almost three-fifths of the nonunanimous cases, only once in dissent, with three of the four together in 85 of such cases. When the Court opposed defendants' criminal procedure claims, the Nixon bloc was in the majority in all but a very few cases over several terms—but when the court supported defendants' claims, they were in the majority only slightly more than half the time.[88] Apart from the criminal procedure area, "although the Nixon appointees voted together frequently enough to reorient the Court, they disagreed among themselves often enough to ensure that they could not dominate the Court as thoroughly as had Brennan and his allies in the late Warren Court."[89]

The most common pattern in nonunanimous cases was the four Nixon appointees plus White and Stewart. Those two had begun to help the Nixon appointees control the Court starting with the 1971 Term, when they had voted together in 70 percent of the Court's cases. In part because they were in the centrist position but also because they arrived there by somewhat different routes (Stewart was more liberal than White on criminal procedure, more conservative on race relations), they voted together less often than the justices closer to the Court's extremes.

The last half of the 1970s showed a Court with fluid blocs: only Brennan and Marshall had an interagreement score over 90 percent. Although Burger and Rehnquist voted together almost 90 percent of the time, Rehnquist disagreed with Powell and Blackmun in more than one-fifth of the cases. Powell, Blackmun, the Chief Justice, and Justice White formed a marginally cohesive bloc (interagreement just over 80 percent). Powell, now occupying the place held earlier by Brennan, was the center of gravity in civil liberties decisions. Justice Stevens, the Court's newest member, added to the fluidity of the Court's alignments, "dissenting regularly in the company of both libertarian and conservative justices" although inclining more to the former.[90]

When Justice O'Connor joined the Court in the 1981 Term, she had an interagreement rate with Justice Rehnquist of over 85 percent, slightly exceeding that of Rehnquist and Burger, thus leading to the formation of the "Arizona Twins" (or the "Phoenix Pair"); they did not, however, match the interagreement of Brennan and Marshall (almost 95%). Justice Blackmun's movement away from Burger, accelerated when Justice O'Connor joined the Court—in order,

Blackmun has said, to maintain the Court's balance[91]—was evident in his voting with Brennan more than twice as often as with Rehnquist. These patterns were also evident in the 1983 Term when, in cases decided by one-vote margins, O'Connor and Rehnquist were together 26 of 29 times but Stevens and Blackmun joined Rehnquist only eight times each.

We can get a different look at the same essentials if we examine alignments in cases in which two justices of widely differing ideology disagreed. Thus in 63 cases in the 1979 Term in which the Chief Justice and Justice Brennan were on opposite sides, Burger and Rehnquist were together in 61 but Brennan and Rehnquist voted together only *twice*. In the 1984 Term, when Burger opposed Brennan 56 times, Rehnquist joined Burger in 51 of those cases (White, 47; O'Connor, 46), while Marshall voted with Burger only twice.

Another view of the recent Burger Court comes from examination of the data presented in Table 7.5, covering the last five Burger Court terms. At least three of the four Nixon appointees were together in three-fourths or more of the Court's nonunanimous cases throughout the period, with O'Connor joining them 70 percent or more of the time after her first term. The voting record of the Minnesota Twins varied considerably, ranging from a high of almost 70 percent to below two-fifths; however, Burger and Rehnquist were regularly together over three-fourths of the time, and Rehnquist and O'Connor voted together even more frequently in four of the five terms. Blackmun's movement to the liberals could be seen in his voting with Brennan and Marshall more than half the time in all but one of the five terms; Brennan and Marshall were a pair at least three-fourths of the time and in two terms were at the 90 percent interagreement level.

The importance of civil liberties cases to the change from the Warren Court to the Burger Court leads us to look more closely at them. Comparison of justices' votes on all civil liberties cases with their votes on *close* cases when their votes were more important indicate that the more conservative and more liberal justices had more extreme voting patterns in the close cases than for all cases. (See Table 7.6.) Thus on close cases Burger and Rehnquist almost never supported civil liberties claims, and Marshall and Brennan almost never opposed the claims. Centrist justices like Powell showed relatively little difference between support for civil liberties claims in all cases and those in close cases.

Studies of the Court's alignments based on Guttman scaling have produced findings comparable to those derived from bloc analysis. The basic scales that regularly appeared were the "C" and "E" scales.[92] The C scale covers civil liberties cases, matters of personal rights and freedoms such as the First Amendment, fair trial, and racial equality. In some terms of the Court, the C scale was a general civil liberties scale; at other times it had subcomponents. The E scale includes economic regulation matters: government regulation of business, antitrust, and labor-management cases. In some years, other scales, including one encompassing questions of federalism and another for judicial activism in reviewing decisions of the other branches of government, have also been identified.

Table 7.5 Vote Patterns, 1981–1985—Nonunanimous Cases
(frequency with which particular groupings of justices vote together)

	1981	1982	1983	1984	1985
Nixon Four or 3 of the 4	74.5%	87.6%	89.7%	78.3%	75.2%
Above + O'Connor	64.9	69.1	77.0	71.1	76.2
"Minnesota Twins"	38.3	60.6	69.0	63.9	44.6
Burger + Rehnquist	73.4	75.2	75.9	78.3	80.2
Rehnquist + O'Connor	79.8	89.6	81.6	79.5	72.3
Brennan + Marshall	91.4	76.2	82.8	89.2	74.2
Brennan, Marshall and Blackmun	62.8	62.9	41.4	53.0	58.4
Brennan, Marshall and Stevens	52.1	50.5	50.5	44.6	39.6
	n = 94	n = 97	n = 87	n = 83	n = 101

Table 7.6 Civil Liberties Claims: Selected Recent Terms
(proportion of times favoring the claim)

	1981		1983		1985	
	All	Close	All	Close	All	Close
Rehnquist	21.7%	3.8%	19.7%	-0-	12.7%	3.8%
Burger	23.5	3.8	36.4	5.9	21.5	7.7
O'Connor	32.9	15.4	22.5	12.5	31.6	19.2
Powell	34.1	30.8	33.3	31.3	31.6	38.4
White	45.1	53.8	36.0	43.8	30.3	19.2
Stevens	50.6	76.9	64.0	81.3	57.7	72.0
Blackmun	60.5	84.6	45.2	75.0	66.7	84.0
Marshall	79.0	92.3	82.2	93.8	88.4	96.2
Brennan	78.0	96.2	81.6	100.0	83.5	96.2

By combining justices' positions on the political (C) and economic (E) scales, Schubert identified four categories of justices; further classification produced three ideological dimensions. One was Equalitarianism/Traditionalism; someone liberal on both C and E scales would hold the Equalitarian ideology, a belief in greater equality of opportunity for all. The Authoritarian/Libertarian dimension dealt with the scope of freedom as opposed to the scope of authority; those holding the Authoritarian ideology were political conservatives and economic liberals. The third policy dimension was Collectivism/Individualism, involving emphasis on the individual human being as against emphasis on society as such, with a political liberal and economic conservative an Individualist. A fourth dimension cut across the others: Dogmatists, those who believed

Figure 7.1 Judicial Ideologies (based on Schubert)

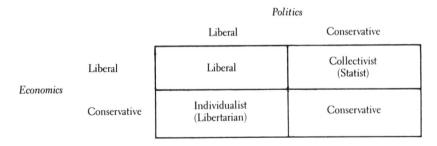

highly in the authority of precedent, and Pragmatists, those less concerned about precedent and more concerned about decisions' effects.

In the 1946–62 period, Traditionalism, Collectivism, Authoritarianism, and Equalitarianism were dominant at different times. The conservatives, but not the liberals, were divided into Pragmatists and Dogmatists. Six of the seven justices who scored positive on the political liberalism dimension also were positive on economic liberalism; four other justices were neutral as to political liberalism but negative as to economic liberalism. Their limited support of civil liberties led them in 1956 and 1957, when the Court was under political attack, to support another cluster of five justices—neutral on economic matters but negative on political liberalism—in limiting the liberals.[93] Because only three justices—including Chief Justice Warren, who became more liberal—changed ideological positions once they joined the Court, shifts in domination of the Court had to come through changes in personnel that altered the three clusters of justices.

Using some different categories to examine a period including the Warren Court and extending into the Burger Court, other scholars found that more than 85 percent of the Court's rulings could be explained in terms of two major dimensions related to civil liberties and one dimension, New Dealism, based on economic activity. The first civil liberties dimension, freedom, covered cases involving criminal defendants and those in political "crimes," such as the loyalty oath cases; the other, equality, covered political, economic, or racial discrimination. Two other relatively minor dimensions—privacy (libel and obscenity) and taxation—also helped explain Warren Court rulings.[94] Six justices—Warren, Douglas, Brennan, Goldberg, Fortas, and Marshall—were liberal, that is, positive on the three major dimensions. Seven, the four Nixon appointees, Frankfurter, Whittaker, and Harlan, were conservatives, negative on all three. Justices Stewart and White were considered Moderates, Black was a Populist—negative as to equality but positive as to freedom and New Dealism—and Clark was a New Dealer, positive only on economic matters, negative on the other two dimensions.

Guttman scaling studies have also suggested whether the Court's decisions have been based on the justices' attitudes toward a situation (AS) or toward an object (AO), that is, whether they would vote in terms of their attitude toward that type of person regardless of the situation. In the Warren Court's last eleven terms, AS was found to be more determinative in cases involving labor unions and persons exercising freedom of communication, while AO was more important in security risk cases and physically injured employees.[95] For the 1971–73 Terms, the attitude toward object—support for the individual or for the government—dominated situational variables for eight of the nine justices in both criminal and noncriminal cases. Only Justice Powell differed between criminal and noncriminal cases, supporting the government to a statistically significant degree in the former but not the latter. That the other Nixon appointees favored the government over the individual in both criminal and noncriminal situations indicated clearly that their voting resulted from broader ideology, not a narrower and isolated "law and order" stance.[96]

All these studies are helpful in understanding the Court and its members, but they are also limited. They show only justices' positions relative to each other, not in absolute terms. Thus we cannot tell from scale positions either where the judges on the extremes are going to fall or exactly where the division between majority and minority will occur. Because they are based only on nonunanimous cases, the scales also cannot explain why the Court achieves unanimous decisions not only on noncontroversial legal questions but on important matters of law such as school desegregation and the Nixon tapes. They show overwhelmingly that attitude and ideology affect justices' votes but not the other factors that also influence the result and that help to explain why not all justices can be located easily on all scales.

A related problem is that, although scaling may indicate a relatively clear alignment of the justices in a broad subject matter, such patterns do not always hold for more specific issue areas. For example, during the 1972–80 period in cases involving freedom of the press, the more liberal and more conservative justices demonstrate consistent attitude-based voting patterns; however, mid-Court justices cast some anti-press and some pro-press votes without an apparently coherent pattern. Such a picture does not mean that random choices are at work, but only "that the Justices differ markedly in their approach to the cases," stressing different elements of "models" of press-government relations, with "detailed examination of [their] votes and opinions" necessary if we are "to isolate the factors which influence each Justice's votes."[97]

Perhaps most significant is that these studies are based only on votes rather than on the justices' opinions and generally do not take into account the fact that justices who vote together do not necessarily write together. Because they capture only the Court's final product, its decision, these studies miss such important matters as interaction among the justices and the changes in written opinions and even results that may occur between the initial conference vote and final announcement of a decision. The result in a case as determined by the vote is perhaps the most important to the litigants, but the doctrine of an opinion is generally thought to be more important for the Court's role as a policymaker. It is to these considerations that enter into writing an opinion that we now turn.

Notes

1. David M. O'Brien, "Managing the Business of the Supreme Court," *Public Administration Review* 45 (Special 1985): 671.

2. Rehnquist's statement is at 409 U.S. 824 (1972). See John MacKenzie, *The Appearance of Justice* (New York: Scribner's, 1974).

3. *Laird v. Tatum,* 107 S.Ct. 309 (1986).

4. See *Board of Education of City of Los Angeles v. Superior Court of California,* 448 U.S. 1343 at 1346–47 (1980) (Justice Rehnquist).

5. See *Woodard v. Hutchins,* 464 U.S. 377 (1984).

6. See *Autry v. Estelle,* 464 U.S. 1 (1983), stay granted by Justice White on different grounds, 474 U.S. 1301 (1983); *Maggio v. Williams,* 474 U.S. 46 (1983).

7. *Wainwright v. Adams,* 466 U.S. 964 (1984) (Marshall); *Maggio v. Williams,* 464 U.S. 46 at 56 (1983) (Brennan). On the Court's procedures for handling stays pending lower court disposition of appeals, see *Barefoot v. Estelle,* 463 U.S. 880 (1983).

8. *Whalen v. Roe,* 423 U.S. 1313 at 1317 (1975).

9. *Holtzman v. Schlesinger,* 414 U.S. 1304 and 414 U.S. 1316; *Schlesinger v. Holtzman,* 414 U.S. 1321 (1973). The court of appeals later ordered the case dismissed.

10. Stuart Taylor, Jr., "Lawyer Wins Vindication Over 1982 Burger Opinion," *New York Times,* August 10, 1986, p. 24.

11. This section draws on Stephen L. Wasby, Anthony A. D'Amato, and Rosemary Metrailer, "The Functions of Oral Argument in the U.S. Supreme Court," *Quarterly Journal of Speech* 62 (December 1976): 410–22.

12. Quoted in Commission on Revision of the Federal Court Appellate System, *Structure and Internal Procedures,* pp. 104–5.

13. Milton Dickens and Ruth E. Schwartz, "Oral Argument Before the Supreme Court: Marshall v. Davis in the School Segregation Cases," *Quarterly Journal of Speech* 57 (February 1971): 39.

14. Anthony Lewis, "Supreme Law of the Land Still Rests in High Court," *Portland Oregonian,* July 14, 1974, p. F3.

15. Dickens and Schwartz, "Oral Argument," pp. 36–37.

16. Woodward and Armstrong, *The Brethren,* pp. 170–72, 179–81, 187–89, 417–22.

17. Ibid., pp. 63, 288–347.

18. For examples see Alexander Bickel, ed., *The Unpublished Opinions of Mr. Justice Brandeis* (Cambridge, Mass.: Harvard University Press, 1957); and Bernard Schwartz, *The Unpublished Opinions of the Warren Court* (New York: Oxford University Press, 1985). See also Schwartz, "More Unpublished Warren Court Opinions," *The Supreme Court Review 1986,* eds. Philip B. Kurland, Gerhard Casper, and Dennis J. Hutchinson (Chicago: University of Chicago Press, 1987), pp. 317–93.

19. See Saul Brenner, "Reassigning the Majority Opinion on the United States Supreme Court," *Justice System Journal* 11 (Fall 1986): 186–95, for the 1946–1952 Terms (the Vinson Court).

20. See Schwartz, *Super Chief,* pp. 410–24.

21. Saul Brenner, "Fluidity on the United States Supreme Court: A Reexamination," *American Journal of Political Science* 24 (August 1980): 526–35, and "Fluidity on the Supreme Court, 1956–1967," *American Journal of Political Science* 26 (May 1982): 388–90.

22. David Danelski, "Explorations of Some Causes and Consequences of Conflict and Its Resolution in the Supreme Court," *Judicial Conflict and Consensus*, eds. Goldman and Lamb, pp. 29, 21–22.

23. Don E. Fehrenbacher, *The Dred Scott Case: Its Significance in American Law & Politics* (New York: Oxford University Press, 1978), p. 321.

24. The original text reads as follows: "In dispensing these items, the pharmacist performs three tasks: he finds the correct bottle; he counts out the correct number of tablets or measures the right amount of liquid; and he accurately transfers the doctor's dosage instructions to the container. Without minimizing the potential consequences of error in performing these tasks or the importance of the other tasks a professional pharmacist performs, it is clear that in this regard he no more renders a true professional service than does a clerk who sells lawbooks." The ultimate opinion covered the same ground in one sentence: "In dispensing these prepackaged items, the pharmacist performs largely a packaging rather than a compounding function of former times." *Virginia State Board of Pharmacy v. Virginia Citizens Consumers Council*, 425 U.S. 748 at 774–75 (1976).

25. Charles W. Nihan and Russell R. Wheeler, "Using Technology to Improve the Administration of Justice in the Federal Courts," *Brigham Young University Law Review* 1981: 667n.

26. Data through the first Burger Court term from Donald D. Gregory and Stephen L. Wasby, "How to Get an Idea from Here to There: The Court and Communication Overload," *Public Affairs Bulletin* 3, no. 5 (November–December 1976); later data developed by the present author.

27. See Bernard Schwartz, "Felix Frankfurter and Earl Warren: A Study of a Deteriorating Relationship," *Supreme Court Review 1980*, eds. Phillip Kurland and Gerhard Casper (Chicago: University of Chicago Press, 1981), pp. 115–42.

28. Bernard Wolfman, Jonathan L. F. Silver, and Marjorie A. Silver, *Dissent Without Opinions: The Behavior of Justice William O. Douglas in Tax Cases* (Philadelphia: University of Pennsylvania Press, 1975).

29. Danelski, "Explorations of Some Causes and Consequences," p. 34.

30. *Manual Enterprises v. Day*, 370 U.S. 478 at 519 (1962).

31. See Steven A. Peterson, "Dissent in American Courts," *Journal of Politics* 43 (1981): 412–34. For an interesting, extended discussion of dissents in various situations, see Maurice Kelman, "The Forked Path of Dissent," *The Supreme Court Review 1985*, eds. Phillip B. Kurland, Gerhard Casper, and Dennis J. Hutchinson (Chicago: University of Chicago Press, 1986), pp. 227–98.

32. An important examination of the Court's efforts to remain unanimous is Dennis J. Hutchinson, "Unanimity and Desegregation: Decisionmaking in the Supreme Court, 1948–1958," *Georgetown Law Journal* 68 (October 1979): 1–96.

33. William J. Brennan, Jr., "In Defense of Dissents," *Hastings Law Journal* 37 (1986): 427–38; *Colorado v. Connelly*, 107 S.Ct. 515 at 533 (1986).

34. See Robert F. Williams, "In the Supreme Court's Shadow: Legitimacy of State Rejection of Supreme Court Reasoning and Result," *South Carolina Law Review* 35 (Spring 1984): 374–75.

35. Danelski, "Explorations of Some Causes and Consequences," p. 42.

36. David Lauter, "A New Polarization for the High Court," *National Law Journal*, August 11, 1986, p. S–3.

37. *Will v. Calvert Fire Insurance Co.*, 437 U.S. 655 at 670 (1978).

38. *Columbus Board of Education v. Penick*, 443 U.S. 449 at 493 (1979).

39. *Florida v. Royer*, 460 U.S. 491 at 529-30 (1983).

40. *Federal Energy Regulatory Commission v. Mississippi*, 456 U.S. 742 at 761 n. 25 and 767 n. 30.

41. *Oregon v. Elstad*, 105 S.Ct. 1285 at 1299, 1301 (1985). See also *United States v. Sharpe*, 105 S.Ct. 1568 at 1584–85 (1985).

42. Russell W. Galloway, Jr., "The Taft Court (1921–29)," *Santa Clara Law Review* 25 (Winter 1985): 2.

43. Stephen C. Halpern and Kenneth N. Vines, "Institutional Disunity, The Judges' Bill and the Role of the U.S. Supreme Court," *Western Political Quarterly* 30 (Fall 1977): 471–83.

44. S. Sidney Ulmer, "Exploring the Dissent Patterns of the Chief Justices: John Marshall to Warren Burger," *Judicial Conflict and Consensus*, eds. Goldman and Lamb, p. 55.

45. Russell W. Galloway, Jr., "The Roosevelt Court." *Santa Clara Law Review* 23 (1983): 513.

46. Arthur D. Hellman, "Preserving the Essential Role of the Supreme Court," *Florida State Law Review* 14 (1986): 29–30.

47. Harold J. Spaeth and Michael Altfeld, "Influence Relationships Within the Supreme Court: A Comparison of the Warren and Burger Courts," *Western Political Quarterly* 38 (March 1985): 70–83.

48. Frank H. Easterbrook, "Agreement Among the Justices: An Empirical Note," *The Supreme Court Review 1984*, eds. Phillip B. Kurland, Gerhard Casper, and Dennis J. Hutchinson (Chicago: University of Chicago Press, 1985), pp. 389, 392.

49. See John M. Scheb II and Lee W. Ailshie, "Justice Sandra Day O'Connor and the 'Freshman Effect,'" *Judicature* 69 (June–July 1985): 9–12.

50. Saul Brenner, "Minimum Winning Coalitions on U.S. Supreme Court," *American Politics Quarterly* 7 (July 1979): 384–92.

51. David W. Rhode, "Policy Goals and Opinion Coalitions in the Supreme Court," *Midwest Journal of Political Science* 16 (May 1972): 218–19; Micheal W. Giles, "Equivalent Versus Minimum Winning Opinion Size: A Test of Two Hypotheses," *American Journal of Political Science* 21 (May 1977): 405–8.

52. Peter G. Fish, "The Office of Chief Justice of the United States: Into the Federal Judiciary's Bicentennial Decade," *The Office of Chief Justice* (Charlottesville, Va.: University of Virginia, 1984), p. 59.

53. See Schwartz, *Super Chief*. Schwartz does not emphasize Brennan's role, but provides the evidence for that role. I am indebted to my colleague Phillip Cooper for this point.

54. See Ulmer, "Exploring the Dissenting Patterns," p. 54.

55. David Danelski, "The Influence of the Chief Justice in the Decisional Process of the Supreme Court," in *Courts, Judges, and Politics*, eds. Walter F. Murphy and C. Herman Pritchett, 2d ed. (New York: Random House, 1974). p. 503.

56. On this and other problems, see Kelman, "Forked Path of Dissent," pp. 290–97.

57. William P. McLauchlan, "Ideology and Conflict in Supreme Court Opinion Assignment, 1947–1962," *Western Political Quarterly* 25 (March 1972): 16–27.

58. David W. Rohde, "Policy Goals, Strategic Choice and Majority Opinion Assignments in U.S. Supreme Court," *Midwest Journal of Political Science* 16 (November 1972): 667; see also S. Sidney Ulmer, "The Use of Power in the Supreme Court: The Opinion Assignments of Earl Warren, 1953–1960," *Journal of Public Law* 19 (1970): 49–67.

59. Harold J. Spaeth, "Distributive Justice: Majority Opinion Assignments in the Burger Court," *Judicature* 67 (December–January 1984): 299–304, for the 1969–1980 Terms.

60. See Saul Brenner and Harold J. Spaeth, "Issue Specialization in Majority Opinion Assignment on the Burger Court," *Western Political Quarterly* 39 (September 1986): 520–27.

61. Elliott E. Slotnick, "The Chief Justices and Self-Assignment of Majority Opinions: A Research Note," *Western Political Quarterly* 31 (June 1978): 224. See also Slotnick, "Who Speaks for the Court?: Majority Opinion Assignment from Taft to Burger," *American Journal of Political Science* 23 (February 1979), particularly pp. 68–72; and Slotnick, "Judicial Career Patterns and Majority Opinion Assignment on the Supreme Court," *Journal of Politics* 41 (May 1979): 640–48.

62. Jeffrey A. Segal, "Predicting Supreme Court Cases Probabilistically: The Search and Seizure Cases, 1962–1981," *American Political Science Review* 78 (December 1984): 891–900, and Segal, "Measuring Change on the Supreme Court: Examining Alternative Models," *American Journal of Political Science* 29 (August 1985): 461–79.

63. As a small example, see Justice Stevens' admission of incorrectly characterizing a case, *Spaziano v. Florida*, 104 S.Ct. 3154 at 3197 (1984).

64. H. N. Hirsch, *The Enigma of Felix Frankfurter* (New York: Basic Books, 1981), pp. 5–6.

65. Ibid., pp. 136–37.

66. Ibid., pp. 9, 153, 176.

67. Ibid., p. 188. See Dennis J. Hutchinson, "Felix Frankfurter and the Business of the Supreme Court, O.T. 1946–O.T. 1961," *Supreme Court Review 1980*, eds. Phillip B. Kurland and Gerhard Casper (Chicago: University of Chicago Press, 1981), pp. 143–209.

68. Hirsch, *Felix Frankfurter*, p. 211.

69. See Woodward and Armstrong, *The Brethren*, pp. 357 ff.

70. See Glendon Schubert, "Aging, Conservatism, and Judicial Behavior," *Micropolitics* 3 (1983): 135–79.

71. S. Sidney Ulmer, "The Longitudinal Behavior of Hugo Lafayette Black: Parabolic Support for Civil Liberties, 1937–1971," *Florida State University Law Review* 1 (Winter 1974): 131–53. See also Ulmer, "Parabolic Support of Civil Liberty Claims: The Case of William O. Douglas," *Journal of Politics* 41 (May 1979): 634–39; and H. Frank Way, "The Study of Judicial Attitudes: The Case of Mr. Justice Douglas," *Western Political Quarterly* 24 (March 1971): 12–23.

72. See *Dun & Bradstreet v. Greenmoss Builders*, 105 S.Ct. 2939 at 2950 (1985).

73. See Russell W. Galloway, Jr., "The Early Years of the Warren Court: Emergence of Judicial Liberalism (1953–1957)," *Santa Clara Law Review* 18 (1978): 613–22.

74. David Danelski, "Values as Variables in Judicial Decision-Making: Notes Toward a Theory," *Vanderbilt Law Review* 19 (1966): 721–40; and Danelski, *A Supreme Court Justice is Appointed* (New York: Random House, 1964).

75. Still more sophisticated methods are used by some scholars. See Glendon Schubert, *The Judicial Mind* (Evanston, Ill.: Northwestern University Press, 1965), for use of "smallest space analysis"; and S. Sidney Ulmer, "The Discriminant Function and the Theoretical Context for Its Use in Estimating the Votes of Judges," in *Frontiers of Judicial Research*, eds. Joel B. Grossman and Joseph Tanenhaus (New York: John Wiley, 1969), pp. 335–69.

76. Joel B. Grossman, "Dissenting Blocs on the Warren Court: A Study in Judicial Role Behavior," *Journal of Politics* 30 (November 1968): 1083, 1089.

77. Hirsch, *Felix Frankfurter*, pp. 129–30.

78. Russell W. Galloway, Jr., "The Court That Challenged the New Deal," *Santa Clara Law Review* 24 (Winter 1984): 86.

79. Schubert, *Quantitative Analysis of Judicial Behavior*, pp. 192–210. See also Russell W. Galloway, Jr., "The Roosevelt Court: The Liberals Conquer (1937–1941) and Divide (1941–1946)," *Santa Clara Law Review* 23 (1983): 495–96.

80. For Roberts' explanation, see Glendon Schubert, *Constitutional Politics* (New York: Holt, Rinehart and Winston, 1960), pp. 168–71.

81. Another bloc that has been identified is a "Truman bloc" in the late 1940s consisting of Truman appointees Vinson, Clark, Burton, and Minton and Roosevelt appointee Reed. David N. Atkinson and Dale A. Neuman, "Toward a Cost Theory of Judicial Alignments: The Case of the Truman Bloc," *Midwest Journal of Political Science* 13 (May 1969): 271–83. See also Russell Galloway, Jr., "The Vinson Court: Polarization (1946–1949) and Conservative Dominance (1949–1953)," *Santa Clara Law Review* 22 (Spring 1982): 375–418.

82. Edward V. Heck, "Changing Voting Patterns in the Warren and Burger Courts," *Judicial Conflict and Consensus*, eds. Goldman and Lamb, pp. 71–74.

83. Glendon Schubert, *The Constitutional Polity* (Boston: Boston University Press, 1970), pp. 124–25. See also S. Sidney Ulmer, "Toward a Theory of Sub-Group Formation in the United States Supreme Court," *Journal of Politics* 27 (1965): 133–52.

84. Russell W. Galloway, Jr., "The Third Period of the Warren Court: Liberal Dominance (1962–1969)," *Santa Clara Law Review* 20 (1980): 789.

85. Edward V. Heck, "Justice Brennan and the Heyday of Warren Court Liberalism," *Santa Clara Law Review* 20 (Fall 1980): 845–46, 858–59, and Heck, "Changing Voting Patterns," pp. 77–78.

86. Heck, "Changing Voting Patterns," p. 84.

87. Russell W. Galloway, Jr., "The First Decade of the Burger Court: Conservative Dominance (1969–1979)," *Santa Clara Law Review* 21 (1981): 908.

88. David W. Rohde and Harold J. Spaeth, *Supreme Court Decision-Making* (San Francisco: W. H. Freeman, 1975), p. 109.

89. Heck, "Changing Voting Patterns," p. 82.

90. Edward V. Heck, "Civil Liberties Voting Patterns in the Burger Court, 1975–1978," *Western Political Quarterly* 34 (June 1981): 199.

91. See John A. Jenkins, "A Candid Talk with Justice Blackmun," *New York Times Magazine*, February 10, 1983, pp. 20–24 ff.

92. What follows is drawn primarily from Schubert, *The Judicial Mind*.

93. Glendon Schubert, *The Judicial Mind Revisited: Psychometric Analysis of Supreme Court Ideology* (New York: Oxford University Press, 1974), summarized in "The Judicial Mind Reappraised," *Jurimetrics Journal* 15 (Summer 1975): 279.

94. Rohde and Spaeth, *Supreme Court Decision-Making*, pp. 137–38.

95. Harold J. Spaeth et al., "Is Justice Blind?: An Empirical Investigation of a Normative Ideal," *Law & Society Review* 7 (Fall 1972): 119–37.

96. S. Sidney Ulmer and John A. Stookey, "Nixon's Legacy to the Supreme Court: A Statistical Analysis of Judicial Behavior," *Florida State University Law Review* 3 (Summer 1975): 331–47.

97. Paula C. Arledge and Edward V. Heck, "Freedom of the Press: Decision-making Models in the Burger Court," *Whittier Law Review* 4 (1981): 10–11.

8 The Court's Opinions: Basic Considerations

In the previous chapter, we examined the justices' voting patterns and dissensus within the Court, emphasizing the part played by justices' *values*. Those values are but one consideration entering into reaching a decision and then writing an "opinion of the Court" through which the Court's policy is most explicitly stated. The justices' views of their roles as justices and of the Supreme Court's place in the American political system also play a significant part in the decisions they reach and in their opinion-writing, just as they do in decisions to accept or reject cases. Even if justices' initial reactions to a case are affected by their personal value positions, the decision reached by the Court and the ultimate content of the Court's opinion are also affected by an understanding of what the Court's audiences or attentive publics expect. This is not surprising when we realize that the Court's basic impact on other government units comes through its opinions. The breadth of an opinion, its doctrinal bases, and the other content it contains—including precedent and history to establish continuity with the past as well as social science materials, generally used sparingly—affect not only an opinion's immediate policy effects but also its value as precedent. Whether an opinion is framed narrowly, staying within the grounds urged by the parties or seemingly applicable only to the facts of the particular case, or departs from those facts to embrace other situations, and whether it is confined to a statute rather than reaching a constitutional question, are thus quite important.

There are some problems in examining the Court's opinions. One is that there have been important changes over time in the Court's decision-making style—the way the justices have made decisions as well as the overall matrix in which the potential elements of an opinion, or factors influencing it, are taken into account. Giving the Court the power to decide which cases to accept had an important effect on such decision making. When the Court had to decide all cases brought to it but its caseload was still small, the justices could decide each case carefully and deliberately—that is, they could engage in rational decision making. With time to consider each case, the likehood that they would depart from precedent would be greater than otherwise.[1] When the Court had an increased caseload but was still operating under the pre-1925 requirement of hearing all cases, decision making was incremental. Changes from past cases were limited, with precedent serving as a cue to allow prompt disposition. Instead of making law, the Court was more likely to be engaged in interpretation of existing doctrine.

Once it obtained the power to turn away cases, the Court could return to rational decision making, at least for those cases it accepted, thus allowing more policy innovation. With the caseload again growing, "mixed-scanning" decision making is produced. A quick glance is given to most cases before they are rejected, while those accepted get more extended and careful treatment. Here the justices' basic doctrinal attitudes affect not only the Court's full decisions but its decisions to grant review as well. The Court's ability to innovate may, however, be hindered if docket size gets too large and approaches "overload chaos," an unmanageable situation that some justices suggest now exists (see pages 194-98).

What justices write is not necessarily a "true" reflection of their reasons and motives in voting for a particular result. Judges' opinions are not "stream of consciousness" writing leading from premises through rethinking to the ultimate product; they thus seldom indicate the process by which the judge has reached the conclusions presented, the serial iterations in the judge's writing process, or changes resulting from interaction with colleagues.[2] A justice's solo dissent may accurately reflect his or her motivations, although not even such a judge may provide a fully accurate account of how that opinion came to be written. However, the author of an opinion of the Court, because that justice must accommodate colleagues' views, is likely to be constrained in what is ultimately issued under that justice's name. Justice Frankfurter once observed, "The compromises that an opinion may embody, the collaborative effort that it may represent, the inarticulate considerations that may have influenced the grounds on which the case went off, the shifts in position that may precede final adjudication—these and like factors cannot . . . be brought to the surface."[3] Instead the opinion is likely to state conclusions along with justifications for those conclusions—the "reconstituted logic" of explanation.[4]

Does this mean, to paraphrase one cynic, that a judge shoots an arrow at a target and then draws the bullseye around the place where the arrow struck, or that opinions are only an elaborate display of erudition serving as window dressing to mask initial gut reactions? Certainly what Justice Oliver Wendell Holmes, Jr., called a judge's "inarticulate major premises" affect the judge's written opinions. Thus the justice writing for the majority and justices writing concurring or dissenting opinions can write equally persuasive opinions, for each reasons from different premises. Nonetheless, despite the crucial importance of unstated premises, justices *are* affected by having to write opinions, by the expectation that they will justify their actions, will include certain material in their opinions, and will address certain problems. In short, whatever the role of personal values in justices' decision making, the justices are affected by being *judges*, who are expected to justify their decisions through opinions: the process of writing justificatory essays (one way of characterizing the opinions) serves as a constraint, to a greater or lesser degree, on the unfettered operation of their values. So does the fact that the function of an opinion is to persuade people outside the Court—first, the parties to the case, and then others, the legal community and other "court-watchers"—that the decision is a reasonable one, reasonably arrived at, with sufficient guidance in the court's opinion to allow those affected to control "primary conduct."

In the course of reaching a decision and arriving at the ultimate scope, content, and tone of an opinion, the Court is expected to consider a number of important matters. When the Court decides cases and writes its opinions, it is expected to reach toward *neutral principles*. It is also expected to develop policy incrementally and to rely on precedent. The justices must also consider whether the Court should exercise its power of *judicial review* (see pages 278-81), a problem because of the importance of the Court's relations with the other branches of government and the tension between judicial review and democracy. An aspect of judicial review is the extent to which the Court will defer to the states as part of *federalism*. Another consideration related to, but not the only aspect of, judicial review, is whether the Court should exercise *self-restraint* or engage in *judicial activism*, the latter being at the heart of criticism of the federal courts for being unnecessarily interventionist (see pages 3-6). All these matters, while not fully *governing* the Court's decisions or justices' opinions, do have some effect and thus can legitimately be called "considerations" in the justices' work. Indeed, if they are not taken into account, criticism is sure to result, coming from inside the Court and from outside.

Still another matter, undergirding the others but not likely to be discussed openly by the justices, is whether and how the Court, in attempting to achieve its goals, and the individual justices, in attempting to achieve *their* goals, will engage in strategy—already an element in the Court's choice of cases for review and in the decision to give cases summary or full-dress treatment (see pages 201-16). After a discussion of all these matters, we conclude the chapter with an examination of another important aspect of the justices' behavior—a reflection of their strategic concerns and role concepts: their off-the-court activities concerning judicial and nonjudicial matters.

Neutral Principles

People who see the Court as finding law, and even many who recognize that it makes policy, expect of the Court that its decisions should be *principled*.

Compromises deriving from pragmatism are for legislators and political executives; courts, on the other hand, must stand for principle, deliberateness, the use of rationality and logic, and detachment from the turmoil and passion of political conflict. Instead of being "engaged in the hurly-burly of legislative activity," they must be a "detached observer engaged in unpressed reflection."[5] As former Solicitor General Archibald Cox put it, "In expounding the Constitution, the Court's role is to discern principles sufficiently absolute to give them roots throughout the community and continuity over significant periods of time, and to lift them above the level of the pragmatic political judgments of a particular time and place."[6] Or, in Bickel's words:

> The root idea is that the process is justified only if it injects into representative government something that is not already there, and that is principle, standards of action that derive their worth from a long view of society's spiritual as well as material needs and that command adherence whether or not the immediate outcome is expedient or agreeable.[7]

In the most noted statement on the subject, Herbert Wechsler said judicial determinations should rest on "reasons that in their generality and their neutrality transcend any immediate result that is involved." Criteria for decisions had to be exercises of reason, "not merely . . . an act of willfulness or will."[8] But Wechsler had demanded too much even for some advocates of the Court's "passive virtues." Bickel argued that if the Court were to have to rest its decisions "only on principles that will be capable of application across the board and without compromise, in all relevant cases in the foreseeable future," with any flexibility built into the principle itself "in equally principled fashion," there would be few such principles; thus few decisions of other branches of government would be overturned, and the "neutral principles" position ends up being restraintist. Moreover, because few cases would be decided in the absence of such neutral principles, the Court would fail to meet the public's demand that it resolve issues. As some judges are fond of saying, it is better that some cases be decided than that they be decided right.[9] It should be enough, Bickel said, to have "an intellectually coherent statement of the reason for a result which in like cases will produce a like result, whether or not it is immediately agreeable or expedient," or a "principled process of enunciating and applying certain enduring values of our society," with the values having "general significance and even-handed application."[10] Thus the "neutral principles" idea is important because it proposes a goal—principled and reasoned opinions—to which judges should aspire even if they are not able to achieve it.

Precedent

Judges, in making decisions, must consider to what extent precedent should limit their actions. An expectation in the legal community, much stronger than that of "neutral principles," is that the justices will adhere to the doctrine of *stare decisis* (literally, to stand on the decision), at the heart of the Anglo-American legal tradition. Precedent performs important functions. It is "the means by which we ensure that the law will not merely change erratically, but will develop in a principled and intelligible fashion."[11] Beyond that, it "serves the broader societal interests in even-handed, consistent, and predictable application of legal rules," in short, "in stability, and in the orderly conduct of our affairs."[12] Judges must take care in departing from precedent, because when they do or the Court "makes new law out of whole cloth," "the holy rite of judges consulting a higher law loses some of its mysterious power."[13]

The importance of precedent is demonstrated by the time and effort justices devote to explaining why their opinions follow precedent or why their colleagues' opinions depart from precedent; such comments may be stimulated by the justices' respective value positions (in Justice Holmes' words, their "inarticulate major premises"), but if precedent were not considered important, they would not use it as either justification or weapon, nor would they spend so much time engaged in extended effort to persuade each other—and the publics who read their opinions—of their "readings" of the relevant cases. In addition, there is the element we might call *personal precedent*, in which a justice is committed, at least within limits, to a position adopted earlier. This is part of a striving for internal consistency, which may reinforce adherence to a position the Court has adopted and with which, at the time, the justice has agreed, which may lead a justice to hold to his or her own views once adopted in a dissent in the face of contrary rulings by the other justices.

The expectation that courts base their decisions on precedent, which involves taking the present case, finding past cases that are similar, and then applying the rules from those past cases, creates a number of problems. How does one know which cases are "similar"? On what competing precedents should one rely? How should legal doctrine of the relevant cases be interpreted? And, at the level of the Supreme Court, should precedent be followed as closely as lower courts are expected to follow it? The Court's place as the nation's highest and last court has led it to feel *less* bound by precedent than do the lower courts. As Justice Powell recently observed, "When governing decisions are badly reasoned, or conflict with other, more recent authority, the Court 'has never felt constrained to follow precedent.'"[14] Likewise, said Justice White, the Court "has not hesitated to overrule decisions, or even whole lines of cases, where experience, scholarship, and reflection demonstrated that their fundamental premises were not to be found in the Constitution."[15] The lessened constraint of precedent is more important when the Constitution is being interpreted, because changes in constitutional rulings can be overturned only through the very difficult process of amending the Constitution itself. Because Congress has the power to rewrite statutes and thus correct the Court's interpretation of those statutes (see pages 309-12), the justices are more reluctant to alter precedents based on statutory interpretation even when they recognize that those precedents may be in error.

Illustrating this point is the Court's disposition of Curt Flood's challenge to the reserve clause in professional baseball, the only major professional sport exempted from antitrust coverage. (Hi there, sports fans!) The baseball exemption stems from the Court's 1923 ruling, based on a narrow interpretation of the Commerce Clause, reaffirmed in 1953, that baseball was not commerce and therefore was not subject to the Sherman Antitrust Act. Later, before Flood's antitrust challenge, other courts, on the basis of the Supreme Court's post-1937 broader definition of commerce, held other sports, particularly professional football and professional basketball, subject to the antitrust laws. In ruling on *Flood v. Kuhn* (1972), the majority agreed that professional baseball was a business in interstate commerce and that the antitrust exemption for baseball was "in a very distinct sense, an exception and an anomaly," with the earlier cases "an aberration confined to baseball." Nonetheless, said Justice Blackmun, "the aberration is an established one" recognized by Congress, which had "by its positive inaction" allowed the earlier baseball decisions to stand and had shown no intention of placing professional baseball within the scope of the antitrust laws. Thus "if there is any inconsistency or illogic in all of this, it is an inconsistency and illogic of long standing that is to be remedied by the Congress and not by this Court."[16]

The *Flood* case does not mean that the Court is invariably resistant to changing its interpretation of statutes when it reads legislative history differently from earlier readings. If the legislature has not relied on the Court's past rulings, if those past rulings are out of step with still earlier rulings, and if the challenged ruling is out of phase with more recent statements of legislative intent, the Court will be more willing to overrule precedents interpreting statutes. Most notable in recent years was the Court's decision in the *Monell* case, only 16 years after initially holding that municipalities could not be sued under the Civil Rights Act of 1871 (42 U.S.C. §1983) (see page 169) and only five years after reaffirming the initial decision, that the courts *would* entertain such suits; the reversal was justified both on the basis of inconsistency with other civil rights rulings and of the Court's having inadequately considered its earlier position before adopting it.

Justice Rehnquist's comment in the *Monell* case that "this Court is surely not free to abandon settled statutory interpretation at any time a new thought seems appealing" suggests that criticism is likely when the Court does overrule a precedent. Such criticism, from other justices and from outside the Court, occurs whether the precedent is new or old: if old, the Court is said to be interfering with the "settled ways" of the law; if new, the Court is not allowing the law to develop properly. The argument that precedent has recently been overturned is also used to block further changes in the law, as we can see in Justice Rehnquist's comment in a post-*Monell* case that "the law in this area has taken enough 90-degree turns in recent years" and therefore should not be changed further.[17] Such comments should also indicate that one's desire to uphold, or abandon, precedent is in part a function of one's like, or dislike, of the precedent itself. Even if this is the case, failure by the majority to explain effectively departure from recently established precedent gives dissenting justices' criticism more force. An example of this situation is provided by the Burger Court's rulings on leafletting in shopping centers. The Warren Court had said in 1968 that picketing of a particular store in a large, privately owned shopping center had to be allowed. In 1972, without overruling that earlier case, the Burger Court, saying the cases were different, allowed antiwar leafletting to be banned because the protest was unrelated to the shopping center or its stores. Then in 1976 the Court banned picketing of a shopping center shoestore by workers whose basic dispute was with the store's warehouse. Here the Court explicitly overruled the 1968 case but in doing so said the overruling had really taken place in 1972 because the 1968 case had not "survived" the 1972 ruling. The inadequacy of this explanation, which conceded that the first opinion had been overruled *sub silentio*, was so obviously at variance with the majority's own 1972 statements that Justice Marshall was prompted to complain that the first case had "been laid to rest without ever having been accorded a proper burial."[18] That the Court does appear to overrule cases without saying so indicates that it does have ways other than overturning precedent to bring about changes in the law. One is to state a new test for judging cases; another is to write into opinions "subtle suggestions or leading remarks that may be cited later for new legal propositions."[19]

Still another way to avoid the thrust of precedent without stirring up as much criticism as an explicit overruling would provoke is "strategic differentiation" or the *distinguishing* of cases from one another, emphasizing their differences and limiting the application of precedent by saying new cases contain facts not identical to those in the older cases. As one can see from the leafletting cases, the Burger Court used this technique in its erosion of Warren Court rulings. It did so particularly in the criminal procedure area, even doing it to some of its own cases. For example, in order to allow police to conduct warrantless searches of cars *and* any containers and packages that might contain contraband (*United States v. Ross*, 1982), the Court distinguished cases in which it had invalidated searches of a locked footlocker and a suitcase, saying those containers had only a "purely coincidental" connection with the automobiles in which they were seized and that the police had lacked probable cause to search anything but the cars themselves. This effort to cut away at precedents by attempting to distinguish them provoked Justice Marshall to comment that the Court had "effectively overruled" rather than distinguished the earlier cases. However, even with precedents that are expandable and contractable, limits are established, so that some opinions stating new policy "won't write." This is undoubtedly one reason the Burger Court remained more liberal than had been expected; Warren Court precedents led to more liberal results than if President Nixon's appointees had been able to write on a clean slate.

The effect of precedent is clear in the statements of individual justices. For example, in *Runyon v. McCrary* (1976), Justice Powell went along with the

Court's outlawing racial discrimination in admission to private schools, which involved application of the Court's 1968 *Jones v. Mayer* decision applying post-Civil War antidiscrimination statutes to private housing sales, because the Court had considered application of those civil rights statutes to private acts "maturely and recently." Although Justice Stevens indicated he would vote differently "were we writing on a clean slate," he said that "the interest in stability and orderly development of the law" and the fact that the precedent "accords with the prevailing sense of justice today" had "greater force" than the argument that the earlier case was wrongly decided. Stevens repeated the argument a few years later in talking "about the potential damage to the legal system that may be caused by frequent or sudden reversals of direction that may appear to have been occasioned by nothing more significant than a change in the identity of this Court's personnel."[20]

When justices agree to abide by particular precedents, even though they dislike them, they are sending "mixed messages"—one part of which may be an invitation to lawyers to challenge the disliked precedent. At times they go further, openly calling for reversal of disliked precedents. Justice Rehnquist, joining the majority in a major parental consent abortion case in upholding precedent because "literally thousands of judges cannot be left with nothing more than the guidance offered by a truly fragmented holding of this Court," announced he would "be more than willing to participate" when "this Court is willing to reconsider" its decision.[21] Rehnquist and Chief Justice Burger also joined in making long arguments for overturning the exclusionary rule with respect to improperly seized evidence. And Justice White, dissenting when the Court invalidated a state "moment of silence" statute, said he "would support a basic reconsideration of our precedents" on the Establishment Clause. However, he noted that his argument was "not surprising" because he had "been out of step with many of the Court's decisions dealing with this subject matter"[22]—perhaps an example of a justice adhering to personal precedent.

The Court does indeed overturn decisions. There are times when the need for consistency in the law leads the Court to abandon past rulings in favor of a new, clear, and up-to-date standard; this may also be made necessary by the presence of competing lines of cases, each of which has developed in a somewhat different way so that, taken together, they are not easily reconciled. It may also occur when the Court has ventured into an area of law for the first time and found that later cases cast a different light on the subject. This appears to have happened with the Burger Court's dealing with double jeopardy claims; in 1978 the Court overturned a 1975 opinion with the same justice (Rehnquist) writing both opinions, and in another 1978 ruling, the Court decided no longer to follow some earlier decisions.[23] The Court's overrulings on the subject of Congress' extension of the minimum wage to state and local government employees took only slightly longer, and also illustrate the overturning of an overturning. The Court first ruled, in 1968 (*Maryland v. Wirtz*) that Congress had the authority to extend the law to certain state and local government employees; then in 1976, in *National League of Cities v. Usery*, in what looked like a resurrection of the Tenth Amendment, the Court overturned Congress' authority, only to have the *National League of Cities* case in turn overruled in 1985 (*Garcia v. San Antonio Metropolitan Transit Authority*). As in those situations, some rulings may be overturned rather quickly, while others are reversed only after a somewhat longer time, as when the Burger Court, in the course of reconsidering the exclusionary rule, overturned two Warren Court rulings on informants' tips used as the basis for obtaining warrants.[24]

The Court, throughout its history, has engaged in some 175 reversals of precedent. From 1958 through 1980, the Court overruled 57 decisions, all but three by closely divided votes. The average life of the precedents before overruling was just under 20 years, and in only a few cases did the overruling take place in less than five years from the date of the original ruling. At the other extreme, some cases that had stood for more than 70 years were overturned.[25] Perhaps the period of most frequent reversal was that of the Roosevelt Court, 1937–46, when "the Supreme Court changed its mind about thirty-two precedents," not counting some cases not overruled but in effect ignored. Of the cases reversed, only nine came from the early 1930s; most (17) were from the previous two decades (1911–30), and four came from prior to 1900. Because of their age, these cases— roughly one-fourth of which dealt with intergovernmental tax immunity— "could fairly be described as constitutional relics" doomed as soon as FDR was reelected.[26] (The Roosevelt Court also overturned two of its own cases.)

Change in the Court's doctrine does occur even when precedent and ways of interpreting previous cases have exerted a brake on the Court's actions. However, the Court has seen the need to move gradually and to make its rulings appear incremental and to stress continuity even when considerable change is taking place. In general, because law develops in response to new circumstances, filling in gaps, abrupt turns (and overturnings) are seldom necessary. Too many sharp deviations and departures, too many unpredictable results disturb the general public and particularly those "opinion leaders" who watch the Court most closely.

Gradual movement might well characterize the Court's decisions even without precedent, as a result of deciding narrow questions before large ones or making summary disposition of appeals instead of rulings with full opinions. As this suggests, the sequence in which cases come to the Court—and particularly the first case on which the Court decides to issue a full-opinion ruling, is quite important. Dealing with one aspect of a topic first may head the Court down a somewhat different road from the one it would have constructed had another aspect of the subject been decided first. Most policymakers do not make radical departures from past policy but operate incrementally, developing policy a bit at a time and making changes "at the margin." As Shapiro has argued, "The theory of incrementalism may explain, or at least describe, the phenomena of stability and gradual change in law just as well as or better than stare decisis."[27] The school prayer decisions, where the Court first struck down a state-written prayer in *Engel v. Vitale* before eliminating all recitation of school prayer and Bible reading in *Abington School District v. Schempp*, provides an example of incremental action. So does reapportionment, where the Court first demanded equally populated districts for the U.S. House of Representatives (*Wesberry v. Sanders*) and invalidated the Georgia "county unit" system (*Gray v. Sanders*) before ruling, in *Reynolds v. Sims*, that both houses of all state legislatures had to be apportioned on the basis of population. In the area of criminal procedure,

> The Court would typically approach a new issue warily, issuing first a narrowly limited decision which contained a hint of the result that might finally be required. A few criminal lawyers would get that hint, cases would develop, and lower court decisions would result. These decisions would usually not be consistent with each other, which could be a boon to the Supreme Court; it could deny petitions for certiorari in all of these appeals, leaving the lower court rulings in effect without indicating whether it approved or disapproved of the results. Over the years experience would develop in the lower courts as to the best way to proceed with the problem, and any warning signs would be detected before the Supreme Court had to take its position.[28]

Although policy may be developed incrementally, it may also be developed in "big pieces" and *applied* incrementally, as successive litigation brings the various parts and pieces of a problem to the Court. Thus the Court first provided a broad definition for obscenity in its 1957 *Roth* decision, gradually adding elements to the definition in later cases. After the Court said in *Brown v. Board of Education* that "separate but equal" was not to apply to education, the Court applied this rule to other public facilities (golf courses, swimming pools, and the like) through a series of *per curiam* opinions shortly afterward. These examples also show the incremental development of what *seems* to be a major policy change, as the important elements of the *Roth* obscenity definition were derived from earlier lower court rulings, and *Brown* built on *Sweatt v. Painter*, invalidating segregation in graduate education because "intangible" factors were not equal.

Strategy

Expectations that the Court seek neutral principles and rely on precedent are traditional, one might say conservative, considerations in developing opinions. Quite different is the possibility that the Supreme Court engages in strategy. Changes in the Court's positions—from liberal to conservative, from activism to self-restraint (see below), from the center of the political arena to the periphery and back—are not accidental. Those changes result in part from external forces, such as the arrival of new justices chosen for their ideological proclivities and cases brought to the Court, and in part from internal factors, such as individual justices' attitudinal changes. Through their strategies, individual and collective, the justices contribute another important element to the decision-making process.

Those who believe that justices find law or who seek to have them apply neutral principles find unseemly any talk of judicial strategy. Issues are to be confronted directly, regardless of cost to the Court, and not for other concerns is justice for litigants to be sacrificed. There is, moreover, no doubt that conflicts between strategy and "justice" do exist and can be quite disturbing. Examples are the refusal in the 1950s to decide a challenge to a cemetery's refusal to bury a Native American, or to rule on the validity of antimiscegenation (anti-mixed-marriage) laws even when a black woman went to prison for marrying a white man, or, more recently, avoidance of persistent challenges to the constitutionality of the Vietnam War, despite the increasing death rate during that conflict.[29] Nonetheless, almost by definition the Court must act strategically, because it is a *political* body acting in an often hostile—or at least nonsupportive—environment.

Courts, no less than other governmental institutions, cannot ignore their environments and must understand them. Because the Court's relevant publics may shift their willingness to support civil liberties, for example, the Court needs to be able to recognize changes in such support if the justices wish their decisions to be accepted. If it is to survive and achieve some of its goals, the Court may have to avoid some controversies. To be avoided where possible are "self-inflicted wounds" like the *Dred Scott* decision legitimating slavery and, some would add, the Warren Court's criminal procedure rulings. A justice's 1954 comment, "One bombshell at a time is enough," made when the Court turned away a miscegenation case,[30] was a recognition of the need to concentrate on achieving school desegregation—affecting a large number of people—rather than damage that effort by angering the South with a decision on the mixed-marriage laws, affecting relatively few individuals. However, some members of the Court may complain that turning away cases is *not* appropriate even if the issues in the cases would produce discomfort for the justices; as Justice Rehnquist observed, the Court's discretionary jurisdiction should not be used "as a sort of judicial storm cellar to which we may flee to escape from controversial or sensitive cases."[31]

That the Court does take actions based on strategy is clear from the evidence provided by the justices themselves. For example, the decision in *Brown v. Board of Education* was delayed to get a vote that was unanimous or more nearly so.[32] When Justice Frankfurter was assigned to write the Court's opinion striking down the "white primary," the Chief Justice was told that, because the ruling was likely to be received negatively in the South, it would be wiser if the opinion were *not* written by a Jewish immigrant who had taught at Harvard Law School—and the case was reassigned to Justice Stanley Reed, a Kentuckian. Similarly Justice Byrnes, also a southerner, was assigned the opinion in *Taylor v. Georgia* (1940), holding that a Georgia statute violated federal prohibitions against peonage, in order to give it more force.[33]

The justices' demonstrated awareness of their political environment makes it quite likely that, acting on the basis of strategic considerations, they take that environment into account even when they claim not to do so. Justice Powell, upholding school financing through the property tax in *San Antonio School District v. Rodriguez* (1973), said, "Practical considerations, of course, play no role in the adjudication of the constitutional issues presented," but commented that to rule otherwise "would occasion . . . an unprecedented upheaval in public education." More recently, Justice Blackmun said he could attribute his colleagues' abandonment of past positions concerning state assistance to parochial school education only to "concern about the continuing and emotional controversy and to a persuasion that a goodfaith attempt on the part of a state legislature is worth a nod of approval."[34] In the past, the Court has acted strategically in responding to threats, as in changing its policy position on economic regulation after FDR's attempt to pack the Court and on internal security matters (loyalty oaths and congressional investigations of subversives) after congressional efforts in the 1950s to limit its jurisdiction (see pages 308-9), by refusing to decide more cases on a controversial issue or by deciding cases with larger majorities (see page 240).

Perhaps justices' taking into account the effect of their rulings has been most obvious in the field of criminal procedure. For example, Justice Stewart justified a new restriction on admissibility of seized evidence by pointing out that the FBI and the federal courts had remained effective although operating under the exclusionary rule for many years. In the 1976 death penalty decisions, several justices said that the fact that 35 states had reenacted death penalty legislation after statutes had been struck down in 1972 was an indication that the penalty was not "cruel and unusual punishment." And Justice Clark asserted that to apply the exclusionary rule of *Mapp v. Ohio* to past cases "would tax the administration of justice to the utmost."[35] One of several criteria the Court regularly used in deciding whether to apply its criminal procedure rules to past convictions was the effect such application would have upon the administration of justice. (The Court was also unwilling to apply a ruling retroactively because of its perceived effects on the equalization of men's and women's pension benefits, where the financial burden from retroactivity was involved.[36]) The retroactivity problem has been said to have been guided largely by strategic considerations such as placating those opposed to the Court's new rules.[37] In evaluating these particular instances, one should, however, keep in mind findings that, in the related matter of setting its agenda, that is, deciding what cases to review, the Court "does not respond to increases in the general level of public concern about crime" and does not use public opinion—"either general levels or increments"—as an input into that decision.[38]

To say that the Court acts strategically does not mean that the justices have a complete blueprint to guide their actions. It is more likely that individual justices act strategically than that there is a "strategy of the Court." Justices appear to share the goal of preserving the Court as an institution, and one may find that at least some justices share a general sense of direction. Nonetheless, the Court is perhaps best seen as a "mixed-motive" or "mixed-strategy" group. Strategy encompasses efforts to affect the political world outside the Court or to fend off attacks from outside (*external* strategy) as well as persuasion and bargaining among justices while a case is under advisement (*internal* strategy), necessary to achieve external effects.

A justice wishing to accomplish any external goal must attract enough colleagues to get a case accepted for review, then to constitute a majority for affirmance or reversal, and, finally, the most difficult task, to constitute a majority supporting an opinion advancing that goal. The goal seeker must be careful not to take so strong a position that the potential majority is lost, said to have occurred with Justice Blackmun in the sodomy case (*Bowers v. Hardwick*). We do, however, know of at least one instance where a justice intentionally took a strong position in an opinion circulated within the Court *in order to* force the hands of his colleagues so they would join *another* justice's more limited opinion.[39]

If unanimity is sought, extended discussions—and potential caution to keep potential "mavericks" from "wandering off the reservation"—may be necessary to retain it. This was apparently true after the 1954 school desegregation ruling, when the justices were highly uncertain about the proper way to enforce it or even about its precise meaning. In this situation, unanimity as a conscious strategy "masked the uncertainty" and also "provided a more solid defense to critics," although, because it deprived the Court of the opportunity to be persuasive, unanimity "operated in time to obscure rather than enhance the Court's decisions"[40]—thus providing an illustration of the difficulties that can result from operating strategically.

A range of tools is available to judges wishing to engage in strategy. Such tools, usually used in combination, are applied not only to a justice's immediate colleagues on the Court but also to the lower court judges so important in implementing the Supreme Court's opinions. At times a justice can assist in the process of selecting new colleagues. Most important, however, and most frequently used are devices necessary to the everyday resolution of cases before the Court. Of the available tools, perhaps force of intellect, demonstrated to lower court judges through carefully reasoned and written opinions and to colleagues through draft opinions and arguments in conference, is the one closest to "the law" and furthest from "politics." Personal intellect is, however, often not a sufficient strategic mechanism. Judges must thus resort to other strategems— including endearing themselves to colleagues, important in obtaining votes in cases of lesser importance to those colleagues, and threatening to vote against the majority. When dissenting views are stated strongly in public, it may damage the Court. Negotiation and compromise, at the core of internal strategy, are most upsetting to those who accept the myth of the Court as apolitical. One needs to ask, however, whether one could expect anything *other than* bargaining and compromise as part of the activities of the nation's highest court charged with interpretation of the Constitution, once that court is recognized to be a political actor acting in a political environment. Nonetheless, despite impressions created by *The Brethren's* focus on bargaining between the justices, examination of the process of accepting cases for review suggests that "in fact, the Court tends to be almost like nine separate law firms that go about their own business with relatively little interaction or wheeling and dealing."[41]

Strategy-related behaviors are brought to bear as the Court chooses issues for decision and the opinions to be written. One way in which the Court has demonstrated strategic concerns is its grouping of cases on a single subject. The Court decided five school segregation cases together in the early 1950s (*Brown* and four others), six cases on reapportionment when the Court first dealt with that subject on the merits, and four cases on confessions obtained without warning defendants of their rights (the *Miranda* decision), although it seems to engage in this action less now than a couple of decades ago. This is a way of focusing on broad issues and avoiding being "trapped" by the specific facts of a particular case, although the individual cases still have to be resolved.

In the process of granting review to a case, *issue fluidity*, a shift in the issues to which the Court gives attention in a case, can occur (see pages 203-4); it can occur as well during postargument consideration of a case and development of the Court's opinion. For example, in *California v. Grace Brethren Church* (1982), the issue changed from the constitutionality of collecting unemployment insurance taxes from religious schools not affiliated with a church—the issue on the basis of which the case was decided in the lower court—to whether the Tax Injunction Act permitted declaratory judgments—the issue decided by the Supreme Court. An instance in which the Court appeared to have changed the issue to be decided and then, somewhat embarrassedly, changed its mind again occurred in *Illinois v. Gates* (1983). Certiorari had originally been granted to consider whether a magistrate could properly issue a search warrant on the basis of a partially corroborated anonymous tip. After briefing and oral argument, the Court asked the parties to address whether the exclusionary rule should be modified when evidence was obtained "in the reasonable belief that the search and seizure at issue was consistent with the Fourth Amendment" (the "good-faith exception" issue). Because some justices' hostility to the exclusionary rule was well known, the request did not surprise observers. However, after the case was reargued, the Court decided to rule on only the original issue, not the newer one, which a majority found had not been addressed by the state court.

As they focus on a case's principal issues, the justices may decide not to deal with some issues that litigants have briefed and argued (*issue suppression*). That the Court has accepted a case to resolve an issue does not mean it will do so; indeed, it may yet avoid decision of the issue. Most recently, that has occurred with the question of whether a zoning regulation constituted a "taking" requiring compensation by the government: in a series of cases, the Court said there was insufficient information in the lower court rulings about the use that could actually be made of the land in question, and so declined to answer the question that was the reason for taking the case,[42] although the Court finally decided the question in the 1986 Term. The Court may not be well served when it obviously avoids an issue, as in its use of a procedural device that precludes reaching the merits—an example is the Court's ruling that the *DeFunis* affirmative action case was moot—although this does insulate it, at least for the time being, from the issue.

On the other hand, as justices examine briefs or listen to oral argument, they may be prompted to consider issues not earlier thought to be present in a case (*issue discovery*), to alter their views of issues' relative importance, or to consider grounds for an opinion that were not discussed by the parties.[43] This occurs because lawyers' arguments may be based on any matter appearing in the record and appellants may use any appropriate arguments in support of the lower court's judgment. Thus arguments may be made on appeal that were not made in the trial court or lower appellate court. Although the Court does not often decide a case on the basis of an issue not presented, and particularly if it has not been presented in the lower courts, issues *are* added to allow the Court to decide a case the way a majority considers appropriate. Thus, "An order limiting the grant of certiorari does not operate as a jurisdictional bar. We may consider questions outside the scope of the limited order when resolution of those questions is necessary for the proper disposition of the case."[44] Furthermore, if a precedent is thought necessary "to cover a large number of detailed questions being posed in the lower courts" when no case is available posing the question with appropriate breadth, the justices may use issue transformation to develop such a question and then decide it. As this suggests, "The question(s) to which the Court will respond in any given case cannot be known with certainty until the Court's opinion in the case is announced. . . . The Court can expand, contract, suppress or replace issues posed by the litigating parties at various points between initial issue framing and final issue resolution."[45]

Once it has been decided that the Court will issue a full, signed opinion, important additional elements in decision making come into play. Pragmatism, evangelism, and the milieu of advocacy are among the factors that diminish the effect of attitude and ideology, particularly with respect to the opinions the justices write. Pragmatism involves the question of "strategic judgments about what professional and lay traffics would bear." It can be seen when a justice withholds a dissent even when opposed to the result or limits himself to a concurring opinion rather than a dissent, perhaps so that the Court's decision can have greater force through a larger majority. Evangelism, the attempt to persuade publics outside the Court of the correctness of the Court's doctrine, certainly influences not only the justices' votes but also what they say. Thus "the demands of persuading colleagues and countrymen in trailblazing cases coalesce with professional habits and personal antagonisms to transform opinion-writing into argument and over-statement."[46]

There are a number of options for the Court and the opinion writer. It is wise for the Court to sound as much as possible like a "law court," with its opinions drawing heavily on precedent and history where possible and avoiding social science evidence, which tends to provoke criticism. The Court may wish to avoid a broad opinion that looks more "legislative" as well as a ruling so narrow it does not illuminate the law for other lawyers and judges and thus leads to the filing of many more cases. However, narrow rulings may be useful as a delaying tactic or as a device to clear away the underbrush before an unmistakable direct attack is mounted on a particular practice. A narrow opinion may also be necessary because a broad opinion may also lose judges from the majority, with the ultimate opinion often the lowest common denominator the justices can produce. Taking aspects of a problem one case at a time also allows the Court more flexibility. Such was the argument against the Court's overturning the legislative veto (see pages 304-5), in which the majority outlawed *all* legislative vetos in one blow instead of restricting itself to the particular, limited type of legislative veto before it. The latter action would have allowed consideration of variants as they appeared before the Court and would have allowed "fine-tuning" in the Court's doctrine on the subject. On the other hand, if the justices were clear about how they would rule in cases known to be "in the pipeline," they may have decided they might as well get the matter over with, a matter of docket management.

Opinions vary in their clarity, in their breadth and narrowness, and in the directness with which issues are approached. Ambiguity may be used strategically, to help keep control of policymaking in the Court's hands because unclear decisions force others to come back to the Court to obtain the justices' clarification. Thus ambiguous decisions, while producing "repeater" cases that may cause docket management problems, allow the Court to "monitor" the action of lower courts.

With respect to the breadth of opinions, the Court can achieve its goals without broad opinions, particularly if negative reaction to a straightforward doctrinal ruling is forseen; limited doctrinal grounds—basing a case on its facts or relying on statutory interpretation—can be used instead of dealing with larger, "tougher" constitutional questions. A narrowly focused ruling may be advantageous for the Court, for such a ruling may lead the public to focus on the issue decided rather than on more global matters that might be likely to provoke controversy. Yet there are times when reaching the principal issues directly is not only what the judges want to do but is also important strategically—to satisfy the demands and expectations of the Court's constituencies. If much of the Court's strategy seems based on avoiding issues or minimizing the degree to which they are confronted, one must remember that this is done so that on the issues the Court considers most important it can act forthrightly.

If a variety of tools are available to aid the exercise of judicial strategy, there are also numerous constraints on a judge's ability to accomplish strategic aims. Two basic constraints serving to limit the degree to which judicial policymaking can be explicit and to which strategy can be openly considered are the strongly held myth that the Court finds and does not make law and the special legal framework within which the justices operate. Beyond those constraints, even if all justices were simultaneously concerned about strategy, each might focus on different aspects of a case or wish to pursue different strategies. Moreover, although a "policy-oriented judge" is "aware of the impact which judicial decisions can have on public policy, realizes the leeway for discretion which his office permits, and is willing to take advantage of this power and leeway to further particular policy aims," not all justices may fit this description: "Probably relatively few justices have had a systematic jurisprudence; more but probably still relatively few have been so intensely committed to particular policy goals as to establish rigid priorities of action that dominated their entire lives; probably few have been able to act only rationally in seeking to achieve their aims." In addition, each judge "has only a finite supply of time, energy, research assistance, and personal influence."[47]

Strategic considerations often compete and there are standard operating procedures (SOPs) and "bureaucratic routines" that courts, like any other organization, follow. The justices respond to self-imposed deadlines like the one that all cases argued within a term are to be decided by the end of that term, as well as to rules for handling caseload, including technical ones on timely filing and judicial doctrines on the standing of a party to raise an issue (see pages 170-73). These rules can be ignored when it is felt necessary, but if the Court is to function effectively, that cannot be done often. Other constraints on the Court's exercise of strategy include the judges' own positions, interpersonal relations within the Court, the Court's prestige at the time, and external pressures—from interest groups, Congress, and the president.

Requiring particular attention in the Court's exercise of external strategy, and thus constituting serious potential constraints, are lower court judges. A major strategic question is whether—and to what degree—the Court should defer to those judges, particularly state judges. Such deference, like that shown the legislative and executive branches, is necessary because the Supreme Court depends on the lower court judges to carry out its mandates, something the latter would be less likely to do if the justices interfered frequently with their work. The deference may allow the lower courts to move ahead of the Supreme Court in applying a new doctrine, creating a base on which the Court itself can later build. However, it may also produce delay or noncompliance, with the case being brought back to the Court for further action and thus interfering with docket management. Particularly when the Court has remanded a case with only limited instructions, evasion may also result. This allows the lower court to find an alternative basis for reaching the result it had reached earlier, while keeping the case out of the Supreme Court's hands. [48]

Judicial Review

If the reach toward "neutral principles" and respect for precedent are two matters with which the Court must concern itself, another is when to engage in judicial review, for at least two related reasons: judges engaging frequently in judicial review will find themselves criticized for being part of an "imperial judiciary" (see pages 3-6) and they will be criticized for being nondemocratic officials encroaching on democratic institutions. The latter concern leads us to look at some fundamental arguments about the propriety of judicial review in a democratic system. (See below.) These arguments change somewhat in form over time but are seldom far from the surface; in recent years, they have turned on the extent to which, in interpreting the Constitution, the justices should follow the "original intent" of the framers of the Constitution and its amendments. Among arguments that judicial review is undemocratic, [49] we find judicial review disparaged because justices appointed for life, who often remain on the Court long after they are out of tune with the nation's views, can overrule acts of periodically elected representatives and acts of the executive branch, whose head, the president, is also elected. One response is that when the Court strikes down statutes as "void for vagueness," Congress, because it is not being told that it cannot act, only that it must act more clearly, can rewrite the statutes with clearer prescriptions. Even when the Court invalidates statutes as unconstitutional, such rulings can be overturned. Although some Court actions can be reversed only by constitutional amendment, at times only a statute is necessary to do so. Thus when state action is invalidated for intruding on the federal government's domain in violation of the Commerce Clause, Congress can restore state authority through legislation granting the states authority over the contested subject matter. [50] Enacting constitutional amendments to overturn the Court is difficult but not impossible, as we see from the Eleventh (no suits against states by citizens of another state), Sixteenth (income tax), and Twenty-sixth (18-year-old vote) Amendments and the post-Civil War amendments eliminating slavery, redefining citizenship, and protecting civil rights. [51]

Another response to the claim that judicial review is undemocratic is Alexander Hamilton's, in *Federalist* #78, that through judicial review, the Constitution—the people's will—is enforced over the will of the people's representatives. However, the people whose will is being enforced are long dead, with the ideas of constitution makers of the distant past pitted against views of much more recent legislators. Frequent exercise of judicial review will also, we are told, make it less likely that those seeking policy changes will press legislators and political executives for action, and will put a damper on legislators' willingness to meet their responsibilities to deal with social problems. In Chief Justice Burger's words,

"When this Court rushes in to remedy what it perceives to be the failings of the political process, it deprives those processes of an opportunity to function. When the political institutions are not forced to exercise constitutionally allocated powers and responsibilities, those powers, like muscles not used, tend to atrophy."[52] On the contrary, the Court's action can also help establish an agenda of issues given active consideration by the other branches and can stimulate activity to deal with otherwise ignored problems. For example, after the Court's reapportionment rulings, state legislatures learned to deal with redistricting; those rulings also opened up, rather than restricted, the political process.

At the center of the debate about judicial review and democracy is the argument that courts must protect the minority rights that are as much a part of democracy as is majority rule, and can make an important contribution to democracy by enforcing rights of free speech and press, assembly, and petition. In a particularly significant statement, Justice Harlan Fiske Stone suggested, in Footnote #4 in the *Carolene Products* case, that the usual presumption of validity for challenged statutes might be given less weight when the statutes affected the subject matter of the Bill of Rights. Moreover, heightened judicial scrutiny might be given legislation that "restricts those political processes which can ordinarily be expected to bring about repeal of undesirable legislation" and laws directed at "discrete and insular" racial, ethnic, and religious minorities who were the object of prejudice, because that prejudice would limit use of the political process. Examples are a city charter amendment requiring approval only of open housing ordinances by referendum and passage of a state referendum that limited busing for desegregation (but not for other purposes). Both were held invalid for restructuring the political process to the disadvantage of minorities.[53]

Justice Stone's cautious statement recently became the focus of John Hart Ely's further-reaching "representation-reinforcing theory of judicial review."[54] Ely argued that, in the exercise of judicial review, judges should not search for fundamental values to be enforced, or substantive results to be imposed, but should focus on restrictions on "the opportunity to participate either in the political processes by which values are appropriately identified and accommodated, or in the accommodation those processes have reached." The Constitution, by seeing to it that "everyone's interests will be actually or virtually represented . . . at the point of substantive decision" and that application of substantive policy "will not be manipulated . . . to reintroduce discrimination," "has sought to assure that [an effective] majority not systematically treat others less well than it treats itself." Thus "unblocking stoppages in the democratic process is what judicial review ought preeminently to be about."[55]

This basic position that the Court must use judicial review, even if incompatible with majority rule, to protect individual rights, is at the heart of another recent argument that the Supreme Court should limit and better focus its exercise of judicial review. Because, "almost by definition," Jesse Choper asserts, "the processes of democracy bode ill for the security of personal rights and . . .

experience shows such liberties are not infrequently endangered by popular majorities . . . the task of custodianship has been and should be assigned to a governing body that is insulated from political responsibility and unbeholden to self-absorbed and excited majoritarianism."[56] Choper also argues, pragmatically, that judges should abstain from exercising judicial review in other situations so that they can be more effective when they do exercise it in cases involving political rights, which are likely to provoke and offend other political actors. Although Choper would have the court "pass final constitutional judgment on questions concerning the permissible reach and circumscription of 'the judicial power'," he would have the Court avoid ruling on conflicts between president and Congress, because judicial action lessens the incentives for the two branches to work out matters on their own, and on states' allegations that Congress has interfered with their authority, although it should review state acts violating the Supremacy Clause.

Despite the effectiveness with which such positions have been developed, arguments that judicial review is undemocratic may be misdirected. For one thing, other governmental institutions may be no more responsive to the public than is the Court, with no one (except perhaps the president) accountable to a majority of the nation's voters. Moreover, our government's institutions operate by means of a system of checks and balances in which each participates in the work of the others and thus limits them. The Court's involvement in these political processes, engaging in strategic actions as a policymaker, thus makes it to some extent a democratic institution; only if it were fully insulated from those processes and if it found the law in total independence of other government bodies would it be undemocratic.

Related to, but not the same as, the argument over judicial review and democracy, is the contemporary argument over how the Constitution should be interpreted. The two matters are related in that those urging justices to give close attention to the "original intent" of the Constitution's framers criticize others for injecting their own views into the Constitution and thus acting undemocratically. The argument over reliance on "original intent" has produced much rhetoric without much understanding. The primary participants in the mid-1980s battle were, on the one side, Attorney General Edwin Meese, and, on the other, Justices Brennan and Stevens. The problem with trying to decipher opposing positions is that the issue is not really about the use or nonuse of "original intent" but about specific value positions. Justice Brennan, at least, makes this clear: "A position that upholds constitutional claims only if they were within the specific contemplation of the Framers in effect establishes a presumption of resolving textual ambiguities against the claim of constitutional right."[57] Thus the term "original intent" becomes a "praise word" if one likes certain results and a "swear word" ("He didn't follow original intent. Shame!") for disliked results.

The value position of Attorney General Meese can be seen in his view that the idea the Fourteenth Amendment "incorporated" the provisions of the Bill of

Rights as prohibitions against the states was on shaky legal ground—although he later claimed he was not calling for overturning cases incorporating portions of the Bill of Rights, cases through which state criminal defendants have received much protection. Meese's view is that judges should restrict themselves to the Constitution's "original intention," not to its "spirit," because use of the latter would turn the Constitution into a "chameleon." Although he has conceded that the "Constitution is not a legislative code bound to the time in which it was written," "neither. . . is it a mirror that simply reflects the thoughts and ideas of those who stand before it."[58]

For Brennan, ambiguity in the Constitution "calls forth interpretation, the interaction of reader and text." He stresses that the Constitution "places certain values beyond the power of any legislature," taking them away from the majority. History must be examined, but later interpretation given to provisions must also be considered, as must the "ultimate question": "what do the words of the text mean in our time." As he added, "We current Justices read the Constitution in the only way that we can: as Twentieth Century Americans." Brennan also argues that from the late twentieth century one could not "gauge accurately the intent of the Framers on application of principle to specific contemporary questions."

Federalism

The Court has among its roles that of arbiter of the federal system—of conflicts between states and between the national government and the states, and much of the history of the Supreme Court can be viewed as a history of the treatment of federalism-related concerns.[59] While the justices vary in the extent to which they defer to the "sovereign" states, issues of federalism are often present. For example, does Congress have the power to lower the voting age to 18 in both national and state elections? (In *Oregon v. Mitchell*, the Court said it could in national but not in state and local elections, provoking passage of the Twenty-sixth Amendment.) Or should states, because of their "police power" over matters of health, welfare and morals, be given more flexibility than the federal government in dealing with obscenity? (The Court, in the *Roth* and *Alberts* cases, treated both levels of government the same; no one else would follow Justice Harlan's lead in pressing for different treatment depending on whether the national or state government was acting.)

In addition to cases directly and explicitly raising federalism issues, there are others in which federalism questions come into play beneath the surface even when the focus is on a substantive issue (abortion, obscenity, the death penalty) rather than on federalism itself, particularly where an important aspect of the case is whether states may take certain action the national government is not permitted to take.

Of particular significance have been the Court's rulings "incorporating" the provisions of the Bill of Rights as prohibitions against the states through the inclusion of those provisions in the Due Process Clause of the Fourteenth

Amendment. The Court never adopted the "full incorporation" position—that all provisions of the Bill of Rights were automatically and at once included in the Due Process Clause—but during the Warren Court period most of the Bill of Rights was incorporated through a process of "selective incorporation." This nationalized the Bill of Rights, particularly because most justices interpreted the "due process" required of the states under the Fourteenth Amendment to be identical with the Bill of Rights provision that is being incorporated. (An exception is the size of a criminal jury trial, which the Court allowed to be as small as six in the states although it remained at twelve in federal court.[60]) One reason for the Supreme Court's "nationalization" of criminal procedure rulings was that the states did not heed relatively quiet warnings from the Court about such matters as the voluntariness of confessions or providing attorneys to criminal defendants; had the states themselves shown greater concern about protecting defendants' rights, the Warren Court criminal procedure rulings might not have been issued.

When actions of state *courts* are under review, questions of federalism and of deference to other judges may reinforce each other. Thus the justices have resisted having federal courts engage in close supervision of state courts, whether the issue is alleged racial discrimination in those courts' actions (see *O'Shea v. Littleton*, 1973) or federal court review of state court criminal cases through federal habeas corpus (see pages 86-87). Another issue concerning Supreme Court deference to state courts is whether the state court has explicitly indicated reliance on state law, which the Supreme Court has now required if the justices are to accept the state ruling as having an "adequate and independent" state ground precluding Supreme Court review (see page 210). In particular, when state courts decided in favor of a criminal defendant, the rhetoric of respect for state court rulings has not been accompanied by a "hands-off" approach that one might expect to accompany the rhetoric (see page 25).

If questions of federalism have *largely* been settled and thus are less frequently the source of conflict within the Court than they once were, they are not *completely* settled. This can be seen most obviously in the line of cases starting with *National League of Cities v. Usery* (1976), limiting Congress' power to force state and local governments to pay their employees the minimum wage, through intervening decisions to the *Garcia* ruling in 1985 removing the constraints on Congress—and indeed, relegating the states to their representatives in Congress for their protection from such congressional commands. The Supreme Court's other rulings on Congress' power to regulate commerce—and on the states' authority to regulate commerce when Congress has not done so (the "dormant Commerce Clause" cases)—have been particularly important. Indeed, the Court's interstate commerce rulings were among those to which the Reagan administration pointed in complaining in 1986 that the Supreme Court had undermined state sovereignty.

Other cases directly posing federalism questions and particularly significant are those, occurring throughout the Court's history, involving the question whether the national government has "preempted" state action on a particular subject. Especially controversial was the decision in *Pennsylvania v. Nelson* (1956), in which the Court set aside a state conviction of a person for attempting to overthrow the government of the United States because the national government had indicated its intention to preempt the field through enactment of the Smith and McCarran Acts. Intense negative reaction led the Court to rule in *Uphaus v. Wyman* (1959) that the states could regulate subversion directed at the states themselves. More recent preemption rulings contributed to the Reagan administration's attack on the Court for undermining state power.

That issues of this sort have been present does not, however, mean that conceptions of federalism have been the primary influence in the Court's rulings generally. Examination of the 1969–77 Terms shows that despite occasional statements about leaving matters to the states, the Burger Court was *not* "an overwhelming example of judicial restraint." The justices deferred less to the states on questions of economic regulation than they did to federal government regulatory actions, and some of the justices' decisions were definitely affected by whether the state policy they were reviewing was probusiness or antibusiness: of four justices who supported probusiness decisions most strongly (three being appointees of President Nixon), three "become remarkably unsupportive" when the state policy is antibusiness. Marshall and Brennan adopted converse positions, and only Justice Rehnquist "defers to the states enough to qualify. . . as an advocate of judicial restraint," although his "conservative economic bias" showed nonetheless. The pattern of greater support for the federal government than for state governments also appeared in civil rights and civil liberties cases extending through early 1979, whether the subject was the First Amendment, double jeopardy, or poverty law, with support for state policy roughly equal to support for the federal government only in search and seizure cases.[61]

Activism and Restraint

A major consideration in Supreme Court decisions, closely related to judicial review and the question of the deference the Supreme Court should give to lower courts, is the extent to which the Court, in dealing with other actors in the political system, should be "self-restrained" or "activist." (See pages 3-6.) Because of the absence of clear definitions, controversy over whether the Court has been sufficiently "self-restrained" or too "activist" has been almost continuous; that each concept has several dimensions further complicates communication about them. Despite the absence of fixed definitions, there is some general agreement on some basic dimensions of the terms. There are "two major premises that serve as underpinning [for] . . . a limited role for the courts": that judicial policymaking "conflicts with the very essence of a democratic society" and "that courts simply are not equipped to make wise policy."[62]

As a federal judge has observed, "Appropriate judicial humility weighs against judicial activism" because on policy questions "the judge can never be justifiably certain that he or she is right even when the judge happens to be right."[63] And, as Chief Justice Burger commented, "We trespass on the assigned function of the political branches under our structure of limited and separated powers when we assume a policymaking role." He added, "It is not the function of the judiciary to provide 'effective leadership' simply because the political branches of the government fail to do so."[64] Thus when congressional legislation is not as polished, or complete, as some justices might wish it to be, "it is not the function of this Court . . . to apply the finishing touches. . . . Our job does not extend beyond attempting to fathom what it is that Congress produced, blemished as the Court may perceive that creation to be."[65] That such statements are not made only by conservative judges can be seen in a recent opinion for the Court by Justice Marshall, who argued, "The fact that Congress might have acted with greater clarity or foresight does not give the courts a *carte blanche* to redraft statutes. . . . Nor is the judiciary licensed to attempt to soften the clear import of Congress' chosen words whenever a court believes those words lead to a harsh result."[66]

There has also been a change over time in the meaning and effect of self-restraint and activism. The pre-New Deal (Taft) Court had "used judicial power actively to police the legislative and executive branches of federal and local government, in order to enforce the Justices' commitment to laissez faire economic policies," while assuming "an almost entirely passive posture in civil liberties cases in striking contrast to its constitutional activism in economic cases."[67] In that situation, "activism" produced a "conservative" result (assistance to the business community). "Self-restraint" meant not disturbing legislation regulating the economy, producing "liberal" results, as it did after Franklin Roosevelt won his battle with the Court, which began to uphold New Deal legislation. On the other hand, in the area of civil liberties, a "hands-off" approach preserved statutes and other actions infringing individual freedoms, while "activism" generally protected civil liberties, at least through the end of the Warren Court.

The Court's basic operational rules of self-restraint were spelled out most explicitly by Justice Louis Brandeis in his opinion in the *Ashwander* case. The Court will not rule on challenged legislation in a nonadversary proceeding nor will it decide a complaint made by someone not injured by the statutes or by someone who has benefited from the action being challenged. A constitutional issue will not be decided if other bases for decision, such as statutory construction, are available; in short, the Court will not anticipate a constitutional question unnecessarily nor will it formulate a rule broader than required by the facts of the case.[68] Thus the Court exercises self-restraint by approaching cases cautiously—by denying review to some cases and, perhaps more important, by developing rules as to who may bring cases and under what conditions they may be brought (see chapter 5).

Considerable disagreement has, however, occurred over whether the Court has followed such "rules" of self-restraint and whether it has heeded Justice Stone's admonition that "the only check upon our own exercise of power is our own sense of self-restraint."[69] For example, Justice Stevens has complained, "The Court seems determined to decide these cases on the broadest possible grounds; such determination is utterly at odds with the Court's traditional practice as well as any principled notion of judicial restraint."[70] There are, however, situations when some justices argue that although the *Ashwander* rules should usually be followed, some departure from them is sensible, for example, not deciding the statutory question before the constitutional one where one would have to "torture" the statute to save it. Thus Justice White complained that the majority in a case had stretched too far to avoid an important First Amendment issue: "our duty to avoid constitutional questions through statutory construction is not unlimited: it is subject to the condition that the construction adopted be 'fairly possible.'"[71]

Richard Nixon had pledged to appoint "strict constructionist" judges who would not encroach on areas belonging to Congress and the president; he criticized judges for having "gone too far in assuming unto themselves a mandate which is not there, and that is, to put their social and economic ideas into their decisions."[72] However, his remarks about Supreme Court decisions setting free "patently guilty individuals on the basis of legal technicalities" meant he did not want self-restrained judges when activism could aid the "peace forces" rather than the "criminal forces." And it is clear that his appointees took actions that aided the "peace forces," whether police, prosecutors, or prison administrators.

When pro-law enforcement policy goals would be aided by so doing, Nixon's appointees deferred to legislative and executive actions, that is, they adopted a "self-restrained" posture. For example, the Court talked of its "reluctance to review legislatively mandated terms of imprisonment" even though a defendant thus received a life sentence for three felonies that had netted a total of less than $250.[73] And the Court also stated in the *Goodwin* case (1982) that "a prosecutor should remain free before trial to exercise the broad discretion entrusted to him to determine the extent of the social interest in prosecution," even when he had reindicted the defendant on higher charges after the defendant had refused to plead guilty.

The Burger Court was deferential and "self-restrained" toward those in charge of institutions, particularly in prison cases, where the Court moved back toward the "hands-off" doctrine on prison policy. For example, Justice Rehnquist, sustaining prohibition of a prisoners' union, criticized the district court for "not giving appropriate deference to the decisions of prison administrators and appropriate recognition to the peculiar and restrictive circumstances of penal confinement." He also asserted, in a case involving conditions for pretrial detainees, that "prison administrators . . . should be accorded wide-ranging deference in the adoption and execution of policies and practices that in their judgment are needed to preserve internal order and discipline and to maintain institutional security." The same deference to institutional administrators was evident in the Court's ruling that decisions concerning the training of the mentally retarded were "presumptively valid" if a professional made the decision.[74]

When deference did not work, however, the Court's majority was unabashedly (although not explicitly) activist, particularly in reaching out to overturn state court rulings that favored defendants' rights—and its rulings were met by criticism from the Court's liberal members (see page 25). Yet it was not only in the area of criminal procedure that the Burger Court was not self-restrained. In terms of statutes invalidated, it was no more deferential than its predecessor to Congress or to state regulatory efforts affecting commerce, and its rulings "significantly constrained" what the states could do. Perhaps more important is that because the Court enforced the underlying premises of many Warren Court precedents, the Warren Court's activism was "solidified" rather than undercut.[75] As a result, those unhappy with that legacy recognize that judicial restraint, in the sense of adherence to precedent, will not assist them in achieving their political agenda; they need some "negative activism" on the school prayer and abortion rulings. Apart from their rhetoric, justices' votes raise questions about whether they *practice* self-restraint to the extent they *advocate* it, whether it actually motivates those who make claims in its behalf or whether ideology is the actual determinant of their actions. For example, the breadth of the Court's criminal procedure doctrine has been related to the justices' goals. Confronting broad rules favoring law enforcement, liberal justices have argued that cases should be decided on the basis of the "totality of the circumstances," rather than in terms of broad rules they had earlier espoused when in the majority. In the 1969–77 Terms of the Court, out of a possible 40 situations—10 justices deciding cases in four categories (regulatory commissions, federalism, access, and civil rights and civil liberties)—in only 10 situations did activism or restraint influence justices' voting, and only Justice Douglas "manifested activism or restraint in more than a single category."[76]

Of particular interest is Justice Felix Frankfurter, the Court's foremost advocate of judicial self-restraint in recent times. He argued in the 1962 reapportionment case, *Baker v. Carr*, that the Court should stay out of the reapportionment issue because it involved "political entanglements" and the "clash of political forces in political settlements." Civil liberties and labor cases in which Frankfurter participated often included questions of jurisdiction and issues of deference to other units of government, questions closely related to self-restraint. With such Denial of Judicial Responsibility (DJR) matters present, Frankfurter's vote was always against the civil liberties claim in civil liberties cases and against the liberal position in 16 of 18 labor cases. However, with DJR-related cases removed, Frankfurter's position relative to that of the other justices remained to the right of center in civil liberties cases. Thus, even if the DJR factor, when present, appeared to control Frankfurter's civil liberties ideology, in other cases he was obviously a conservative rather than an apostle of self-restraint, posing the question of whether self-restraint explains even cases where the DJR issue was present.[77]

The argument for self-restraint has been made forcefully in recent years, but the argument for "affirmative activism" is also a strong one, particularly when such activism takes the form of "an effort by the Court to redress minimally the political imbalance between bureaucrats and those who are subject to bureaucratic power but are typically impotent to reform or influence it."[78] Such a position is closely related to Justice Stone's *Carolene Products* footnote and to use of the courts by those unsuccessful in achieving their goals in other political arenas or who need governmental assistance to prevent being deprived of their rights. Just as government has grown, so has the possibility of challenges to government action and thus judicial activism to restrain that action.

Adoption of a strongly activist position with respect to individual freedoms is not necessarily realistic for the Court as a political actor. Despite approval from some segments of the public, the Warren Court's decisions were frequently attacked and often disobeyed. Indeed the Court almost lost some of its jurisdiction and perhaps would have suffered severe damage had it not avoided some issues and retreated on other occasions. The absence of attacks on the Burger Court, a result of the greater congruence of its decisions with the nation's civil liberties orientation, suggests the virtues of its actions, whether self-restrained or activist, and the advantages flowing from its being able to persuade most people that it is indeed acting from a self-restrained position.

Off-the-Court Activity

The Court's opinions—and the justices' separate concurring and dissenting statements—may provide the principal mechanism by which the justices participate in policymaking, and the principal way in which they carry out their strategies, but they are not the only one. There is also judicial participation in matters outside the Court, where we can see off-the-bench "activism" related to justices' on-the-bench activism.

A justice who has been politically active is not likely to slacken interest in political issues once his or her Supreme Court nomination has been confirmed nor to sever all contacts with the political world, for example, to cease contacts with the president. Thus justices have informally continued as presidential advisers, as Chief Justice Vinson did with President Truman and Justice Abe Fortas did with President Lyndon Johnson on such topics as Vietnam, steel price increases, and strikes. It is not, however, clear whether, as alleged, Vinson advised Truman that the latter had the authority to order an emergency seizure of the steel mills, an action the Court later determined to be invalid (see page 320). Even when prior personal contact has been limited, as in Richard Nixon's acquaintance with Warren Burger during Burger's Justice Department service, contact may later expand, particularly in the case of the Chief Justice. Thus Burger apparently met on occasion with the president or with Attorney General

Mitchell, but whether these discussions went beyond matters of judicial selection and judicial administration to comments about the school busing cases is unresolved. Whatever its scope, the role of presidential adviser is likely to be submerged and kept screened from the public to avoid the considerable criticism generated by public knowledge of such relations.

By comparison with activities in the Court's early years, justices' present political activities, such as contacts with the president, are very limited. Over the course of the Court's history, roughly two-thirds of the justices have engaged in some such activity, "either informally or in response to official government requests," and the justices were viewed "as valuable resources to be employed in a wide variety of public services bearing little or no relationship to their judicial function."[79] There has, however, been considerable variation in the general level of that activity, with some, like Chief Justice Melville Fuller (1888–1909), taking the equivalent of the veil, even avoiding Washington social contact. There has also been variation in the norms about the extent of such activity and in justices' sensitivity to those changing norms. Changes in the norms are in part a function of public reaction to the exent of previous extrajudicial activity, with the norm generally moving toward lessened out-of-Court involvement, relaxing somewhat after criticism abates, and then, in something of a ratchet effect, tightening further in the next similar cycle. However, in times of war and crisis the norm of noninvolvement tends to recede to allow the justices to "undertake any necessary informal extrajudicial tasks that might be useful to the nation."[80]

Before the Court's traditions were established, justices were often active participants in partisan activity, and spoke openly on partisan subjects, particularly when they were "on circuit." Some of the justices used the occasion of giving charges to grand juries "to issue political broadsides and thus enter into the heated debates raging between Federalists and Jeffersonian Republicans."[81] Indeed, it was activities of this type that led to the impeachment and trial (but not conviction) of Justice Samuel Chase. Also participating was Chief Justice John Marshall, who, using a *nom de plume*, wrote essays defending his decision in *McCulloch v. Maryland*. From 1810 to the Civil War, judges' extra-Court speeches and public letters were less partisan. Perhaps to help repair the damage from the *Dred Scott* case, they became even more quiet after the Civil War, but at the end of the nineteenth century, when the Court's prestige again improved, there was an "explosion" of speeches and writing. After the Depression, the level of oratory again fell and has generally remained low, but there are exceptions— pehaps the most extensive being Justice Douglas' book writing and statements on conservation and the environment.

Not until after the Civil War did judges themselves begin to look askance at justices' close ties to political parties or interest groups. Indeed, up to that time, justices had failed even to adhere to a norm of not talking about the Court's cases outside the Court; and until late in the nineteenth century, justices had regularly courted high political office from their positions on the Court. There have been few such instances in the twentieth century, with Charles Evans Hughes' departure from the Court to run unsuccessfully for president the best known; that his nomination came while he still sat on the Court was thought to injure its nonpartisan image. There was off-and-on-again discussion of the candidacy of Justice William O. Douglas, who also offered to resign from the Court to campaign for President Truman if Truman had decided to run in 1952, but an indication of changed norms is that the very discussion provoked criticism.

After the justices cut most political party ties, it took longer before they could be weaned from contacts with interest groups. Most twentieth century out-of-Court activity not concerning judicial administration has focused on issues rather than partisan elections. Examples are provided by the extrajudicial activities of Justices Louis Brandeis and Felix Frankfurter. Before he joined the Court, Brandeis had been committed to advancing a wide variety of political positions. Once he became a justice, he maintained his interest in those issues, both political (such as the concentration of big business) or more specifically religious (Zionism), and he continued to meet and to talk about them with those involved in politics and government. Did he wish to feed an insatiable appetite for knowledge of "current events," or did he continue to influence legislative policy indirectly, for example, pressing against what he thought was the New Deal's excessively pro-big business orientation? Did he simply express concerns to friends to orchestrate political battle plans? We cannot be sure.

We do know that between 1916 and 1938, Brandeis, an extremely wealthy man, provided to then Harvard law professor Felix Frankfurter regular payments totaling roughly $50,000 (worth many times that amount in current dollars) to assist Frankfurter's engaging in political activity. Because of Frankfurter's medical expenses for his chronically ill wife, such activity would otherwise have been difficult for him, and the payments did allow Frankfurter to remain politically active. Whether they made him a "paid political lobbyist and lieutenant"[82] is another conjectural matter, about which we may be properly dubious. Many communications passed back and forth between Brandeis and Frankfurter; Brandeis' political positions apparently appeared in print as editorials in *The New Republic,* for which Frankfurter regularly wrote; Frankfurter served as Brandeis' representative at Zionist conferences; and Frankfurter apparently worked on legislation of interest to Brandeis, including legislation on subjects that had been before the Court or would come before it. Moreover, a number of Frankfurter's protégés (the "Happy Hot Dogs") went to work for the Roosevelt administration and could there espouse Brandeis' positions as transmitted to them from Frankfurter, but they were politically active in their own right and hardly acted solely as Frankfurter's agents.

All this may indicate no more than a commonality of interests between the two men or the professor's working on matters of joint concern as a result of Brandeis' intellectual and personal influence, rather than Frankfurter's taking direction from Brandeis. Frankfurter also worked on matters of primary interest to himself, including some—most notably FDR's Court-packing plan—on which the two disagreed. Thus Frankfurter "cannot be viewed solely as Brandeis's agent, in that he became involved in a wide circle of issues and causes célèbres on his own and in which the justice expressed no strong interest."[83]

The question also remains of whether—and to what extent—Brandeis' actions, even if it is clear they could not be ethically acceptable for a Supreme Court justice in the 1980s, exceeded the bounds of propriety. His strong (if behind-the-scenes) efforts to correct the injustice of the Sacco-Vanzetti conviction put him in a position of having to disqualify himself when attorneys brought the case to him and then to the Court. It is, however, at best a matter of interpretation as to whether Brandeis took specific positions on New Deal policies that would have hindered his performance as a justice. Brandeis did deal with major political figures through intermediaries, perhaps as a matter of personal style, perhaps as a smokescreen to conceal his activity. When cases involving statutes on which he had given advice came before the Court we are told that he did not recuse but instead took "only a very minimal role in the ultimate judicial decision,"[84] perhaps a result of his view of the cases rather than a function of efforts to conceal political activity.

Frankfurter's political activity also did not cease when he became a member of the Court and indeed it was more open than Brandeis'. He continued his interests in affecting the staffing of particular government departments, and also put considerable effort into the American war effort and into helping develop the international order for the postwar years. After World War II, and particularly as a result of President Roosevelt's death, Frankfurter's ability to affect the executive branch declined, and so did his efforts, although his involvement in the political battle can be seen in his continuing conflict, off the Court as well as on, with the equally strong-minded Justice Douglas.

It is, however, difficult not to be concerned about recent revelations by Philip Elman, a former clerk of Frankfurter's, about conversations he and the justice had during the Court's consideration of the *Brown* school desegregation case, because at the time Elman was a senior attorney in the solicitor general's office and was principal author of the government's briefs in the case. Justice Frankfurter told Elman about his colleagues' concerns about the case, and this led Elman to write into one of the government briefs an argument he says he would not otherwise have made. Although Elman says the conversations took place before the government entered the case as *amicus curiae*, both he and the justice could have anticipated such action in a cases of such importance. The problem of a justice revealing in-Court confidences remains serious, despite the closeness that does develop between justices and some of their clerks.[85]

If Brandeis tried to limit public knowledge of his extrajudicial political interests, Frankfurter used "strong arguments, indignantly put" to stifle criticism.[86] He seems to have been far more concerned about his activities than Brandeis had been. Did this result from different personalities, with Brandeis simply more sure of himself, or did Brandeis not believe he had committed improprieties? Or did standards change between Brandeis' accession to the Court during World War I and Frankfurter's arrival there over 20 years later? Whatever our evaluation, we should be careful not to read 1980s standards—on matters of political activity and recusal, justices' financial interests, or their participation in judicial selection—back into an earlier era.

The involvement of justices in nonjudicial governmental positions has been a source of continuous controversy because their absence from the Court can produce an evenly divided Court, or it can involve a justice in a matter that would later come before the Court.[87] When the Court's workload was not heavy, outside activity did not interfere with the Court's work. Both Chief Justice John Jay and Justice Oliver Ellsworth were involved in treaty negotiations, and Jay, who was also a candidate for governor of New York, served as secretary of state. In the nineteenth century, Melville Fuller and David Brewer arbitrated a boundary dispute between Venezuela and British Guiana, five justices served on the commission to help resolve the disputed 1876 Hayes-Tilden presidential election, and Stephen Field served on a commission to revise state laws in his native California. Earlier in this century, Charles Evans Hughes served on a commission to determine second-class postal rates.

More recent "calls" from the president to take on extra-Court jobs have encountered more objections because such jobs interfere with disposition of the Court's increased workload and because it has been feared that the Court's independence would be injured if it appeared that justices would readily serve at the president's bidding. During Franklin Roosevelt's presidency, Justice Reed chaired a committee to improve the civil service, Owen Roberts conducted an investigation of Pearl Harbor, and Robert Jackson was chief U.S. prosecutor at the war crimes trials in Nuremburg. Jackson's extended absence brought conflict within the Court as well as criticism for thrusting a judge into a simultaneous prosecutorial position and led Chief Justice Stone to turn down Roosevelt's requests to assume other tasks, such as investigating the nation's rubber supply. (During Taft's chief justiceship, Stone, a former attorney general, had been willing to serve on the Wickersham Commission investigating crime, but Taft had resisted.) Chief Justice Warren, who generally stayed away from most extra-Court activity as a matter of propriety, headed the commission to investigate the assassination of President Kennedy, but he did so only after resisting President Johnon's request. Subsequent questions about the commission's report, including Senate Intelligence Committee revelations that the FBI and CIA withheld information, reinforce the case against this type of extrajudicial activity.

Most recently, Chief Justice Burger became chairman of the Commission on the Bicentennial of the American Constitution—a topic that was close to his heart—and he remained in that position after stepping down as chief justice; indeed, he said he left the Court so that he could devote his energies to the Commission. However, even a subject as neutral-sounding as the Constitution's bicentennial provoked controversy when the Commission, whose staff director was Burger's former Supreme Court administrative assistant, held meetings in private and was sued for violating the law requiring advisory committees to hold public meetings.

Although no one challenged Burger's chairing the commission, challenges were made to having federal judges sit on other government bodies. The membership of the President's Commission on Organized Crime included Judge Irving R. Kaufman from the Second Circuit and retired Justice Potter Stewart; in May 1985, a panel of the U.S. Court of the Eleventh Circuit said that those two appointments were unconstitutional because they cast doubt on the impartiality of the two as judges, although several months later the Third Circuit held that their participation was proper because the work was nonjudicial and the justices' service was voluntary.[88] The same issue was raised concerning the United States Sentencing Commission, a body created by the 1984 Crime Control Act to develop uniform guidelines for sentencing federal offenders. Judges were to be named to this commission, but Chief Justice Burger indicated that naming them raised constitutional questions because this was an appointment to an executive commission; nonetheless, he suggested 12 names and the president appointed three of them to the Commission. (There was also concern that services by active-duty judges would deprive their courts of needed personnel.[89]) Although neither commission had a sitting Supreme Court justice among its members (Justice Stewart had retired from the Court), were one to be named to such a governmental agency, the question of the constitutionality of that justice's so serving—as well as the question of what such service meant for the justice's impartiality—would certainly be raised.

Justices' off-the-Court activity has included teaching in law school (Justice Story taught at Harvard and both the first Justice Harlan and Justice Brewer taught at the predecessor to George Washington Law School) and at seminars for judges. The "flap" over Justice Fortas' receiving $15,000, raised by friends, to teach a law school seminar, plus judges' increased public speaking, led the Judicial Conference in 1969 to adopt rules prohibiting the acceptance of fees unless the circuit judicial council approved after determining that the services to be rendered would be in the public interest, were justified by exceptional circumstances, and would not interfere with judicial duties. Such Conference rules, however, do not bind Supreme Court members, although several justices said they would follow them voluntarily.

Drafting legislation affecting the courts and commenting on matters directly affecting the Supreme Court are activities more directly related to the justices' regular tasks. Justice Willis Van Devanter drafted the Judiciary Act of 1915 modifying the Court's appellate jurisdiction and Justice McReynolds, helped by Justices Van Devanter and Day, drafted the 1916 Judiciary Act. Chief Justice Burger, instrumental in initiating examination of the need for a new level of national appellate court (see pages 62-63), and his colleagues all responded to the

Hruska Commission's preliminary proposal for a National Court of Appeals, with several making statements supporting or opposing the creation of the new court; at the hearings on Justice Rehnquist's nomination to be chief justice, he strongly supported its creation and suggested how its judges were to be chosen (see page 63). Although justices do take public positions on matters such as a major restructuring of the court system, an issue on which they are thought to be expert, any activity on the justices' part is likely to be more informal and more covert the more the topic departs from judicial administration. And even on matters directly relating to the judiciary, there is a view that judges should restrict their comments to institutionalized channels, such as having the Judicial Conference convey views to Congress. There has, however, been departure from this norm to the extent individual judges disagree with the Judicial Conference's position; their unhappiness about their pay (see pages 89-90) led to the formation of the Federal Judges Association, which lobbies on behalf of its members' interests.

Perhaps coming to be more and more expected as a form of extra-Court activity—and certainly permissible under the Code of Judicial Conduct—are the Chief Justice's comments about the "state of the judiciary," and proposals have been made that such an address be made to Congress. Chief Justices William Howard Taft and Charles Evans Hughes appeared at bar association meetings and at the American Law Institute (ALI) to discuss the "state of the judiciary." Such presentations were revived by Chief Justice Warren, who preferred the ALI as his forum because of ABA criticism of the Court's decisions. However, as noted earlier (see page 26), Chief Justice Burger, in addition to making numerous appearances to stress the importance of court administration, regularly delivered a State of the Judiciary address at ABA meetings, a practice continued by Chief Justice Rehnquist.

Within the last few years, we have seen what amounts to an outpouring of public commentary by other justices as well—including television interviews with former Chief Justice Earl Warren, Hugo Black, and Justice Potter Stewart (before and after he left the Court), and extended newspaper interviews with Justices Blackmun, Rehnquist, and Brennan. Justice Stewart's comments were general in nature and uncontroversial, indeed almost platitudinous, in their support of upholding the Constitution, although a later speech on freedom of the press was more substantive[90]; Justice Black talked of his "constitutional faith"—his doctrinal beliefs. Justice Blackmun, however, spoke openly of relations among the justices, alignments within the Court, and particularly about his relationship with the Chief Justice; Justice Rehnquist, although less open about matters of internal strategy, was not hesitant to talk about the Court's decision-making process; and Justice Brennan, in an interview with one of his law clerks, discussed his appointment to the Court, his reputation as a "playmaker" (consensus-builder), his close relationship with Chief Justice Earl Warren, Justice Douglas' independence, how a new justice is courted by other justices, and the role of a justice's religion in his decisions.[91]

Justice Blackmun appeared as a panelist on a Public Broadcasting System series on difficult choices in health care in America; while being careful not to make any statements reflecting a position on matters that might come before the Court in cases, he did discuss doctor-lawyer relationships and problems of trying medical questions in court, and expressed his confidence in American physicians. (Justice Scalia, shortly after joining the Court, *did* discuss a hypothetical case about unauthorized disclosure of government secrets, at a university panel discussion.) The bicentennial of the Constitution has produced even more public appearances by some of the justices. Justice Blackmun appeared at the end of "Superior Court," urging people to read the Constitution, and he was interviewed for a full hour by Bill Moyers as part of the PBS "In Search of the Constitution" series, as were Justices Brennan, Powell, and O'Connor.

There has even been commentary on specific Court cases. In particular, in speeches at the Second Circuit Judicial Conference, in open criticism of his colleagues, Justice Marshall applauded important Second Circuit civil liberties rulings that Marshall's Supreme Court colleagues had reversed, and Justice Stevens, at a law school dedication, criticized the Court's majority for overreaching to achieve results in civil rights and defendants' rights cases. Other justices also used speeches at universities to make important points about the judiciary. Attracting particular attention, because of its obvious political implications, was Justice Rehnquist's speech at the University of Minnesota Law School during the 1984 presidential campaign, in which he said there was nothing wrong with presidents trying to name justices who shared their views. Although he mentioned neither President Reagan nor Democratic candidate Walter Mondale, and although he noted that nominees do not always act as predicted, the speech produced criticism—from the liberals, predictably—for intruding the Court into partisan politics.

We cannot be sure what explains the recent increase in justices' speaking out, not merely to other judges, but to bar associations and the broader public. One suggestive explanation for the recent outpouring is that *The Brethren*, with its revelations of the justices as "real, live" people, engaging not only in bargaining but also in bickering—instead of causing them to put on the "false face" of congeniality—may have actually lowered the barriers to communicating what "actually" goes on in the Court. Thus, despite the considerable initial unhappiness at the exposure the volume produced, the justices may have felt less restraint in addressing the realities of the situation.[92] An earlier examination found that, despite the end-of-nineteenth century outpouring of commentary by judges, there seemed to be no relation between the level of off-Court commentary and either the Court's prestige, the policy direction of its decisions, or the judges' own liberal or conservative tendencies.[93] However, the content of the recent spate of remarks is clearly tied to the speaker's ideology. Justices have, without doubt, had strong feelings in the past but have nonetheless muzzled them, and we can expect that restraint still has an important effect.

Notes

1. The argument is that of S. Sidney Ulmer and John Alan Stookey, "How Is the Ox Being Gored: Toward a Theory of Docket Style and Innovation in the U.S. Supreme Court," *University of Toledo Law Review* 7 (Fall 1975):1–28.

2. See Thomas B. Marvell, *Appellate Courts and Lawyers: Information Gathering in the Adversary System* (Westport, Conn.: Greenwood Press, 1978), pp. 106–16.

3. Quoted by Cannon and O'Brien, *Views from the Court*, p. xiv.

4. The phrase was suggested to me by William Haltom.

5. *Marsh v. Chambers*, 463 U.S. 783 at 815 (1983) (Brennan).

6. Justice Powell, in the *Bakke* case, 438 U.S. 265 at 299 (1978), quoting Cox, *The Role of the Supreme Court in American Government* (1976), p. 114.

7. Alexander Bickel, *The Least Dangerous Branch* (Indianapolis: Bobbs-Merrill, 1962), p. 58.

8. Herbert Wechsler, "Toward Neutral Principles of Constitutional Law," *Harvard Law Review* 73 (November 1959): 19, 11.

9. *Burnet v. Coronado Oil & Gas Co.*, 285 U.S. 393 at 406 (1932) (Justice Brandeis).

10. Bickel, *The Least Dangerous Branch*, p. 59. See also Bickel, "The Supreme Court's 1960 Term, Foreword: The Passive Virtues," *Harvard Law Review* 75 (November 1961): 40–79.

11. *Vasquez v. Hillery*, 106 S.Ct. 616 at 624–5 (1986) (Marshall).

12. *Thomas v. Washington Gas Light Co.*, 448 U.S. 261 at 273 (1980) (Justice Stevens); *Thornburgh v. American College of Obstetricians*, 106 S.Ct. 2169 at 2189 (Stevens).

13. Walter F. Murphy, *Elements of Judicial Strategy* (Chicago: University of Chicago Press, 1964), p. 204.

14. *Vasquez v. Hillery*, 106 S.Ct. at 626.

15. *Thornburgh*, 106 S.Ct. at 2193.

16. The first part of Justice Blackmun's opinion contains a history of baseball, "Casey at the Bat," and a list of Blackmun's favorite players, from which he may have omitted at least one. See Woodward and Armstrong, *The Brethren*, pp. 189–92. The second part of the opinion begins with Flood's batting and fielding averages. At the end of the opinion, there is the following notation: "The Chief Justice and Mr. Justice White join in the judgment of the Court, and in all but Part I of the Court's opinion." Did they have no sense of humor? Don't they like baseball (White played professional football)? Or did they have a different "All-Star Team"?

17. *City of Oklahoma v. Tuttle*, 105 S.Ct. 2427 at 2434 n. 5.

18. The three cases are *Food Employees v. Logan Valley Plaza*, 395 U.S. 575 (1968); *Lloyd Corp. v. Tanner*, 407 U.S. 551 (1972); and *Hudgens v. National Labor Relations Board*, 424 U.S. 507 (1976). See also *Solem v. Helm*, 463 U.S. 277 at 312 (1983) (Burger), on the Court's ignoring *Rummel v. Estelle*, 445 U.S. 263 (1980) (life sentences for repeat offenses). See also *Press Enterprise Co. v. Superior Court of California*, 106 S.Ct. 2735 at 2752 (1986) (Stevens), overturning part of *Gannett v. DePasquale*, 443 U.S. 368 (1979) (open pretrial hearings).

19. Phillip J. Cooper, "Due Process, the Burger Court, and Public Administration," *Southern Review of Public Administration* 6 (1982): 78, 79.

20. *Florida Department of Health v. Florida Nursing Home*, 450 U.S. 147 at 154 (1981).

21. *Bellotti v. Baird*, 443 U.S. 622 at 652–53 (1979). The earlier case was *Planned Parenthood of Central Missouri v. Danforth*, 428 U.S. 52 (1976).

22. *Wallace v. Jaffree*, 105 S.Ct. 2479 at 2508 (1985).

23. *United States v. Scott*, 437 U.S. 82 (1978), overruling *United States v. Jenkins*, 420 U.S. 358 (1975); *Burks v. United States*, 437 U.S. 1 at 12 (1978).

24. *Illinois v. Gates*, 462 U.S. 213 (1983), overruling *Aguilar v. Texas*, 378 U.S. 108 (1964), and *Spinelli v. United States*, 393 U.S. 410 (1969).

25. David J. Danelski, "Causes and Consequences of Conflict and Its Resolution in the Supreme Court," *Judicial Conflict and Consensus*, eds. Goldman and Lamb, p. 38.

26. Robert Harrison, "The Breakup of the Roosevelt Supreme Court," *Law and History Review* 2 (Fall 1984): 215.

27. Martin Shapiro, "Stability and Change in Judicial Decision-Making: Incrementalism or Stare Decisis?" *Law in Transition Quarterly* 2 (Summer 1965): 155.

28. Fred Graham, *The Self-Inflicted Wound* (New York: Macmillan, 1970), p. 171.

29. *Rice v. Sioux City Memorial Cemetery*, 349 U.S. 71 (1955): *Jackson v. Alabama*, 348 U.S. 888 (1954); Anthony D'Amato and Robert O'Neil, *The Judiciary and Vietnam* (New York: St. Martin's Press, 1972). Full discussion of this point and most of the argument in this section can be found in Stephen L. Wasby, Anthony A. D'Amato, and Rosemary Metrailer, *Desegregation from Brown to Alexander: An Exploration of Supreme Court Strategies* (Carbondale, Ill.: Southern Illinois University Press, 1977).

30. Murphy, *Elements of Judicial Strategy*, p. 193. Murphy's discussion of strategy remains the best available.

31. *Ratchford v. Gay Lib*, 434 U.S. 1080 at 1081 (1978).

32. S. Sidney Ulmer, "Earl Warren and the Brown Decision," *Journal of Politics* 33 (August 1971): 697.

33. Alpheus Thomas Mason, *Harlan Fiske Stone: Pillar of the Law* (New York: Viking Press, 1956), pp. 614–15; Chief Justice Burger, 409 U.S. xxviii (1972).

34. *Committee for Public Education v. Regan*, 444 U.S. 646 at 665 (1980).

35. *Elkins v. United States*, 364 U.S. 206 (1960) (search); *Gregg v. Georgia*, 428 U.S. 153 at 180 (1976) and *Woodson v. North Carolina*, 428 U.S. 280 at 299 (1976) (death penalty); *Linkletter v. Walker*, 381 U.S. 618 (1965) (*Mapp* retroactivity).

36. See *Arizona Governing Committee v. Norris*, 463 U.S. 1073 at 1106–1107 (1983).

37. G. Gregory Fahlund, "Retroactivity and the Warren Court: The Strategy of a Revolution," *Journal of Politics* 35 (August 1973): 570–93.

38. Gregory A. Caldeira, "The United States Supreme Court and Criminal Cases, 1935–1976: Alternative Models of Agenda Building," *British Journal of Political Science* 2 (1981): 461; in italics in original.

39. The case was *Bell v. Maryland*, 378 U.S. 226 (1964), on the constitutionality of the sit-ins. Justice Clark circulated an opinion reaching the merits and reversing the convictions of those who had participated in the sit-in, but his real intent was to obtain a majority for Justice Brennan's opinion avoiding the merits (because Congress was considering "public accommodations" legislation). The strategic action was successful. See Schwartz, *Super Chief*, pp. 522–24. Recently, discussing the sit-in cases, Justice Brennan said, "We decided to wait and see what Congress would do." Bill Moyers, Interview with Justice Brennan, "In Search of the Constitution," PBS series, May 19, 1987.

40. See Dennis J. Hutchinson, "Unanimity and Desegregation: Decision-making in the Supreme Court, 1948–1958," *Georgetown Law Journal* 68 (October 1979): 87.

41. H. W. Perry, Jr., "Agenda-Setting in the U.S. Supreme Court," paper presented to Midwest Political Science Association, 1985, p. 23 n. 10.

42. See *MacDonald, Sommer & Frates v. Yolo County*, 106 S.Ct. 2561 (1986); *Williamson Planning Commission v. Hamilton Bank*, 105 S.Ct. 3108 (1985); *San Diego Gas & Electric Co. v. San Diego*, 450 U.S. 621 (1981); *Agins v. Tiburon*, 447 U.S. 255 (1980).

43. For an example, see *Batson v. Kentucky*, 106 S.Ct. 1712 (1986) (prosecutors' use of peremptory challenges to eliminate racial minorities), and Chief Justice Burger's complaint, at 1732–33.

44. *Piper Aircraft v. Reyno*, 454 U.S. 235 at 246 n. 12 (1981) (Justice Marshall).

45. S. Sidney Ulmer, "Issue Fluidity in the U.S. Supreme Court: A Conceptual Analysis," in *Supreme Court Activism and Restraint*, eds. Stephen C. Halpern and Charles M. Lamb, (Lexington, Mass.: Lexington Books, 1982). p. 322.

46. J. Woodford Howard, "The Fluidity of Judicial Choice," *American Political Science Review* 62 (March 1968): 49–50.

47. Murphy, *Elements of Judicial Strategy*, pp. 4–5.

48. See Note, "State Court Evasion of United States Supreme Court Mandates," *Yale Law Journal* 36 (1947): 574–83, and Jerry K. Beatty, "State Court Evasion of United States Supreme Court Mandates During the Last Decade of the Warren Court," *Valparaiso University Law Review* 6 (Spring 1972): 260–85.

49. For an extended treatment, see Howard Dean, *Judicial Review and Democracy* (New York: Random House, 1966).

50. For example, see the regulation of insurance: *United States v. South-Eastern Underwriters Association*, 322 U.S. 533 (1944) (interstate insurance a form of commerce); the passage of the McCarran-Ferguson Act confirming state authority to regulate insurance; and *Prudential Insurance Co. v. Benjamin*, 328 U.S. 408 (1946), sustaining the act.

51. Reversing, respectively, *Chisholm v. Georgia*, 2 Dall. 419 (1793); *Pollack v. Farmers Loan & Trust Co.*, 157 U.S. 429 (1895); *Oregon v. Mitchell*, 400 U.S. 112 (1970); and *Dred Scott v. Sanford*, 19 How. 393 (1857).

52. *Plyler v. Doe*, 457 U.S. 202 at 253 (1982).

53. *Hunter v. Erickson*, 393 U.S. 385 (1969) (housing ordinances); *Washington v. Seattle School District No. 1*, 458 U.S. 457 (1982) (busing).

54. John Hart Ely, *Democracy and Distrust: A Theory of Judicial Review* (Cambridge, Mass.: Harvard University Press, 1980), p. 181.

55. Ibid., pp. 77, 100–101, 117.

56. Jesse Choper, *Judicial Review and the National Political Process* (Chicago: University of Chicago Press, 1980), p. 68.

57. William J. Brennan, Jr., "The Constitution of the United States: Contemporary Ratification," speech at Georgetown University, October 12, 1985, pp. 4–5.

58. Quoted in *Washington Post*, November 16, 1985, p. A2 (speech of November 15).

59. John C. Schmidhauser, *The Supreme Court as Final Arbiter in Federal-State Relations, 1789–1957* (Chapel Hill, N.C.: University of North Carolina Press, 1958).

60. *Apodaca v. Oregon*, 406 U.S. 404 (1972), and *Johnson v. Louisiana*, 406 U.S. 356 (1972).

61. Harold J. Spaeth and Stuart H. Teger, "Activism and Restraint: A Cloak for Judicial Policy Preferences," in *Supreme Court Activism and Restraint*, eds. Halpern and Lamb, pp. 283, 296; data at pp. 288–94.

62. Charles M. Lamb, "Judicial Restraint on the Supreme Court," ibid., pp. 9, 12.

63. J. Clifford Wallace, "The Jurisprudence of Judicial Restraint: A Return to the Moorings," *George Washington Law Review* 50 (1981): 6.

64. *Plyler v. Doe*, 457 U.S. at 243.

65. *Federal Bureau of Investigation v. Abramson*, 456 U.S. 615 at 644 (1982) (O'Connor, dissenting).

66. *United States v. Locke*, 105 S.Ct. 1785 at 1793 (1985).

67. Russell W. Galloway, Jr., "The Taft Court (1921–29)," *Santa Clara Law Review* 25 (Winter 1985): 1.

68. For a recent discussion and application of these rules, see *United States v. Locke*, 105 S.Ct. 1785 (1985).

69. *United States v. Butler*, 297 U.S. 1 at 79 (1936).

70. *United States v. Leon*, 468 U.S. 897 at 962 (1984).

71. *Lowe v. Securities and Exchange Commission*, 105 S.Ct. 2557 at 2574–75 (1985).

72. James Simon, *In His Own Image: The Supreme Court in Richard Nixon's America* (New York: David McKay, 1973), p. 227.

73. *Rummel v. Estelle*, 445 U.S. 263 at 275, 276 (1980). However, three years later the Court overturned a life sentence without the possibility of parole for a multiple offense. *Solem v. Helm*, 463 U.S. 277 (1983).

74. *Jones v. North Carolina Prisoners' Labor Union*, 433 U.S. 119 at 125 (1977); *Bell v. Wolfish*, 441 U.S. 520 at 548 (1979), citing *Jones*; *Youngberg v. Romeo*, 457 U.S. 307 at 323 (1982).

75. Blasi, "The Rootless Activism of the Burger Court," in *The Burger Court*, pp. 198–99.

76. Spaeth and Teger, "Activism and Restraint," p. 296.

77. Joel B. Grossman, "Role-Playing and the Analysis of Judicial Behavior: The Case of Mr. Justice Frankfurter," *Journal of Public Law* 11 (1962): 285–309. See also Harold J. Spaeth, "The Judicial Restraint of Mr. Justice Frankfurter—Myth or Reality," *Midwest Journal of Political Science* 8 (February 1964): 22–38, and Harold J. Spaeth and Michael F. Altfeld, "Felix Frankfurter, Judicial Activism, and Voting Conflict on the Warren Court," *Judicial Conflict and Consensus*, eds. Goldman and Lamb, pp. 86–114, particularly pp. 93, 95.

78. Stephen C. Halpern, "On the Imperial Judiciary and Comparative Institutional Development and Power in America," in *Supreme Court Activism and Restraint*, eds. Halpern and Lamb, p. 225.

79. Bruce Allen Murphy, *The Brandeis/Frankfurter Connection: The Secret Political Activities of Two Supreme Court Justices* (New York: Oxford University Press, 1982), p. 7; Fish, "The Office of Chief Justice," p. 112.

80. Murphy, *The Brandeis/Frankfurter Connection*, p. 352.

81. "Preface," *Views from the Bench*, eds. Cannon and O'Brien, p. xv.

82. Murphy, *The Brandeis/Frankfurter Connection*, p. 10. This is one of several instances in which serious criticism has been raised about Murphy's use of source material and interpretations and inferences drawn from those materials; another is the question of judicial impropriety by Brandeis, discussed below. Murphy's account should thus be approached with caution. See, for example, Robert Cover, "The Framing of Justice Brandeis," *The New Republic*, May 5, 1982: 17–21, and David J. Danelski, Review, *Harvard Law Review* 96 (November 1982): 312–30.

83. Murphy, *The Brandeis/Frankfurter Connection*, p. 43.

84. Ibid., p. 55.

85. Philip Elman, "The Solicitor General's Office, Justice Frankfurter, and Civil Rights Litigation, 1946–60: An Oral History," *Harvard Law Review* 100 (February 1987): 817–52.

86. Murphy, *The Brandeis/Frankfurter Connection*, p. 253.

87. Russell Wheeler, "Extra-Judicial Activities of the Early Supreme Court," *Supreme Court Review 1973*, ed. Phillip Kurland (Chicago: University of Chicago Press, 1973), pp. 122–58.

88. *In Re Scaduto*, 763 F.2d 1191 (11th Cir. 1985); *In Re President's Commission on Organized Crime, Subpoena of Scarfo*, 783 F.2d 370 (3rd Cir. 1986).

89. Stephen S. Trott, "Implementing Criminal Justice Reform," *Public Administration Review* 45 (Special 1985): 798.

90. Potter Stewart, "Or of the Press," *Hastings Law Journal* 26 (1975): 631–37.

91. John A. Jenkins, "A Candid Talk with Justice Blackmun," *New York Times Magazine*, February 20, 1983, pp. 20–24 ff.; John Jenkins, "The Partisan: A Talk with Justice Rehnquist," *New York Times Magazine*, March 3, 1985, pp. 28–33 ff.; Jeffrey T. Leeds, "A Life on the Court," *New York Times Magazine*, October 5, 1986, pp. 24–27, 74–79.

92. See Ronald J. Fiscus, "Studying *The Brethren*: The Legal-Realist Bias of Investigative Journalism," *American Bar Foundation Research Journal* 1984 (Spring): 487–503.

93. Alan F. Westin, "Out-of-Court Commentary by United States Supreme Court Justices, 1789–1962: Of Free Speech and Judicial Lockjaw," in *An Autobiography of the Supreme Court: Off-the-Bench Commentary by the Justices* (New York: Macmillan, 1963), pp. 28–29.

9 The Supreme Court and the Other Branches

As our examination of judicial review should make clear, one of the Supreme Court's major tasks is to rule on issues concerning the separation of powers between legislative, executive, and judicial branches. Indeed, the Court has done so in some important cases, and, in other instances, it has been content to let lower court rulings on the subject stand. Increasingly, the courts are being called upon to resolve conflicts between Congress—or at least certain members of Congress, who have brought suits challenging executive action (or inaction)—and the president and his subordinates. Judicial review is, however, not the only situation in which the Supreme Court (and the remainder of the federal judiciary) interact and conflict with Congress and the executive. Judicial rulings interpreting statutes or administrative regulations are far more frequent, and there has also been friction, even conflict, over those rulings. It is the interaction between the judiciary and other branches of government, including the other branches' response to the courts' actions, that we examine in this chapter. That examination should help us understand to what extent the Supreme Court is an independent force within our governmental system or a dependent institution.

After examining the branches' interaction over operation of the judiciary, we turn to the Supreme Court's overall treatment of congressional actions, followed by an analysis of Congress' responses to those decisions and to other rulings by the Court with which it disagreed. We then turn to the Supreme Court's rulings on the presidency, with particular attention to how the Court has dealt with the war power and foreign policy and to the substantial litigation involving the Nixon administration. The chapter ends with a discussion of judicial rulings on regulatory agency decisions.

The Court and Congress

Apart from judicial rulings on legislation, judges and legislators are in frequent contact over matters of judicial administration. For the most part, those contacts are institutionalized, with the judiciary approaching Congress through the Judicial Conference of the United States (see pages 68-69). Matters at issue include the number of judgeships and administrative support positions, judges' salaries, the courts' jurisdiction, and rules of procedure and evidence—the last generally promulgated by the judiciary under the Rules Enabling Act (see page 75). Lobbying by judges will be quite evident over major legislation affecting the court system, as in the Judges Bill that gave the Supreme Court its discretionary jurisdiction, changes in the bankruptcy courts (see pages 51-53), and the present proposals for a National Court of Appeals (see pages 62-63). There are also judge-legislator contacts about substantive legislation, but such contacts are likely to be informal because of the general judicial position that judges should not get directly involved with the legislature in making the law. Despite existing contacts, communication between members of the two branches is sporadic and imperfect, and members of each feel misunderstood by the other—which has led to some conferences in which judges and legislators have tried to bridge the gap outside the context of discussing particular proposals.

Court Budget

A crucial part of judicial-legislative interaction concerns the judiciary's budget. Because the judicial budget is a very small part of the total federal budget, it is not likely to command legislators' attention, however important—even crucial—it is for the judges. Prior to the 1939 creation of the Administrative Office of the Courts, the judiciary's budget requests were handled by the Department of Justice, but now, while the judicial budget is included in the budget the president sends to Congress, only the courts really deal with the Congress over budget matters because the Office of Management and Budget in the executive branch is prohibited by law from changing the Judicial Conference's recommendations.[1] Indeed, "separation from the Executive Branch has certainly been achieved," creating judicial independence in budget matters. However, despite the Judicial Conference's role, "the process once dominated by civil servants in the Executive Branch has come to be dominated by civil servants in the Third Branch," specifically the personnel of the Administrative Office.[2]

Interaction between judiciary and Congress on budgetary matters, like most other judicial-legislative interaction, is carried out "through well established, institutionalized channels."[3] On the judges' side, the Judicial Conference's Budget Committee is the focal body. To assist the judiciary in attaining its financial goals, the committee's members are chosen because they come from states represented on relevant congressional committees, thus facilitating contact, or because they have legislative (and particularly congressional) experience. The key congressional body is the relevant subcommittee of the Judiciary Committee, as its recommendations are generally enacted without much change. If the Judicial Conference believes the House has cut the judges' requests too deeply, it may ask the Senate to restore some of the funds.

The judiciary's budget for Fiscal Year 1987 (FY 87) was $1,192,592,000. For the FY 1969–85 period (before Gramm-Rudman), the judiciary received—after House cuts and Senate restorations—"an average annual increase of almost 16 percent." That is "a rate higher than the average annual growth in the entire federal budget," perhaps because the judiciary's requests—"an average increase of slightly more than 20 percent over the previous year's appropriations"—were "quite modest."[4]

Judicial budget totals can be explained largely in terms of the number of permanent personnel positions in the budget year, because the judiciary is a "labor-intensive" organization, and the number of cases filed in the courts, a better indicator of the judiciary's *needs*. A better predictor is a three-year lag between caseload and budget dollars, which exists for several reasons: the lapse of time between the beginning of the judiciary's budget process (well before the start of the budget year) and actual caseloads, and Congress' failure to appropriate funds immediately for requested increases, as it perhaps adopts a "wait and see" attitude (Does the increase in caseload continue?) and a related outlook of "See if it keeps up" (Does the increase trend continue?). Moreover, judgeship and staff positions created at one time may not be filled immediately and increases in salaries are not always effective immediately.[5]

Judicial Review: Congress and Its Response

Examining separation of powers between judiciary and legislature requires a look at how far courts intrude into Congress' actions, not only by invalidating statutes but also by examining matters internal to Congress. We find that the Court has:

- ruled on the qualifications of members of Congress—or at least on Congress' right to expel its members;
- defined "legislative" functions subject to protection under the Speech and Debate Clause (Art. I, Sec. 6), which provides immunity for legislators' official activities, and in so doing has constrained legislators by expanding the area of their liability;
- ruled that members of Congress may be held liable for racial discrimination in choosing staff (*Davis v. Passman*, 1979); and
- taken action to control congressional proceedings, particularly committee investigations and the exercise of the contempt power against witnesses at legislative hearings.

In recent years, rulings by the Court have also served to block some cases challenging Congress' actions or failure to act when the Court limited standing to sue (see page 171). In all those actions, the Court has been engaged in interpreting and applying provisions of the Constitution.

Thus, in setting aside Congress' refusal to seat Representative Adam Clay ton Powell—a case held not to fall under the "political question" doctrine (see page 178)—the Court ruled that the Speech and Debate Clause prevented a suit against members of Congress for their votes not to seat Powell but not against Congress' employees, thus providing a basis for the suit. In the *Gravel* case (1972), the Court said that a grand jury could not question a senator's legislative assistant about activities related to the senator's legislative work, but also said that the act of arranging to have a private company publish the Pentagon Papers was *not* legislative activity and thus the senator's assistant, and probably the senator himself, could be questioned about that subject. The *Gravel* decision and the Court's holding in *United States v. Brewster* that acceptance of a bribe—by Senator Daniel Brewster (D-Md.)—was not part of a legislator's official duties and thus could properly be the basis for an indictment not only limited the meaning of "legislative activity" but also restricted the effect of an earlier ruling that a congressman's speech on the floor of the House could not be used against him in a bribery case. Going even further, the Court then held in *Doe v. McMillan* that circulation outside Congress of a House committee report that named specific schoolchildren in connection with an investigation of the District of Columbia schools was not part of the legislative process and could be the basis for an injunction.

The Court strengthened the protections of the Speech and Debate Clause when it said in the *Helstoski* case (1979) that evidence of a representative's legislative acts could not be used in a prosecution of that representative for accepting a bribe, nor had the legislator waived the clause's protection by testifying before the grand jury and voluntarily producing legislative documents. At the same time, in a case stemming from Senator William Proxmire's "Golden Fleece Awards" for what he felt were unnecessary expenditures, the Court, further limiting what constitutes a "legislative" act, ruled in *Hutchinson v. Proxmire* (1974) that senators and their assistants were not protected from libel suits for transmitting allegedly defamatory material in press releases.

Over the years, the Court has handed down decisions affecting the scope of congressional investigations—at times supporting an expansive reading of Congress' authority, at times restricting Congress' power to punish those who have objected to or hindered investigations.[6] In dealing with legislative investigations, in one of its most important internal security rulings, *Watkins v. United States*, the Warren Court invalidated a contempt citation resulting from a witness' refusal to answer the House Un-American Activities Committee's questions because the relationship between the questions and the committee's investigation had not been made clear; in his opinion for the Court, the Chief Justice severely criticized both the committee and Congress for failing to control the committee's activities. However, after Congress had threatened to remove the Court's jurisdiction over internal security matters (see page 309), the Court seemingly backed down, in the *Barenblatt* case (1958), rejecting the claim by a witness at a congressional hearing of a First Amendment right to silence and upholding the contempt citation against him. Despite all these rulings, courts can still be hesitant to deal with internal congressional matters. Some lower courts, even when granting standing to members of Congress to challenge legislative actions, have declined to decide the cases.

Judicial Review of Statutes. Despite the impression left by the conflict between President Franklin Roosevelt and the Hughes Court, neither before that time nor after has the Court regularly struck down many congressional acts in a short period, although the total number—even before the legislative veto case (see below)—is considerable. Prior to the Civil War, decisions invalidating acts of Congress "occurred on an episodic, nonsystematic basis." Over the long run, "periods of aggressiveness toward Congress have not occurred on a very regular basis." Swings from intervention to passivity have, however, grown larger over time, in proportion to increases in the frequency of the exercise of judicial review. There has also been a "very high correlation" between invalidation of congressional acts and those of state legislatures. Interestingly, the greatest judicial activity concerning state legislation occurred not during Warren Court activity concerning civil liberties but early in the twentieth century as part of judicial resistance to state economic regulation.[7] Judicial review has also been "significantly shaped by such political considerations as the degree of party difference between Congress and the Court, the nature of the party in power in the national government, and the party affiliations of the individual judges deciding specific cases."[8] Reexamination of judicial review during periods of partisan realignment has, however, led to the findings that (1) with the New Deal period eliminated because of the extremely high rate at which the Supreme Court invalidated recent legislation, the Court was actually more likely to invalidate a law in periods of partisan stability than during partisan shift; and (2) for the 1930s and 1960s, but not in the post-Civil War and end-of-nineteenth-century realignments, invalidations of state policy contained high proportions of issues "which cut across existing lines of ideological cleavage in the major parties" and were related to political realignment, and that a high proportion of the invalidated policies were enacted by majorities of the political party opposite that controlling the Supreme Court.[9]

Just as judicial review of state legislative acts has continued past midcentury, so the Court has continued since 1937, particularly after 1950, to invalidate a number of federal statutes. The Warren Court used prohibitions against bills of attainder (legislative punishment without trial) and cruel and unusual punishment to invalidate removal of a person's U.S. citizenship for such acts as desertion from the military or remaining abroad to avoid military service, and the Court prohibited courts-martial of civilians in a number of circumstances as well as of service personnel for offenses not service-connected.[10] Restrictions on the rights of Communist Party members were also struck down. The Fifth Amendment was used to void registration provisions that forced people to incriminate themselves under other federal laws or state law.[11] Social Security Act durational residence requirements for welfare benefits were set aside in *Shapiro v. Thompson* as an interference with the right to travel.

Burger Court acts of national judicial review, which at times occurred through summary affirmance of lower court decisions, were scattered across a wide range of policy areas. These included welfare (limits on who could receive food stamps and discrimination in benefits on the basis of gender and illegitimacy) and free speech (Post Office methods for screening obscenity, a ban on demonstrations on U.S. Capitol grounds, and a ban on displaying the flag on the grounds of the Supreme Court itself).[12] Interference with freedom of speech was also the basis, in *Buckley v. Valeo* (1976), for voiding Federal Election Campaign Act limits on individuals' expenditures on behalf of candidates of their choice. In the first instance since FDR's 1937 battle with the Court that regulatory legislation based on the Commerce Clause had been struck down, in *National League of Cities v. Usery* (1976) the justices invalidated the extension of the minimum wage law to state and local government employees, but the Court reversed its position in 1985. As we have seen, the Court also struck down the 1978 bankruptcy statute, leading to a difficult time for both Congress and the courts before new legislation was passed (see pages 51-53).

One of the most sweeping instances of judicial review of legislative action in the Court's history came in 1983, when the Court invalidated the *legislative veto*, a major point of friction between president and Congress, and thus affected both the trend toward increased presidential power and the countertrend of increased assertion of congressional authority. Under legislative veto provisions, enacted as part of over 200 statutes, executive branch actions can be rejected by a resolution of one house of Congress (the "one-house veto") or by a concurrent resolution passed by both Senate and House of Representatives. The president had accepted legislative veto provisions by approving statutes containing them, but those provisions were said to allow Congress to take legislative action not subject to presidential veto. Some of the provisions limited the president's authority to use American troops overseas (War Powers Act of 1973), reorganize the executive branch, or defer expenditure of funds appropriated by Congress (Budget and Impoundment Act of 1974). Many concerned foreign policy matters such as foreign trade, international development, and export of defense technology; others allowed Congress to reject regulations promulgated by agencies such as the Federal Trade Commission or the Department of Education.

In general, availability of the legislative veto allowed Congress to give the president broad authority while retaining controls over exercise of that authority. In 1983, however, the Supreme Court, in *Immigration and Naturalization Service v. Chadha*, ruled that legislative vetos of whatever type violate the separation of powers doctrine and the Constitution's specific provisions concerning enactment of legislation, including *presentment* (presentation to the president) and *bicameralism* (both houses must consider legislation).

The Court's ruling appeared clear, with even dissenting Justice White saying it applied to two-house as well as one-house legislative vetoes. However, there was confusion in Congress as it tried to move toward alternatives such as joint resolutions of approval or disapproval (which require the president's signature). Congress continued to pass bills containing legislative veto provisions, doing so 53 times in the 16 months after the ruling. It did so not out of spite or resistance but because it didn't know what to do; despite some complaints, the president signed the bills. Even where Congress did not include a formal legislative veto requirement, it continued arrangements for "reprogramming" of funds or inserted provisions equivalent to the legislative veto, like requiring agencies to notify congressional committees before taking action or including riders in appropriations bills (which the president can't delete from the bill before signing).[13] All this indicated the conflict between the realities of separation of powers in the everyday working relations of Congress and the president and the Court's formal view of the separation of powers.

This conflict was again evident when the Court invalidated the Balanced Budget and Emergency Deficit Control (Gramm-Rudman-Hollings) Act of 1985, Congress' effort to deal with rising budget deficits by setting targets and providing that, if Congress did not meet those targets, automatic budget cuts would go into effect based on a determination by the Comptroller General of the United States on advice of the Congressional Budget Office (CBO) and Office of Management and Budget (OMB). In an example of members of Congress challenging their colleagues' handiwork, several of them—and a union of government employees—challenged the Act. The Supreme Court ruled by a 7-2 vote in *Bowsher v. Synar* (1986) that execution of the laws could not be placed in the hands of someone responsible to Congress, like the Comptroller General, removable on passage of a joint resolution of Congress and "consistently viewed" by Congress "as an officer of the Legislative Branch." Congressional reaction to the ruling included consideration of placing authority for the automatic budget reduction determination in the hands of the Director of OMB (an executive official) but in the short run Congress did nothing to replace the invalidated provision. Instead, it returned to wrestling directly—and generally unsuccessfully—with budget deficits. The Gramm-Rudman target figures are, however, still in place and serve to push members of Congress toward expenditure reductions.

Despite the difficulties that the legislative veto and Gramm-Rudman ruling created for Congress, most of the Court's decisions affecting Congress involve statutory interpretation—"supplementary lawmaking" as the courts interpret, apply, and flesh out statutes—with the Court emphasizing different modes of statutory interpretation in different policy areas, depending on the number, specificity, and complexity of statutes in the policy area.[14] Statutory interpretation is judicial policymaking although not as explicit as when the Court rules in constitutional cases. Statutory interpretation is not easy work because the least clear statutes are more likely to be litigated, and justices do not agree as to how to interpret statutes. They talk of turning first to a statute's "plain meaning" but must often resort to unclear legislative materials (or *legislative history*) in a search for Congress' intent.

In the course of statutory interpretation, the Court may explicitly suggest what Congress must do to make a statute valid. Overturning a law regulating grain futures transactions, Justice Taft said that Congress could not regulate the transactions unless it saw them as directly interfering with interstate commerce. Congress then placed such an explicit declaration in the Grain Futures Act, which the Court upheld. Even more indicative of the Court's influence are statutes into which Congress has written language the Court has already approved. In enacting the surveillance provisions of the Omnibus Crime Control and Safe Streets Act of 1968, Congress used procedures for wiretapping under a warrant spelled out by the Court in *Berger v. New York*. Similarly, when the Court ruled in *McCarty v. McCarty* (1982) that property settlements in divorces could not include military pensions, but said that Congress could provide otherwise if former spouses were to receive more protection, both houses of Congress took the Court up on the invitation.

At other times, the Court engages in the "trap pass," interpreting a statute so rigidly that the statute looks ridiculous, in the hope that Congress will be provoked to change the law.[15] An example is *Tennessee Valley Authority v. Hill*, a ruling that under environmental protection law, a major dam, largely constructed but still incomplete, would have to be stopped to protect the snail darter fish. Congress then both specifically provided for completion of the dam *and* altered the statute to provide procedural flexibility—probably exactly what the Court had in mind. Of course, not all clear statements by the Court are "trap passes." Many are simply a result of the justices carrying out their function of giving particularity to general statutory provisions.

Congressional Response. What has Congress' response been to judicial review and statutory interpretation? "Supreme Court abrogations of majority-sponsored activities have been the primary source of retaliation, real and seriously threatened, by the national political branches . . . against the federal judiciary."[16] However, as time has passed, there have been fewer broad-gauge congressional attacks on the Court. Action has usually been directed at particular rulings or sets of rulings. Even the efforts of the early 1980s to restrict federal courts' or the Supreme Court's jurisdiction stemmed primarily from the Court's "social issue" rulings—on school prayer, school desegregation, and abortion. In general, conflict between Congress and Court has been more likely to arise on matters where "constitutional language is unclear and . . . on which public sentiment has been largely unsettled"; where interest groups see vital interests at stake; and where the Court has threatened Congress' authority.[17] Action reversing the Court has, at least until the present, occurred more frequently in the economic sphere than in the civil liberties domain, undoubtedly a reflection of the focus of the Court's caseload. Economic regulation issues were involved in four of seven periods (excluding the present one) in which proposals to curb the Court were frequent, but civil liberties issues were involved in only two such periods. Moreover, the presence of intensely held economic or civil libertarian interests meant less success for Court-curbing than occurred in the areas of separation of powers or federalism, where Congress could take into account policy factors outside the Court's concern.[18]

There have also been important reversals with respect to issues of federal-state relations, although they tend to be quite case-specific. Congress acted to reverse the Court's ruling that the offshore oil lands belonged to the national government, passing "quitclaim" legislation giving the lands to the states,[19] and Congress kept state regulation of insurance in force when the Court held in the *South-Eastern Underwriters* case that insurance was part of interstate commerce and thus subject to national regulation. In both instances, the Court then sustained Congress' reversal action, explicitly acknowledging Congress' intent to overturn the Court's initial decisions. At times Congress has also allowed the states to act after the Court has said the federal government had "preempted" an area and prevented state regulation. For example, when the Court said a state could not regulate interstate labor disputes even in the absence of National Labor Relations Board action, Congress rewrote the law to allow such state activity.[20]

Negative congressional reaction to the Court's rulings has taken a wide variety of forms: criticism, attempts to overrule the Court by amending the Constitution or by limiting the Court's appellate jurisdiction, and refusal to provide compensation required by the Court's rulings. The latter occurred in the Yazoo land fraud case (*Fletcher v. Peck*) and much more recently after the Court had struck down, as a bill of attainder, an appropriations bill rider stipulating that three alleged subversives not be paid (*United States v. Lovett*, 1946). In addition, there have been proposals for such basic structural change as requiring that federal or state laws could be declared invalid only by a vote of at least seven justices, allowing Congress to override declarations that a federal or state law was constitutionally invalid, or limiting justices' tenure. Negative reaction is also evident in reluctance or refusal to provide additional judges for the federal courts or to increase the justices' salaries, in attempts to impeach justices—as in the unsuccessful effort to remove Justice Douglas—and in resistance to confirming presidential nominees to the Court.

The Eleventh, Sixteenth, and Twenty-sixth Amendments, as well as the post-Civil War amendments on slavery and the status of blacks—all initiated by Congress—were passed to override Court decisions. After the Court limited Congress' power to regulate the use of child labor either through the power over interstate commerce (*Hammer v. Dagenhart*, 1918) or taxation (*Bailey v. Drexel Furniture*, 1922), Congress submitted for ratification a constitutional amendment prohibiting child labor. The Court's post-1937 shift, which included upholding the Fair Labor Standards (minimum wage) Act with its child labor provisions in *United States v. Darby* (1941), eliminated the need for the amendment, still open to ratification because it contains no termination date (unlike later amendments, including the ERA).

Many more such efforts have also failed. These include attempts in the 1960s to overturn reapportionment and school prayer rulings, the latter effort renewed after 1980 in the drive to allow "voluntary" prayer in the schools. Continuous activity to limit school desegregation through constitutional amendment is part of a larger set of legislative efforts aimed at achieving that goal, including limits on federal judges' power to order busing and prohibitions on executive branch initiation of desegregation. Similarly, extensive effort to repeal the Court's 1973 abortion ruling through constitutional amendment—such as defining when life begins and turning over abortion policy to the states—is only one aspect of legislative action aimed at limiting abortions, perhaps the best known of which is the Hyde Amendment—a ban on Medicaid payments for abortions except in very limited circumstances, upheld by the Court itself in *Harris v. McRae*.

Attempts to limit the Court's jurisdiction have been less successful than efforts to overturn rulings by amending the Constitution. Only once has Congress successfully removed some of the Court's appellate jurisdiction. In the aftermath of the Civil War, the Reconstruction Congress, at odds with President Andrew Johnson and fearful of the Court's potential action concerning questionable detentions of citizens, passed a law removing the Court's jurisdiction over cases arising under the Habeas Corpus Act. The Court complied, in *Ex parte McCardle*, dismissing a case already argued. However, the Court examined congressional action before complying, and its compliance did not foreclose other Court actions to protect the individual. Moreover, when Congress removed the Court's jurisdiction in claims cases involving proof of former Confederate soldiers' present loyalty—ordering the Court to treat acceptance of a presidential pardon as proof of aid to the Confederacy but to ignore the pardon in determining loyalty—the Court struck down the limitation in *United States v. Klein* (1872). That case is said to stand for the proposition that Congress may not withdraw jurisdiction when the intent is to dictate a specific result, as some current congressional efforts are thought to do.

There is little question about Congress' power to withdraw jurisdiction over the lower federal courts, which Congress established, and the Supreme Court has sustained limited withdrawals of such jurisdiction, for example, upholding withdrawal of the power to issue injunctions in labor disputes (the Norris-LaGuardia Act) and approving Emergency Price Control Act procedures under which review of the Price Administrator's actions was routed through the Emergency Court of Appeals, which was deprived of the power to grant injunctions.[21] Removal of *all* federal court jurisdiction, however, like removal of the Supreme Court's appellate jurisdiction, leaves no final authority to resolve disputes over the affected subjects. It thus leaves standing divergent interpretations of constitutional provisions by the lower courts, either state (if all federal jurisdiction is removed) or both federal and state (if only Supreme Court appellate jurisdiction is withdrawn), without a judicial body to reconcile them. No definitive answer is now available to the question of whether such removal of authority, regardless of the subject matter or the effect of such action, is constitutional, and *McCardle*, the most relevant case, does not provide such an answer.

The late 1950s saw a serious attempt by Congress to restrict the Court's jurisdiction. Bills were introduced aimed at the Court's rulings on internal security matters such as legislative investigations, the executive's loyalty-security programs, state control of teachers and admission of lawyers to the practice of law, and federal preemption of state internal subversion legislation. None of these bills passed, although the Senate vote was very close (a one-vote margin) and the Court appeared to retreat in the face of the attack.[22]

Ronald Reagan's election as president and the Republicans obtaining control of the Senate in 1980 led to another substantial attack on the Court's appellate jurisdiction and on all federal court jurisdiction over subjects like school busing, school prayer, and abortion by those who thought state courts would be more favorable to their position. That effort was somewhat undercut when President Reagan's own attorney general, although approving limits on judicial power that would limit only particular federal judicial remedies, argued that Congress could not limit the Court's jurisdiction when the effect is to "intrude upon the core functions of the Supreme Court as an independent and equal branch in our system of separation of powers."

Perhaps because of the lack of consensus about Congress' authority in this area, the legislation has been attacked by many, including legal scholars, the American Bar Association, and even some who strongly oppose the rulings at which the legislation is aimed, as violating the Constitution's spirit and as unwise. For one thing, eliminating Supreme Court review would be short-sighted because it would leave disliked rulings in place and would eliminate the possibility that the Court itself, perhaps with new appointees, would modify or overrule its "errors," as the Reagan administration tried to accomplish with the abortion decision.[23] The Conference of State Chief Justices has also complained that the efforts insult state judges because it is assumed that, free of Supreme Court review, they would not honor the Constitution as the Supremacy Clause requires them to do. (In 1958, by contrast, the then far more conservative state chief justices criticized the Supreme Court's internal security decisions, some of which restricted state authority to deal with subversion, as activist interference with states' rights.) None of the strong efforts by congressional (and particularly Senate) conservatives in 1982 or 1983 prevailed, because of preoccupation with budget matters, the absence of strong presidential support, and the effectiveness of the liberals' filibusters.

Congressional efforts to rewrite or reenact statutes, although affecting only a small proportion of the Court's rulings, have been far more frequent, and far more successful, than efforts either to amend the Constitution or to limit the Court's jurisdiction.[24] Between 1944 and 1960, the Court's actions were revised 50 times. Among the decisions altered were 34 instances in which the Court overturned 60 statutes.[25] Among examples of congressional action to counter action by the Court are protection, provided in the Longshoresmen's and Harbor Workers' Compensation Act (1927), for longshoremen working on vessels and on gangplanks between the vessels and piers, and antitrust immunity for efforts to control activities of nonsigners of "fair trade" agreements, provided after the 1951 *Schwegmann Brothers* ruling that there was no such immunity.

Sponsors of bills introduced in reaction to Supreme Court rulings vary in their aims. Few bills are aimed at writing the judicial decision into law, although there are such instances; for example, legislation was introduced to carry forward the effects of the Supreme Court's *Manhart* and *Norris* rulings on pension benefits for men and women by requiring that all pension and insurance premiums be calculated without respect to sex. That effort failed but a resulting bill required employer-sponsored pension and insurance plans abide by the Court's ruling about equal benefits. Congress has also supported Supreme Court doctrine by preventing the executive branch from arguing for the overturning of that doctrine in the antitrust field, imposing such a restriction in a joint resolution on emergency spending.[26]

Some bills supplement or clarify the Court's rulings, but most bills are intended either to reverse or to modify. However, only a small portion of such efforts are enacted; only 13 percent of 176 bills introduced between 1950 and 1978 to react to Supreme Court decisions handed down between 1950 and 1972 were the subject of any congressional action, and less than one-third of those were enacted.[27]

At times, after the judiciary has altered the law, Congress has returned the law to its original state. Some instances come from the period in which Congress was battling the Court over the New Deal. Thus, after the Court held the 1934 version of the Railroad Retirement Act unconstitutional as a taking of property in violation of the Fifth Amendment and as exceeding Congress' Commerce Clause power,[28] Congress enacted a new version in 1935 under the power to tax and spend for the general welfare. After a district court enjoined that statute, Congress enacted still another version, the Railroad Retirement Act of 1937.

When the Supreme Court held in the *Wunderlich* case that judicial review in certain government contract cases could be based only on a fraud by a government contracting officer, Congress responded by providing that government contracts must allow an appeal by the contractor to the court of appeals. This not only reinstated the status quo ante after the Court had disturbed a "preexisting 'common understanding,'" true in other instances as well, but provided a broader basis for judicial review than had existed before the Court's action.[29]

There are, however, other occasions on which, subsequent to the Supreme Court's ruling, Congress has acted with the intent to restore an earlier situation but the result has been to leave intact the basic thrust of what the Court has done. For example, after the *Jencks* ruling that the government must make available to the defense all records used by a witness so that the witness' credibility could be tested, Congress in the Jencks Act said that only such records as a judge had determined were relevant to the witness' testimony had to be produced.

Congress takes some actions, including reenacting statutes with clarified provisions, because the legislators feel the Court has improperly interpreted the statutes. However, a changed balance of legislative power in favor of supporters of an interpretation of the law different from that initially intended can also result in enactment of new provisions. One revision of an intended statutory meaning came after the Court—perhaps as a result of lack of congressional clarity—defined "employee" in the National Labor Relations Act to exclude foremen from the act's coverage. Congress reversed that interpretation when it passed the Taft-Hartley Act. An instance of Court ruling-response-ruling-response also came in the labor field. After the Court upheld "hot cargo" agreements (that workers would not have to handle nonunion goods) voluntarily entered into by labor and management, Congress prohibited them; later, in reaction to the Court's ruling that picketing a general contractor's entire project to protest the presence of a nonunion contractor was an illegal secondary boycott, Congress created a construction industry exception to the ban.[30] The antitrust area saw a recent reversal to protect the interests of local governments. After the Supreme Court ruled that municipalities were subject to the Sherman Act,[31] Congress passed legislation exempting municipalities and their officials and private units acting under their authorization from Sherman Act damage awards.

Some reversals have occurred in the area of civil liberties and civil rights. After the Court in the *Miller* case ruled that a depositor had no Fourth Amendment interest in bank records that the government had subpoenaed, the Right to Financial Privacy Act provided for notification of subpoenas of bank records and the right to challenge them. After the Court's ruling in *Zurcher v. Stanford Daily* (1978), allowing searches of newsrooms without prior notice, Congress reversed the ruling in part by enacting the Privacy Protection Act of 1980, which limited government searches and seizures of documentary material in the possession of journalists not themselves suspected of being involved in a crime. A reversal of considerably greater effect came after the Court ruled, in *General Electric v. Gilbert* (1976), that failing to provide disability benefits to pregnant women was not discrimination based on sex. Congress, after a strong campaign by women's groups, passed the Pregnancy Discrimination Act to make clear that Title VII of the 1964 Civil Rights Act (concerning employment discrimination based on race or sex) covered that situation, and the Court recognized that Congress had sided with the *Gilbert* dissenters.[32] Another instance of Congress' reversing the Supreme Court, with the Court then upholding Congress' action, came in the voting rights area: after the Court had adopted a restrictive test for "discrimination," in renewing the Voting Rights Act Congress returned to an earlier test that was easier for plaintiffs to satisfy.[33]

These instances suggest that Congress has the last word, but even when the Court's rulings permit further legislative action, there are instances when Congress does nothing—perhaps because the forces there are so evenly balanced that no agreement can be reached on a new statute. After the Court's *Grove City College* ruling that the antidiscrimination provisions of Title IX (sex discrimination in education) applied only if a specific program received federal funds, protracted efforts to overturn the rulings failed, in part because of opponents' claims that the "overturning" bill would have subjected many more units to coverage under a variety of antidiscrimination laws. Congress' temporary failure to respond to the Court's invalidation of the new bankruptcy statute resulted from disagreement both over the proper status of bankruptcy judges and over whether further changes in the substantive provisions of bankruptcy law were needed (see pages 51-53).

Nonaction after a Court ruling can itself have consequences. For example, the *Toth* decision preventing courts-martial of ex-members of the armed services for in-service offenses did not preclude a statute allowing them to be tried in federal district court, but such a law was never enacted, allowing some of those involved in the My Lai massacre to remain beyond the government's reach because their involvement was not discovered until after they were discharged from the service. Another example was provided by *Branzburg v. Hayes*, in which the Court said that although the First Amendment directly did not provide protection for news media personnel refusing to reveal confidential sources to a grand jury, federal and state "shield laws" were permissible. Although legislation to provide such protection was introduced in Congress, none has yet been enacted (although it was in many states). Nor did Congress take action after the decision in the *Flood* case that Congress would have to act if professional baseball were to be subject to the antitrust laws, although a few representatives, perhaps hoping to force the return of baseball to Washington, D.C., did introduce bills on the subject. (Yes, sports fans, Washington once did have a team, the Senators, whose performance led to the saying, "Washington: First in War, First in Peace, and Last in the American League.") Congressional action was to become unnecessary when the baseball players themselves forced an arbitration that resolved the issue—largely in their favor. Similarly, after the Lindberg (kidnapping) Act death penalty provisions were invalidated (*United States v. Jackson*, 1968) and other federal death penalty statutes (for murder, treason, and espionage) were rendered inoperable by the 1972 *Furman* death penalty ruling, Congress did not replace them—except for a capital punishment provision in the Antihijacking Act of 1974—in large part because of the difficulty of enacting a new federal criminal code, in which the death penalty was only one element.

Congress' *reaction* to the Court should not make us forget its *use* of judicially developed doctrine. Both point to the question of whether and to what degree Congress should defer to the Court's judgment. Here it is important to remember that although attacks on the Court are not prevented, "reversal bills" have been less likely to pass when arguments about the Court's sacrosanct nature have been used frequently; broad attacks on the Court also produce more arguments that the Court should remain inviolate than do "decision-reversal" proposals. [34]

Members of Congress, in addition to using the Court's legitimacy to support their positions, may find it useful to rely on the Court to resolve difficult problems, although congressional reliance on the Court varies from one policy question to another. When an issue is particularly complex, Congress may stop when it has made a general policy statement—usually a result of legislative compromise—and thus leave it up to the justices to make policy as the Court applies the laws. Views that can be found in Congress include the "tripartite" position, whose holders feel that Congress itself should decide matters of constitutionality and think that such questions are raised seriously, and the "judicial monopoly" position, according to which questions of constitutionality should be referred to the courts for decisions by judicial experts. Those adopting the latter position, who have been more likely to think that constitutional issues are raised primarily as political maneuvers, are particularly likely to wish to refer matters to the courts when the Court has not ruled on them. [35] However, a strong argument can be made that Congress has in fact debated vigorously on constitutional issues, such as the Bank of the United States, Congress' investigative power, the war-making power, removal from office, and the legislative veto, *before* the courts ruled on them. [36] Moreover, in recent years, Congress as a whole has done more to monitor court decisions affecting itself and to provide the capacity to defend its position in court, particularly when the Department of Justice (which usually defends federal statutes and Congress' prerogatives) fails to do so or withdraws as cases approach the Supreme Court. The Senate created the Office of Senate Legal Counsel and there are several attorneys on the staff of the Clerk of the House; both have participated in major recent cases such as that on the legislative veto—when the Ninth Circuit invited Congress to submit briefs in the *Chadha* case.

The Court and the Presidency[37]

A key element of interbranch relations between president and judiciary is, of course, judicial selection. Being able to name individuals to the courts may mean having gained "access" to the judiciary, at least in the sense of having someone there who may be predisposed to one's position. Presidents wishing to have the Supreme Court adopt a particular policy agenda will find themselves at a disadvantage if vacancies do not occur—FDR's problem in the 1930s, when no vacancy occurred during his first term. (No vacancy occurred during Jimmy Carter's presidency but with less apparent effect.)

Once someone is seated on the Court, contacts with the president, probably few to nil beforehand for most justices, become even less frequent. Beyond occasional informal contacts between the president and members of the Court (and their presence at state dinners or at the State of the Union message), most interaction between the president and the Court has been indirect, occurring when the justices have ruled on executive department actions and on challenges to presidential policies after Congress has enacted them into law. The Court's decisions concerning statutes usually come only after a private citizen has challenged executive branch action, promulgation of implementing regulations, or actual or imminent enforcement of the statute or regulations. An increasing number of lawsuits against the executive branch are being brought by members of Congress, particularly over exercise of the war and appointment powers and certain agency activities. Such lawsuits lead to confrontations in which the two elected branches are the primary contestants and the Court an actively involved umpire.

The subject of this section is direct disagreement in the formal relations between Court and president. Famous confrontations between president and Court—which include President Lincoln's rejection of Chief Justice Taney's order to release a person imprisoned by Lincoln after his suspension of habeas corpus—have been few. Even President Andrew Jackson's famous statement, "Mr. Justice Marshall has made his decision; now let him enforce it," seemingly the epitome of resistance, involved not direct defiance but reluctance to assist in enforcing a Supreme Court mandate directed at the State of Georgia. Only five presidents (Jefferson, Jackson, Lincoln, Franklin Roosevelt, and Nixon) have been engaged in direct conflict with the judiciary, and the administration of only one (Nixon) was frequently involved in litigation.

The best-known conflict between Court and president, prior to President Nixon's troubles, involved Franklin Roosevelt and the Hughes Court. Roosevelt, upset (to put it mildly) about the Court's invalidation of New Deal legislation, raised the Court as an issue in the 1936 campaign, but did not indicate what he would do if the Court did not change direction. In 1937, he proposed that for every justice over the age of 70 who did not retire, an additional justice could be named. Although it was clear the president wished to use the new appointments to neutralize justices opposed to his program, he said that the change was needed in the interest of judicial efficiency, a premise undercut by Chief Justice Hughes' letter to the Senate Judiciary Committee that the Court was current in its work. Because Roosevelt, while developing the Court-packing plan with Attorney General Homer Cummings, had paid little attention to signs of potential opposition to the proposal, he was caught unprepared by the strong disapproval that arose even among his own supporters.[38] That disapproval, coupled with the Court's shift in position on major economic regulation issues and Justice Van Devanter's announcement of his retirement, led to the plan's defeat, although it can be said that FDR won his "campaign" because the Court—with new members replacing the conservative justices—sustained a wide variety of economic regulatory measures.

As a candidate, President Reagan inveighed against the Court's "abuse of power." Although there has been no direct conflict between the Supreme Court and the presidency during his administration, some of the president's policies have been rejected by the Court and the lower courts, and the administration's policy concerning enforcement of certain laws brought it regularly into conflict with the lower federal judiciary. Criticism of the Court's position continued almost unabated during the Reagan administration, even increasing in volume in the second term. Of particular note were statements from Justice Department officials. In September 1986, Assistant Attorney General for Civil Rights Bradford Reynolds attacked Justice Brennan for trying to attain "a radically egalitarian society" that was a "threat to individual liberty" and also criticized Brennan's noninterpretivist reading of the Constitution. Most administration criticism focused on specific rulings. Particularly attacked were *Miranda*, which Attorney General Meese said in 1986 should be overturned, and rulings on church-state relations, with the attorney general saying those on school and religion were "bizarre" and Secretary of Education William Bennett complaining that released-time and shared-time decisions failed to recognize the importance of Judeo-Christian values—while he gave school districts a year in which to comply. To these we can add the president's endorsement of a constitutional amendment allowing "voluntary" prayer in the public schools.

The criticism of specific opinions also took the form of the Justice Department's calling for overturning of earlier rulings. While these involve policy and not, at least explicitly, the presidency per se, the association of the president (or his administration) with the policy may be so great that they are seen as an extension of the presidency. Particularly is this so when the solicitor general files briefs directly and clearly embodying positions earlier adopted by the administration apart from the specific case, and when those briefs urge the Court to overturn precedent. When the administration so obviously "puts itself on the line" and the Court rebuffs the administration's position, the Court's ruling is properly seen as a defeat not merely for the policy but for the president.

With Reagan, this occurred particularly with respect to affirmative action and abortion. Efforts to read *Firefighters v. Stotts* (a victory for the administration position) to restrict affirmative action programs that did not involve layoffs was rejected by the Court.[39] Likewise, the Court's strong reaffirmation of *Roe v. Wade* (albeit in a 5-4 decision) in *Thornburgh v. American College of Obstetricians* (1986), after the Court had been urged by the administration to overturn *Roe*, was without doubt a defeat for the president and his aides. Indeed, the Reagan administration may have made a strategic mistake in asking that *Roe* be reconsidered in the 1985 Term instead of waiting until it might have had another vote through being able to name another justice. The Court's reaffirmation of precedent will make it that much more difficult for a later Court, whatever it may do with undecided abortion questions, to overturn *Roe* itself.

Although the Reagan administration urged the Supreme Court to overturn some of its rulings, it has not thumbed its nose at the high court. It did, however, take that action with the lower federal courts. After Congress passed the Competition in Contracting Act, authorizing the General Accounting Office (GAO) to review disputed contracts and Reagan, while expressing doubt about the constitutionality of a provision, signed the bill, the Office of Management and Budget instructed government agencies not to follow the "invalid provisions." When a federal judge ordered the Secretary of Defense and the Director of OMB to comply, Attorney General Meese argued that the administration had the constitutional authority not to obey a statute approved by Congress and signed by the President; that led to criticism of the administration position by the House Government Operations Committee—not only the majority Democrats but 13 Republicans as well.

More frequent executive-judicial conflict occurred because of the administration's policy of "nonacquiescence" in disliked judicial decisions. Here the primary battleground was Social Security disability benefits. When the administration removed large numbers of people from the disability benefit rolls, saying the disabled had the burden of proving they were still disabled, a number of courts ruled against the Department of Health and Human Services (HHS). Other agencies generally follow adverse court of appeals rulings within the same circuit, but under its "nonacquiescence" policy, HHS, while considering rulings binding as to the individual involved in the case, neither appealed defeats to the Supreme Court for a definitive ruling nor considered the lower court rulings binding. Judges blasted the department, saying its position undermined the rule of law and violated the Constitution, with one appellate judge calling it like the discredited policy of "nullification" of disliked laws. The U.S. Attorney for the Southern District of New York, a former Reagan administration Deputy Attorney General, refused to defend the government in some of its Social Security disability cases because of this position, and the House of Representatives passed a bill saying that the government must apply rulings to all beneficiaries within the circuit or appeal to the Supreme Court. Finally Congress passed a bill changing the burden of proof with respect to removing people from disability benefits, and applying the standard to those involved in class actions so the government could not "escape" with respect to those people. The Social Security Administration also changed its policy with respect to judicial rulings, giving somewhat more weight to court of appeals rulings if the agency's own rules would lead to a denial of benefits but it still was unwilling to follow judicial determinations throughout all its own processes.[40] (Another area in which the administration was not doing well in the courts began to develop in 1986, as numerous federal judges invalidated various aspects of the president's program for drug testing of government employees.)

By no means all challenges to executive branch action end in the Supreme Court, but, like the Social Security disability challenge, may be resolved before that point. Even when a case involving a challenge to executive authority is taken to the Supreme Court, there is no guarantee that the justices will accept it. For example, when President Carter's enforcement of wage-price guidelines through government procurement policy—canceling contracts or prohibiting businesses from bidding if they did not comply with the guidelines—was challenged, the Supreme Court refused to grant review after the Court of Appeals for the District of Columbia ruled there was an adequate statutory basis for his action; this case involved a presidential executive order, to which courts have generally shown deference.[41] The Court similarly denied review when members of the House of Representatives argued that the president should have submitted to both houses of Congress the Panama Canal treaty under which our control of the Canal Zone was terminated. After the appellate court ruled that treaties were a constitutionally proper way of disposing of property, the Supreme Court declined to hear the case.[42] The Court came closer to involvement in the challenge to President Carter's unilateral termination of the 1954 Mutual Defense Treaty with Taiwan. After a district judge ruled that a defense treaty could be terminated only by two-thirds of the Senate or a majority of both houses of Congress, the court of appeals promptly ruled in the president's favor. Then the Supreme Court ordered the suit dismissed (*Goldwater v. Carter*, 1979). Four justices said the case posed a "political question," while another said the question was not ripe for review. Only one justice voted to affirm the appeals court and two more would have heard argument.

Overall, presidents have fared well in the federal courts, although presidential power has been supported more in some areas than in others,[43] as we shall see in looking at specific Supreme Court decisions. Of over 400 federal court cases from 1949 through 1984, 70 percent were decided in the president's favor. The most successful president was Lyndon Johnson (92%), while Nixon was the least successful (58%). The third and fourth decades after World War II showed lower support for presidential power than the two decades immediately after the war; the decreased support was accompanied by a long-term upward trend in litigation involving presidential power—a trend that holds even if we remove litigation against the Nixon administration. Foreign affairs issues constituted the largest number of cases, with the war power next, but the foreign affairs area was the one in which the president was most successful (losing only 19 of 100 decisions). Presidential power is likely to be turned aside over issues of spending (where Nixon impoundment actions accounted for many of the cases) and of executive privilege and confidentiality. If one looks at all federal cases, trials and appellate, the judges react to "two presidencies"—one domestic, one foreign—but that distinction does not apply if only district court rulings are examined.

Appointment Power

Franklin Roosevelt's administration was the first in this century during which the Court dealt with important questions of presidential power. The Court first ruled adversely to the president on the question of his right to dismiss employees. Relying on *Myers v. United States* (1926), in which the Supreme Court, speaking through Chief Justice (and former President) William Howard Taft, had upheld the president's authority to discharge a postmaster, FDR tried to assert his authority to remove Federal Trade Commissioner William Humphrey. Upon Humphrey's refusal, FDR removed him anyhow, but the Court ruled, in *Humphrey's Executor v. United States* (1935), that Congress could limit the president's power to discharge members of regulatory commissions simply because he disagreed with them politically, as the commissioners were expected to play a quasi-judicial role requiring independence of the one who appointed them. (It was this decision that most infuriated President Roosevelt.[44])

President Eisenhower produced the same response, in *Weiner v. United States* (1958), when he removed a member of the War Claims Commission to replace him with someone of his own choosing. The Court has also ruled that, although the president cannot insist on the right to remove members of a commission, he is entitled to be involved in the appointment process when commission members have enforcement and administrative powers making them "officers of the United States." As part of its ruling in *Buckley v. Valeo* (1976), the Court therefore overturned the original method designated by Congress for selection of members of the Federal Election Commission.

Delegation of Authority

In the 1930s, Congress turned over considerable policymaking authority to those adminstering the law. The issue of whether Congress could do so without specifying standards to guide the president's actions reached the Court during Roosevelt's first term. In the *Panama Refining* case, with liberal and conservative justices agreeing, the Court overturned Congress' grant of authority to embargo shipments of oil produced in excess of state quotas ("hot oil") because Congress had not provided standards by which the president could determine when to act. "This is delegation run riot," said Justice Cardozo. The Court also ruled in the *Schechter Poultry Corporation* case that the National Industrial Recovery Act, under which "codes of fair competition" were developed by industry groups and promulgated by the president, was infected by improper delegation. Recognizing Congress' need to delegate certain tasks to the executive branch, the Court said, however, that "Congress cannot delegate legislative power to the President to exercise an unfettered discretion to make whatever laws he thinks may be needed or advisable for the rehabilitation and expansion of trade or industry." Because the NIRA was at the heart of Roosevelt's economic program, the ruling was even more important than *Panama Refining*, but as his attention had shifted to other programs by the time of the ruling, he may not have been particularly distressed by the Court's action.

At almost the same time, the Court upheld delegation without standards in the foreign affairs area in the *Curtiss-Wright Export Corporation* case, a challenge to another presidential embargo (on the sale of arms to warring Latin American countries) imposed pursuant to a congressional grant. In so doing, the Court underscored the executive's relative independence in foreign policy under the Constitution. *Curtiss-Wright* is still the law, but *Panama Refining* and *Schechter* are not; in fact, those two cases, for all their strong language, were the Court's only two invalidations of delegation of authority. The Court has repeatedly accepted delegations of authority couched in terms at least as broad/vague as those involved in *Panama*, for example, in *Yakus v. United States* approving the delegation of authority to the administrator of the Office of Price Administration (OPA), under the Emergency Price Control Act, to fix "generally fair and equitable" prices that would carry out the purposes of the law. More recently, the Supreme Court overturned lower court rulings against the president and sustained actions by Presidents Nixon and Ford increasing fees on imported oil. The statute had authorized the presidential action; standards had also been provided; and the president's actions were limited so that he could do only what was necessary to prevent damage to the national security.[45]

War Powers and Foreign Policy

Unlike its rulings on the president's appointment powers and its mid-1930s rulings on delegation of authority, the Court's decisions on the president's authority as commander-in-chief have been favorable. Judges have generally been quite unwilling to challenge the president's war-making authority, at least until after a war is over. As Rossiter observed, "Whatever limits the Court has set upon the employment of the war powers have been largely theoretical, rarely practical," and the impression left by the Court's rulings has generally been that "as in the past, so in the future, President and Congress will fight our wars with little or no thought about a reckoning with the Supreme Court."[46] Even though *Ex parte Milligan*, invalidating the practice of trying civilians at courts-martial when the civilian courts were operating, contained stern words applying the Constitution to the president (Lincoln), it came after the Civil War had ended. Moreover, in *The Prize Cases*, involving the blockade of the South, the Court sustained Lincoln's ability to wage war without a congressional declaration of war, and later, in *Texas v. White*, it upheld his theory of the relation between the seceded states and the Union.

In World War II, the Court sustained use of a military commission to try German saboteurs who had landed in the United States (*Ex parte Quirin*, 1942), and President Franklin Roosevelt's relocation of the Japanese-Americans was held valid in the *Korematsu* case despite the dissenters' claims that the relocation was racist. In fact, the Court sustained the action not only on limited grounds of "military necessity" (the idea that the Court did not have jurisdiction to review military judgments) but also specifically held the action constitutional, although the Court did say that, once found to be loyal, a relocated citizen must be released (*Ex parte Endo*). In the mid-1980s, lower court judges set aside the convictions of the Japanese-Americans tried 40 years earlier under the curfew and relocation provisions, on the grounds that the government had withheld from the courts information bearing on the validity of the underlying orders. That government action was also the basis for a suit for compensation on behalf of those relocated, which the Supreme Court deferred by ruling it had been appealed to the wrong lower court, thus necessitating further action (*United States v. Hohri*, 1987).

There are exceptions to the Court's general deference to the president on wartime matters; for example, in World War II the Court refused to uphold the imposition of martial law in Hawaii, but did not issue that ruling until after the war's end.[47] The Court also reversed a treason conviction of an American who had aided the Germans because the constitutional standard for treason had not been met and also reversed, for insufficient evidence, an Espionage Act conviction of someone found guilty of impairing the morale of the armed forces.[48]

President Truman's 1952 seizure of the steel mills to avoid their shutdown as a result of a labor dispute tied to wage-price control problems was founded in part on the war power; the government's claim was that if the mills closed, our national security would be endangered. In response to the challenge to the seizure, the government also argued the president's "inherent power" to make the seizure. Insistence on such authority not grounded in specific statute or constitutional provision, particularly where there was no real emergency, led the Court to invalidate the seizure in *Youngstown Sheet & Tube Co. v. Sawyer* (1952): Congress had provided means for handling such situations and moreover had refused to enact the broader provisions Truman had requested. Justice Black, in his opinion for the Court, directly rejected the president's "inherent powers" argument, but if one takes the concurring and dissenting opinions together, a majority of justices did not denounce such powers outright, leaving the possibility of their use where Congress had not spoken. Of the president's four appointees to the Court, only two (Minton and Chief Justice Vinson), joined by FDR appointee Stanley Reed, supported his action. Truman's compliance was immediate; the mills were returned to private hands the day after the Court's ruling, which may have taught the president to use with business and labor "several lesser sanctions none of which is as potent as seizure but the cumulative impact of which enables the President to prevail."[49]

Because Congress had not declared war in Vietnam and because the war was said to violate international law, many efforts were made to challenge its constitutionality. Using the "political question" doctrine or ruling that by making appropriations Congress had acquiesced in the war, lower courts refused to interfere. Despite repeated dissents by Justice Douglas, joined occasionally by Justice Stewart and once by Justice Harlan, the Supreme Court consistently refused to grant review, even refusing to do so in *Massachusetts v. Laird*—over dissents from all three—when pursuant to state legislative action Massachusetts' attorney general sought adjudication of the war's constitutionality.

The Supreme Court also avoided a ruling after Representative Elizabeth Holtzman (D-N.Y.) obtained an injunction against further bombing of Cambodia because the bombing lacked congressional authorization. As circuit justice, Justice Marshall would not lift an appeals court stay of the injunction but did say both that the issue might be justiciable and that the president could not wage war "without some form of congressional approval" except in extreme emergencies. He added that "the decision to send American troops 'to distant lands to die of foreign fevers and foreign shot and shell' [quoting Justice Black] . . . may ultimately be adjudged to have not only been unwise but also unlawful." When the plaintiffs persuaded Justice Douglas to vacate the stay, the Defense Department threatened noncompliance, and the entire Court overruled Douglas *the same day* and directly stayed the district court injunction. The result of this maneuvering was the usual one of judicial noninterference in war matters.[50]

The Iran hostage crisis produced litigation on the hostage agreement, which provided mechanisms for resolving claims and obligated the United States to terminate all legal proceedings in U.S. courts involving claims against Iran and its state enterprises and to nullify attachments against Iranian property. Implementing regulations prohibited any attachment of Iranian property in this country or other nonapproved judicial action. The president then allowed judicial proceedings against Iran but no entry of judgment. When a district judge nonetheless issued orders of attachment, the case—*Dames & Moore v. Regan* (1981)—reached the Supreme Court on an expedited schedule and was decided eight days after oral argument and thus more than two weeks before the deadline for transfer of Iranian assets.

The Court, unanimous except for Justice Powell's limited partial dissent, said the question whether nullifying the attachments was a "taking" (subject to compensation) was presented prematurely but upheld the president's broad authority under both the Trading with the Enemy Act and the more recent International Emergency Economic Powers Act. The ruling was confined "only to the very questions necessary to decision of the case," with Justice Rehnquist "freely confess[ing] that we are . . . deciding only one more episode in the never-ending tension between the President exercising the executive authority in a world that presents each day some new challenge with which he must deal and the Constitution under which we all live and which no one disputes embodies some sort of system of checks and balances." The Court, he continued, would not find the president without authority to settle claims when their settlement "has been determined to be a necessary incident to the resolution of a major foreign policy dispute between our country and another, and where Congress acquiesced in the President's action." The ruling is significant not because the Court again did not interfere with the president, but because the Court sustained his action even though that action had restricted judicial power in the name of dealing with a foreign policy emergency. The justices were, however, careful to note that courts were not being stripped of their jurisdiction.

The Court also did not interfere when an individual's passport was revoked on the grounds his activities—revealing the identities of present and former CIA agents—had caused serious damage to the national security and U.S. foreign policy. Although the Passport Act did not explicitly confer such authority, the Court showed its typical deference to the president, saying that "matters intimately related to foreign policy and national security are rarely proper subjects for judicial intervention" and affirming the president's action (*Haig v. Agee*, 1981). The Court, as part of its deference to the president, has looked to congressional acquiescence in past practice as an important basis for sustaining presidential action; it did this in both the *Dames & Moore* case and in *Haig v. Agee*.

We have hardly seen the last conflict before the judiciary over the president's war powers and foreign policy authority. Controversy over the sending of military advisers to El Salvador, the invasion of Grenada, and, in particular, the controversy over our Marines' presence in Lebanon, led some Senate leaders, joined by White House officials, to think about bringing a "test case" to obtain a Supreme Court ruling on the constitutionality of the War Powers Act, although it was not brought. Despite the understandable desire to get a court ruling in a "nonconfrontational context" because it would take too long to obtain a ruling during a time of crisis, such a "test case" would, of course, face the bar on advisory opinions (see pages 174-75).

The foreign affairs area also produced conflict over the president's use of the pocket veto, previously litigated in a domestic context. In 1929, in the *Pocket Veto Case*, the president had been given a bill less than 10 days before adjournment at the end of the first session of Congress, and the Court ruled the bill had been properly pocket-vetoed, because adjournment prevented return of the bill.[51] When President Nixon pocket-vetoed the Family Practice of Medicine Bill during a congressional adjournment for the Christmas holidays—a during-session adjournment—the courts ruled he had acted improperly; the decision was, however, not taken to the Supreme Court.[52] In 1985, the president pocket-vetoed a bill requiring him to certify human rights progress in El Salvador. Members of the House, joined by the Senate, argued that the pocket veto could be used only at the end of a session in an election year, and claimed that an officer was authorized to receive veto messages during an adjournment, so that the president was not prevented from returning the bill with his objections. After the district court upheld the president, the D.C. Circuit ruled against him, but the Supreme

Court said the case had become moot while it was pending, and thus did not decide it.[53]

In any event, the rulings by the courts and their refusal otherwise to decide cases would seem to provide further evidence that "the rare decision" in which the justices "shout 'Check!' at the President" has not "had the presumably salutary effect of keeping the Presidency in rein, to say nothing of rendering it [check]mated. The most effective restraints upon both the Presidency and the Congress have been those imposed by other components of the national political system."[54]

The Nixon Administration

Judicial challenges to actions of the president had been relatively infrequent until the Nixon administration, when the courts regularly were asked to invalidate the president's acts or to force him to do what he had not done. Many of these controversies never reached the Supreme Court because the administration did not appeal adverse lower court decisions, hoping thus to limit their legal effect. Among these cases was a ruling that the president had unconstitutionally failed to submit to the Senate the name of his nominee to be director of the Office of Economic Opportunity (OEO); another, that he had acted improperly in failing to appoint a National Advisory Council on Indian Education after recommending rescission of American Indian education funds; and invalidation of his attempt to terminate the Community Action Program (CAP) element of the War on Poverty because he had not given Congress the statutorily required opportunity to act on a reorganization plan.[55]

The issue of funds allotted or appropriated by Congress and then impounded by the president because he felt priorities must be given to other programs or that the expenditures would be inflationary generated a large number of cases, each over a specific withholding of funds. The government lost over 30 lower court decisions involving funds for education programs, mental health centers, highways, and environmental programs, and then the justices unanimously ruled against the president's actions on the basis that Congress, intending to spend the money to solve what it thought were important problems, would not have undercut itself by giving the president unlimited impoundment power (*Train v. City of New York, Train v. Campaign Clear Water,* 1975). Although the president lost, the decision was in a way anticlimactic, in large part because of enactment of the Impoundment Control Act of 1974, which provided for impoundment or deferral of appropriate funds only after congressional consideration. (When President Reagan tried to defer spending for domestic programs, saying that to block the deferral Congress would have to pass a law subject to his veto, the lower courts eliminated the deferral provision of the 1974 Act, thus defeating the president's efforts.)

Far more serious than impoundment were the continuous confrontations over the release of the Watergate tapes. Prior to the Watergate cases but relevant to them, the administration had been embroiled in litigation over who—the Department of Justice or the courts—should determine the relevance to a prosecution of conversations overheard during electronic surveillance. When the Supreme Court refused to accept the department's own determination of nonrelevance and held, in the *Alderman* case (1969), that a defendant alleging improper interception of conversations was entitled to inspect the "logs" of those conversations, the administration asserted that the Court's ruling would damage the national security and threatened not to tell the courts of the existence of foreign intelligence surveillance the department thought irrelevant. Not intimidated, the Court refused to change its position.

When the administration used electronic surveillance without a court order in a *domestic* security case (the Omnibus Crime Control Act of 1968 allowed it in national security cases), the Court handed the administration another defeat. The Court unanimously ruled in *United States v. U.S. District Court* (1972) that such surveillance could not be conducted without a proper warrant, because Congress had meant to restrict the law's exceptions to the warrant requirement. Perhaps more important, the Court said that surveillance had to be controlled by judges: the executive branch could not be the sole judge of whether surveillance should take place. When the administration again failed to follow statutory procedures for authorization of surveillance orders, the Court also ruled against the government in some cases. [56]

When the president resisted requests to supply material for various Watergate-related investigations and trials, Judge John Sirica ruled that, because the need for information for criminal proceedings was superior to the president's claims of authority to withhold material, a *judge*, not the executive acting alone, must decide the president's claim. The judges of the court of appeals unsuccessfully tried to avoid a constitutional confrontation by suggesting a compromise— inspection of the tapes by the president (or his designee), his counsel, and the special prosecutor—and then sustained Judge Sirica's ruling.

The president at first said he would comply only with a "definitive ruling" from the Supreme Court, which he later indicated meant one with a vote of at least 7-2; this meant the president reserved to himself the power to accept or reject matters of constitutional interpretation. Having ascertained that apparently only Justice Rehnquist and possibly Chief Justice Burger would have voted for his position, the president chose not to appeal to the Supreme Court. Compliance with a lower court ruling came only after the "Saturday night massacre" in which Special Prosecutor Archibald Cox and the attorney general were fired (by Solicitor General Bork, as acting attorney general). (Even the firing of the special prosecutor was found illegal by a lower court because the president had violated Justice Department regulations "having the force of law."[57]

The Supreme Court's definitive ruling in the Watergate tapes matter came when the president refused to comply with Judge Sirica's subsequent order for production of a much larger number of tapes for the Watergate cover-up trial. In *United States v. Nixon*, a unanimous Court, speaking through Chief Justice Burger, rejected the president's arguments. (It did, however, decline to rule on whether the grand jury had acted properly in naming the president as an unindicted co-conspirator in the cover-up.) The justices emphasized their power to determine the constitutionality of claims made by other branches of government, whether pursuant to express or implied constitutional provisions. Chief Justice Burger twice used Chief Justice Marshall's *Marbury v. Madison* language that it is "emphatically the province and the duty" of the Court "to say what the law is."

The Court did legitimize "executive privilege" by recognizing that the president needed "complete candor and objectivity from advisers," which confidentiality of communications would assist. However, balancing that interest against the requirements of the criminal process, the Court struck the balance against the president, who could not be above the law. An undifferentiated claim of privilege not involving protection of special types of secrets "cannot prevail over the fundamental demands of due process of law in the fair administration of criminal justice." The decision, with which the president complied, helped send him from office. The recognition of executive privilege—even though its application in the context of a criminal trial was not in the president's favor—may, however, have been a more far-reaching result of the case.

Closely related to the recognition of executive privilege was the Court's legitimation of absolute immunity for the president from civil damage suits. A result of President Nixon's involvement in the removal of "whistleblower" Ernest Fitzgerald from his Pentagon job, this ruling did not come until long after Nixon had left office. By a 5-4 vote, the Court ruled in *Nixon v. Fitzgerald* (1982) that the president had absolute immunity from civil suits for damages for acts within the "outer perimeter" of his official responsibility, unless Congress authorized such lawsuits. The energies of the president who had to defend himself against such suits, said Justice Powell for the Court, would be diverted from the government's effective functioning; moreover, our system of checks and balances, including impeachment, was available to constrain the president. Because of his "unique status," the president could be treated differently from other executive officials. In the companion case of *Harlow v. Fitzgerald*, on the liability of presidential assistants, the Court, by an 8-1 vote, extended earlier rulings concerning Cabinet members' immunity, holding that most such asssistants were entitled to only qualified (limited) immunity from suit, but left open the possibility of absolute immunity for those involved in national security and foreign policy work. Justice White, dissenting in the *Nixon* case, attacked absolute presidential immunity for placing the president above the law and allowing him "deliberately [to] cause serious injury to any number of citizens." It was, said White, "a reversion to the old notion that the king can do no wrong." The *Fitzgerald* litigation led to failure of some suits against Nixon administration officials for improper electronic surveillance, but the Supreme Court ruled, in a case filed after the *U.S. District Court* wiretap ruling, that the Attorney General was entitled to only qualified immunity when sued for acting unconstitutionally in connection with his national security duties.[58]

After President Nixon's resignation, the issue of his pardon by President Ford did not reach the Supreme Court. A federal judge in Michigan, however, did rule the pardon constitutional, saying it was within the letter and spirit of the presidential pardon power as well as a "prudent public policy judgment."[59] The Supreme Court had also said in late 1974 in *Schick v. Reed* that the president had broad discretion to treat individually each commutation and pardon he chose to issue and to attach conditions, even those not mentioned in the statutes.

Litigation over President Nixon's tapes and papers continued after he left office. Congress set aside his agreement with the General Services Administration (GSA) on disposition of his presidential papers in the Presidential Recordings and Materials Preservation Act, which provided for screening of materials by archivists and return of purely private material, and included safeguards against disclosure of materials affecting confidential communications with the president. Sustaining the Act in *Nixon v. Administrator of General Services* (1977), the Court found no improper intrusion and swept aside the ex-president's barrage of objections: the act did not violate the separation of powers nor the president's privilege to have confidential communications, nor did it improperly invade his privacy or association rights. Nor, said the Court, was the law a bill of attainder; the president was a legitimate "class of one" on which Congress could legislate; moreover, Congress was acting to protect materials, not to punish. Justice Stevens, more forthright, said the statute did implicitly condemn Nixon as an unreliable custodian of his papers, but he approved the legislation because of Nixon's resignation from office and acceptance of a pardon. The Court, relying on procedures in the Presidential Recordings Act, ruled in *Nixon v. Warner Communications* (1978) that neither a common law right of access nor the First Amendment required release of the tapes; the lower courts could use their informed discretion in providing procedures for release of materials that had been used in judicial proceedings and in limiting release of those materials. Even this ruling did not end Nixon's resistance to release of materials, but in 1982 the Court of Appeals for the District of Columbia upheld allowing the public to listen to the president's tapes, including those from the cover-up trial, after archivists had reviewed them in accordance with statutory procedures. With respect to materials other than the tapes, after each new set of regulations concerning their screening and release is issued, court orders have been sought— mostly by Nixon aides—blocking release of material, so that some of the Nixon papers were made available only in late 1986, with many of the most sensitive documents still unavailable.

The Courts and the Regulatory Agencies

The regulatory commissions and executive branch departments performing regulatory tasks handle many more cases than do federal district courts. In the commissions' early years, courts were often hostile to them, but later the lower courts and the Supreme Court have allowed them and executive agencies considerable discretion.

The Supreme Court's earliest response to some agencies was to restrict both their jurisdiction and the weight judges were to give the agencies' determinations. Decisions like the one stating that the Interstate Commerce Commission could only determine whether railroad-proposed rates were reasonable led the ICC to concede that "by virtue of judicial decisions, it has ceased to be a body for the regulation of interstate carriers."[60] Similarly, the ruling in the *Gratz* case that methods of unfair competition unknown before passage of the Federal Trade Commission Act were not within the FTC's jurisdiction and that the courts would identify those methods led the commission to stop trying to prohibit new unfair trade practices. However, when the Court held in the *Winstead Hosiery* case that the FTC could deal with false advertising and misbranding, the commission's level of activity on those subjects increased. The Court's later limitation of the commission through the decision that the FTC could deal with only false advertising that was both unfair *and* a method of competition had to be overruled by Congress. Only in 1934 in the *Keppel Brothers* case did the Court say that it would give weight to the FTC's determination of what practices would be considered unfair. The agencies were also restricted procedurally by the Court. While the Court finally came around to giving administrators greater freedom of action, the Court's restrictive rulings caused reexamination of the agencies' procedures and helped lead to their codification in the Administrative Procedure Act of 1946.

The courts' more deferential approach to agency action resulted both from judges' greater familiarity with the agencies, new judges' more favorable attitudes toward regulation, and a greater recognition of the necessity of letting the agencies operate with less supervision lest the courts be swamped with cases appealed from the agencies. Instead of reviewing agency action with a fine-toothed comb, that is, subjecting even the agencies' factual determinations to *de novo* review, doctrines were developed by Congress and enforced by the courts that decreased judicial oversight of the agencies' work. Judicial review has been ruled unavailable in some situations; in others, courts have insisted that various steps must be followed prior to judicial review (*exhaustion of administrative remedies*); and courts examining agency rulings have generally limited themselves to determining whether "substantial evidence" supports agency actions.

Courts continue to interpret the law applied by the agencies and commissions, so courts determine whether agencies are acting within the scope of authority granted them by Congress. For example, the Supreme Court ruled, in the *Hampton* case, that the Civil Service Commission's exclusion of aliens from federal government employment, far from the commission's core duties, had not been explicitly authorized. (The president then issued an executive order embodying the appropriate authorization.) Because agency and court jurisdictions overlap at times, the courts also have to help distribute responsibilities among agencies, or, as in the field of labor law, among agencies, arbitrators deciding cases closely related to agency jurisdiction, and courts.

Courts have available a battery of rules to assist them in sustaining agency actions that are challenged in court, and the courts sustain agency actions in a high proportion of these cases. One rule is to give great weight to agency interpretations of the statutes under which they operate. Thus, in reviewing Department of Justice "preclearance" decisions under the Voting Rights Act of 1965, concerning changes in voting procedures to determine whether they have the purpose or effect of discriminating against minorities, the Court has shown substantial deference to the attorney general's rulings on the scope of coverage (what types of changes are subject to preclearance) and, with limited exceptions, has tended to adopt Justice Department standards. When the department failed to object to proposed changes, the Court also deferred, holding such inaction not subject to judicial review. That the Court's position and the agency's stance *converged* through interaction made it easier for the Court's majority to draw upon the executive's position. This is similar to the pattern found in appeals court rulings on the Federal Power Commission. In that pattern, the agency, although trying to anticipate the courts' reaction from accumulated judicial rulings, initiates policy changes, and the courts decide whether to accept those changes intact or to require modifications. Throughout, "the typical pattern of interaction . . . has been one of adjustment and accommodation to divergent viewpoints," with cooperation rather than conflict predominating, as the courts learn from the agencies and do not simply tell them what to do.[61] A study of agency policymaking on the Clean Air Act also found that judicial decisions shaped agency programs: not only did specific court rulings have an effect but "anticipation of judicial review . . . influenced the EPA's regulations . . ." Moreover, with division in government about the proper course of policy, judicial rulings assisted some "players" to achieve their goals; in this case, the EPA was able to benefit from judicial rulings. Within the agency, the courts' rulings "helped political executives gain control over lower levels of the bureaucracy."[62]

The Administrative Procedure Act's "substantial evidence" standard and closely related tests, such as whether agency actions are "arbitrary and capricious," generally produce deference to the agencies. As Justice White remarked when the Court sustained a National Labor Relations Board (NLRB) ruling, "Assessing the significance of impasse and the dynamics of collective bargaining is precisely the kind of judgment that [we earlier] ruled should be left to the Board. We cannot say that the Board's current resolution of the issue is arbitrary or contrary to law."[63] Similarly, in ruling on a challenge to a Federal Election Commission decision concerning expenditure agreements between state party organizations and the national party's senatorial campaign committees, Justice White wrote that a court's task in acting against the background of an agency ruling—not the same as acting initially in a judicial proceeding—"was not to interpret the statute as it thought best but rather the narrower inquiry into whether the Commission's construction was 'sufficiently reasonable' to be accepted by a reviewing court." He did, however, concede that "the thoroughness, validity and consistency of an agency's reasoning are factors that bear upon the amount of deference to be given an agency's ruling."[64]

Application of the Freedom of Information Act (FOIA), which has a general policy of disclosure but contains many exemptions, has provided recent tests of the Court's deference to agencies, which use the exemptions to withhold information. In its first FOIA ruling, *Environmental Protection Agency v. Mink* (1973), the Supreme Court upheld the EPA's refusal to provide members of Congress information about an underground nuclear test because the relevant documents, classified Secret or Top Secret, were exempted from disclosure; it also ruled courts could not examine the questioned materials but should accept agency determinations concerning classification. (Congress thereupon limited the materials that could be withheld as classified and provided for judicial examination of the documents, thus giving the courts authority the Supreme Court had declined to exercise.) By and large, the court has continued to reinforce agencies' FOIA positions. The Court has strengthened the agencies' hand by ruling that they need not release documents that were not final opinions. However, the justices have also ruled in favor of disclosure of final opinions and of materials that would not produce a "clearly unwarranted" invasion of privacy, and have decided that private companies, such as government contractors, could not prevent release of information otherwise obtained by the government.[65] The Court has also ruled that when material subject to disclosure is no longer in the agency's possession because an official—in this instance, Secretary of State Henry Kissinger—treating the documents as his own, has taken the documents from the agency, it did not "improperly withhold" them. In the same case the Court also ruled that Kissinger's notes of telephone conversations made when he was the president's assistant for national security were not State Department "agency records" and thus were not subject to disclosure even after Kissinger brought those notes to the State Department when he became Secretary of State.[66]

The Court's deference to agencies does, however, have limits. For one thing, the Court does not always follow agency interpretations of statutes, for example, refusing in the previously noted *Gilbert* case to follow Equal Employment Opportunity Commission guidelines treating pregnancy as a disability. Of particular significance is the Court's invalidation of Occupational Safety and Health Administration's (OSHA) rules on occupational exposure to benzene. Because the Secretary of Labor had not made the threshold determination required by the statute that the particular toxic substance posed a significant workplace health risk and that under the statutory standard of "reasonably necessary or appropriate to provide safe or healthful employment and places of employment," the agency rulings had to fall.[67] (That ruling, coupled with the Reagan administration's emphasis on deregulation and the availability of fewer research dollars for OSHA, was said to have made it extremely difficult to develop the data needed to meet the Court's burden of proof.[68]) Generally, the Court has said that agencies need to explain how they have reached their conclusions, even if they do not produce the ultimate in clarity, and the justices have invalidated agency orders not linking findings and conclusions. This applies to decisions to deregulate by eliminating regulations (which the courts say is not the same as not issuing a regulation in the first place) as well as decisions to regulate, as can be seen in the Court's ruling that the National Highway Traffic Safety Agency had not properly rescinded the "air bag" rule.[69]

The Court says that it does not weigh the evidence presented to an agency, except to see whether there is enough (under the "appropriate" standard) to support the agency's result, and that it does not judge the "wisdom" of the agency's action. Sometimes, however, the justices manage to send an agency "multiple messages" by saying they support the agency position while indicating strong misgivings. For example, in voting to sustain a Federal Communications Commission order, Chief Justice Burger said he was unsure that the FCC had made the right decision, but that as a justice of the Supreme Court, he could not "resolve this issue as perhaps I would were I a member of the . . . Commission."[70]

The Court can also limit agency discretion by requiring due process protections for those affected by agency actions, but the Court has not done this frequently. Typical are procedural rulings in which the Court refused to require full hearings for all aspects of new drug applications, allowing summary proceedings instead, and did not require the Secretary of Transportation to make formal findings even though he had to follow certain procedural requirements in making his determination that there was no "feasible and prudent" alternative route for an interstate highway scheduled to go through a park. The court will also not allow lower courts to demand more procedurally than the Administrative Procedure Act requires.[71] Perhaps the most notable application of due process came in the Court's 1970 *Goldberg v. Kelly* and *Wheeler v. Montgomery* rulings that welfare benefits could not be terminated without a prior evidentiary hearing even though a full HEW "fair hearing" need not be held until after termination. However, in *Mathews v. Eldridge* (1976) the Court refused to extend its earlier rule to termination of disability benefits. The test developed by the Burger Court in that case "balances the harm to legally protected rights of the individual against the costs and burdens on the agency using the criterion of whether increased procedures would improve the accuracy of the fact-finding process."[72] This test and other recent cases contravene the conventional wisdom that the federal courts, including the Supreme Court, interfere with adminstrative agencies and do not allow the managers of those agencies sufficient discretion: "Recent cases indicate an increasing judicial sensitivity to management problems and priorities."[73]

Related to deference to administrative agencies is deference to the lower courts, particularly the courts of appeals, that rule initially on agency actions. In recent controversial cases involving OSHA standards for exposure to "cotton dust," which results in byssinosis ("brown lung"), the Court remarked, in upholding the agency, "Our inquiry is not to determine whether we, in the first instance, would find OSHA's findings supported by substantial evidence. Instead we turn to OSHA's findings and the record upon which they were based to decide whether the Court of Appeals 'misapprehended or grossly misapplied' the test for evaluating agency decisions."[74]

In other cases, the Court has not hesitated to overturn lower court rulings on the basis of its own examination of the relevant statute and administrative action—even when the lower court is the U.S. Court of Appeals for the District of Columbia, the most important court of appeals for administrative law because of the high proportion of appeals from administrative agency decisions it handles. The D.C. court's posture toward the agencies—essentially liberal and activist— has led it on a path different from the Supreme Court's, particularly in the 1970s, making deference by the Supreme Court less likely. For example, after the Federal Communications Commission decided that market forces should prevail and that it would not consider changes in program format (from rock to jazz or from jazz to classical music) in a license renewal application, the D.C. Circuit held that the FCC's policy violated the Federal Communications Act. "Unconvinced" that the lower court's doctrine was "compelled by the Act," the Supreme Court sustained the commission, which had "provided a rational explanation for its conclusion that reliance on the market is the best method of promoting diversity in entertainment formats."[75] As this case indicates, where agency and lower court differ, the Supreme Court can "have its pick" of policies, dressing up its conclusion in the language of deference—to the agency or to the lower court as appropriate.

We can see the relation between the Supreme Court and the agencies in the area of patent law, where the Supreme Court's impact has come less from individual decisions than from their collective force, as the decisions have been reinforced by rulings of the lower federal courts. During the 1930s the Supreme Court quietly changed its standards concerning the patentability of inventions by substantially increasing the rate at which it invalidated patents; it was the results rather than the Court's language that mattered. Those decisions from the 1930s and further Supreme Court rulings in 1941, 1949, and 1950 were frequently cited by both the lower courts and others interested in patent policy. However, without a "clear command" from the Court, the Patent Office chose to follow the Supreme Court's doctrine rather than its actions. The agency thus did not change its decision making even when it was criticized by the Supreme Court for departing from the Court's standards.[76]

One reason for Patent Office resistance was that, although some lower court judges recognized the Supreme Court's change in posture and shifted their positions accordingly, others, among them the Court of Customs and Patent Appeals, resisted the change. This lower court reluctance to recognize what the Supreme Court had done meant that the justices, to try to make their point, had to reverse those courts frequently. When either the appeals courts or district courts found a patent valid, the likelihood of reversal by the Supreme Court was very high. Even when a new patent statute was enacted—partly a result of the Supreme Court's actions—little appeared to change. The Supreme Court's declaration that the new law was in fact a codification of the old law reinforced the pattern of divergent interpretations: some courts of appeals applied Patent Act language, others applied a different standard, and some appeared to apply no particular standard.

Overall Support

The Supreme Court's rate of affirmance of agency rulings has usually been in the vicinity of 70 to 80 percent. During the 1947–56 Terms, average support for the agencies was 69 percent; for the 1960–65 Terms, it was 78 percent; for the 1967 Term, the rate went to 84 percent, a further indication of term-by-term variation. Even with the Burger Court's conservative tendencies in economic regulation, 76 percent of agency actions challenged in the Supreme Court were sustained there in the 1971–73 Terms,[77] but this may reflect a change in the types of cases being appealed. The high level of support is particularly striking because only a very small percentage of the regulatory agencies' rulings are appealed to the courts and even fewer—the "difficult" and controversial decisions—to the Supreme Court, which denies certiorari in most cases. This means that the support level for the agencies is extremely high, with very, very few of their decisions overturned. We must, however, remember that there are situations in which the Court's rulings have no effect, situations in which,

> while administrative lawyers harangue each other concerning the fine points of the Supreme Court's or the D.C. Circuit's most recent procedural ruling, billions of dollars per year are being transferred, for good or ill, by an invisible army of bureaucratic adjudicators to whom court decisions may have absolutely no relevance.[78]

Not all agencies have been supported at the same level, however. During the Roosevelt Court, although the FCC won fewer than half its cases before the Court, the basic range of support ran from a high of 86 percent (NLRB) to a low of 60 percent (FTC). The Federal Power Commission and the Federal Trade Commission were supported at rates of over 90 percent during 1957–68, and the NLRB and Internal Revenue Service won about three-quarters of their cases, but the ICC was supported less than two-thirds of the time and the Immigration and

Naturalization Service won only 56.3 percent of its cases. These differences are explained largely in terms of the agencies' substantive policies. At least through the Warren Court, Schubert has argued, the Court supported the agencies because the agencies decided cases in the same liberal direction to which the justices were favorably inclined. Thus, where agency results were conservative, the Court was more likely to overturn the decisions.

A different look at Warren Court agency support scores shows that when the agency decisions were probusiness, the Court supported the agency just slightly more than half the time (52%), but when the agencies were antibusiness, support increased to almost two-thirds (65%). The Court supported two-thirds of prolabor agency decisions, but only 53 percent of antilabor rulings. The Burger Court, although supporting the agencies over 70 percent of the time—more when unanimous than when divided in the 1969–77 Terms—was more likely to overturn liberal agency actions. When the NLRB was prolabor, the Burger Court supported it only 53 percent of the time, but did so in 89 *percent* of the board's antilabor cases. Support for probusiness or antilabor agency decisions was higher than for prolabor and antibusiness decisions (63% to 51%).[79]

The Court's overall supportive position toward the agencies masks differences among justices. For the 1947–56 Terms, all except Black were consistent in overall support for the agencies. However, justices' value preferences appeared to affect their voting in some situations, for example, Black and Douglas (prounion) and Chief Justice Vinson (antiunion) in labor cases and Black and Douglas in business competition cases. Black, Douglas, and Frankfurter were more likely to oppose an agency ruling when a person's freedom was involved than when it was not. All the justices were more likely to support the agencies when evidentiary questions were involved than when they were not, but some (Jackson, Reed, Burton) were particularly likely to do so; questions of statutory authority and due process of law also affected some voting in the Court. During 1957–68, differences between justices followed the Court's overall pattern. The justices' basic substantive policy attitudes had a greater effect on their voting than "due process" and "statutory authority and interpretation" dimensions of cases[80]—findings supported in a study of the 1953–61 period, where data showed that "justices vote on the basis of their pro- and antiunion attitudes rather than their degree of deference to the NLRB" and that "the justices' economic policy preferences rather than tenets of activism or restraint explain their behavior."[81]

In the Burger Court, one could also find differences among the justices; even among the four Nixon appointees, two (Burger and Powell) showed a relative lack of deference to the agencies, while Blackmun and Rehnquist were more deferential. Looking at the entire Burger Court membership, one can see that some justices were deferential in particular categories of cases—Powell when agency decisions were probusiness, Marshall when they were prolabor—while only two (Blackmun and White) seemed restrained or deferential across all categories of cases.[82]

Overall, the picture we find in examining Supreme Court judicial review at the national level is that the Court only infrequently reverses the actions of Congress, the president, or the regulatory commissions and executive branch agencies. However, it is not hesitant to do so and can have considerable effect when it does. Yet, despite an apparent lack of reaction to many of its decisions and more willing compliance in other instances, Congress rewrites statutes and at times takes more severe reversal action, and the regulatory agencies have shown themselves quite capable of resisting the High Court through delay and persistence. Judicial review certainly did not cease after 1937, although the focus of such actions shifted from economic regulation to other matters, most notably in areas of civil liberties policy. These actions and their aftermath show the Court important but not all-powerful.

Notes

1. Thomas G. Walker and Deborah J. Barrow, "Funding the Federal Judiciary: The Congressional Connection," *Judicature* 69 (June–July 1985): 44–45.

2. Jonathan P. Nase, "Of Dollars and Justice: The Appropriations Process of the Federal Judiciary," *Justice System Journal* 10 (Spring 1985): 72–73.

3. Walker and Barrow, "Funding the Federal Judiciary," p. 46.

4. Ibid., p. 50.

5. Nase, "Of Dollars and Justice," pp. 63–64, 66.

6. See Louis Fisher, *Constitutional Conflicts Between Congress and the President* (Princeton, N.J.: Princeton University Press, 1985), pp. 184–95.

7. Gregory A. Caldeira and Donald J. McCrone, "Of Time and Judicial Activism: A Story of the U.S. Supreme Court, 1800–1973," in *Supreme Court Activism and Restraint*, eds. Halpern and Lamb, pp. 111–13, 120–21.

8. Stuart Nagel, *The Legal Process from a Behavioral Perspective* (Homewood, Ill.: The Dorsey Press, 1969), pp. 248, 259.

9. Bradley C. Canon and S. Sidney Ulmer, "The Supreme Court and Critical Elections: A Dissent," *American Political Science Review* 70 (December 1976): 1215–18; Richard Funston, "The Supreme Court and Critical Elections," *American Political Science Review* 69 (September 1975): 795–811; and John B. Gates, "Partisan Realignment, Unconstitutional State Policies, and the U.S. Supreme Court, 1837–1964," *American Journal of Political Science* 31 (May 1987): 259–80.

10. *Trop v. Dulles*, 356 U.S. 86 (1956), and *Kennedy v. Mendoza-Martinez*, 372 U.S. 144 (1963) (citizenship); *Reid v. Covert*, 354 U.S. 1 (1957), *United States ex rel. Toth v. Quarles*, 350 U.S. 11 (1955), and *O'Callaghan v. Parker*, 395 U.S. 258 (1969) (courts-martial).

11. For example, *Marchetti v. United States*, 390 U.S. 39 (1968) (gambling), and *Leary v. United States*, 395 U.S. 6 (1969) (marijuana tax).

12. *U.S. Department of Agriculture v. Murry*, 413 U.S. 508 (1973), and *U.S.D.A. v. Moreno*, 413 U.S. 529 (1973) (food stamps); *Weinberger v. Wiesenfeld*, 420 U.S. 630 (1975), and *Jimenez v. Weinberger*, 417 U.S. 628 (1974) (benefits); *Blount v. Rizzi*, 400 U.S. 419 (1971); *Chief of Capitol Police v. Jeannette Rankin Brigade*, 409 U.S. 972 (1973); and *United States v. Grace*, 461 U.S. 171 (1983) (free speech).

13. Louis Fisher, "Judicial Misjudgments About the Lawmaking Process: The Legislative Veto Case," *Public Administration Review* 45 (Special 1985): 706.

14. See Beth Henschen, "Judicial Use of Legislative History and Intent in Statutory Interpretation," *Legislative Studies Quarterly* 10 (August 1985): 353–71.

15. Walter Murphy, *Elements of Judicial Strategy*, pp. 129-31.

16. Jesse H. Choper, *Judicial Review and the National Political Process*, p. 143.

17. Nagel, *The Legal Process*, p. 275; Walter F. Murphy, *Congress and the Court* (Chicago: University of Chicago Press, 1962), pp. 257–58.

18. Nagel, *The Legal Process*, p. 266.

19. Lucius J. Barker, "The Offshore Oil Cases," in *The Third Branch of Government*, eds. C. Herman Pritchett and Alan F. Westin (New York: Harcourt, Brace, and World, 1963), pp. 234–74.

20. *Guss v. Utah Labor Relations Board*, 343 U.S. 1 (1957).

21. *Lauf v. E. G. Shinner & Co.*, 303 U.S. 323 (1968); *Yakus v. United States*, 321 U.S. 414 (1944).

22. Murphy, *Congress and the Court*, is an account of Congress' action.

23. For a discussion of some of these points, see Kenneth R. Kay, "The Unforeseen Impact on Courts *and* Congress," *Judicature* 65 (October 1981):185–89; Charles E. Rice, "The Constitutional Basis for the Proposals in Congress Today," ibid., 190–97; Telford Taylor, "The Unconstitutionality of Current Legislative Proposals," ibid., 198–207; and Carl A. Anderson, "The Government of Courts: The Power of Congress," *American Bar Association Journal* 68 (June 1982): 686–90.

24. An earlier version of part of this material appeared in Stephen L. Wasby, *The Impact of the United States Supreme Court: Some Perspectives* (Homewood, Ill.: The Dorsey Press, 1970), pp. 203–13.

25. Samuel Krislov, *The Supreme Court in the Political Process* (New York: Macmillan, 1965), p. 143.

26. Michael W. Dolan, "Congress, the Executive, and the Court: The Great Resale Price Maintenance Affair of 1983," *Public Administration Review* 45 (Special 1985): 718–22.

27. Beth Henschen, "Statutory Interpretations of the Supreme Court: Congressional Response," *American Politics Quarterly* 11 (October 1983): 441–58.

28. *Railroad Retirement Board v. Alton Railway Co.*, 295 U.S. 330 (1935).

29. Note, "Congressional Reversal of Supreme Court Decisions: 1945–1957," *Harvard Law Review* 71 (May 1958): 1336. See *S & E Contractors v. United States*, 406 U.S. 1 at 13–14, 25–26, 48–51, and 69–90 (1972).

30. The cases are, respectively, *National Labor Relations Board v. Denver Building Construction Trades Council*, 341 U.S. 675 (1951) and *Local 1976, United Brotherhood of Carpenters v. N.L.R.B. (Sand Door)*, 357 U.S. 93 (1958). See *Woelke & Romero Framing v. N.L.R.B.*, 456 U.S. 645 (1982).

31. *City of Lafayette v. Louisiana Power & Light Co.*, 435 U.S. 389 (1978); *Community Communications v. City of Boulder*, 455 U.S. 40 (1982).

32. *Newport News Shipbuilding & Dry Dock Co. v. Equal Employment Opportunity Commission*, 462 U.S. 669 (1983). On the campaign to overturn *Gilbert*, see Joyce Gelb and Marian Lief Palley, "Women and Interest Group Politics: A Comparative Analysis of Federal Decision-Making," *Journal of Politics* 41 (May 1979): 385–87.

33. *City of Mobile v. Bolden*, 446 U.S. 55 (1980); *Thornburg v. Gingles*, 106 S.Ct. 2752 (1986).

34. Harry Stumpf, "The Political Efficacy of Judicial Symbolism," *Western Political Quarterly* 19 (June 1966): 293–303; and "Congressional Response to Supreme Court Rulings: The Interaction of Law and Politics," *Journal of Public Law* 14 (1965): 376–95.

35. See Donald G. Morgan, *Congress and the Constitution: A Study of Responsibility* (Cambridge, Mass.: Harvard University Press, 1966), pp. 10–11.

36. See Louis Fisher, "Constitutional Interpretation by Members of Congress," *North Carolina Law Review* 63 (1985): 707–9.

37. For greater detail, see Stephen L. Wasby, "The Presidency Before the Courts," *Capital University Law Review* 6 (December 1976): 35–73, in which some of this material was first presented.

38. See Michael Nelson, "Presidents, Politics, and Policy: A Theoretical Perspective on the Court-Packing Episode of 1937," paper presented to American Political Science Association, 1986.

39. *Local 28 v. E.E.O.C.*, 106 S.Ct. 3019 (1986); *Local 93 v. City of Cleveland*, 106 S.Ct. 3063 (1986).

40. See the Supreme Court's actions concerning stays of lower court rulings, *Heckler v. Lopez*, 463 U.S. 1328 and 464 U.S. 879 (1983), and Susan Gluck Mezey, "Policymaking by the Federal Judiciary: The Effects of Judicial Review on the Social Security Disability Program," *Policy Studies Journal* 14 (March 1986): 343–61.

41. *A.F.L.-C.I.O. v. Kahn*, 618 F.2d 784 (D.C.Cir. 1979), cert. denied, 443 U.S. 915 (1979). For executive agreements, see Phillip J. Cooper, "By Order of the President: Administration by Executive Order and Proclamation," *Administration & Society* 18 (August 1986): 233–62.

42. *Edwards v. Carter*, 445 F.Supp. 1279 (D.D.C. 1978), 580 F.2d 1055 (D.C.Cir. 1973), cert. denied, 436 U.S. 907 (1978).

43. The material in this paragraph is drawn from three papers by Craig R. Ducat and Robert L. Dudley: Ducat and Dudley, "Presidential Power in the Federal Courts During the Post-War Era," American Political Science Association, 1985; Ducat and Dudley, "Federal Judges and Presidential Power: Truman to Reagan," Midwest Political Science Association, 1986; and Ducat and Dudley, "Federal District Judges and Presidential Power: A Multivariate Analysis," American Political Science Association, 1986.

44. See Nelson, "Presidents, Politics, and Policy," p. 12.

45. *Federal Energy Administration v. Algonquin SNG*, 426 U.S. 548 (1976).

46. Clinton Rossiter, *The Supreme Court and the Commander in Chief* (Ithaca, N.Y.: Cornell University Press, 1951), pp. 127–28, 131.

47. *Duncan v. Kahanamoku*, 327 U.S. 304 (1946).

48. *Cramer v. United States*, 325 U.S. 1 (1945) and *Hartzel v. United States*, 322 U.S. 680 (1944). For a fascinating story of the *Cramer* case, see J. Woodford Howard, Jr., "Advocacy in Constitutional Choice: The *Cramer* Treason Case, 1942–1945," *American Bar Foundation Research Journal* 1986 (Summer): 375–414.

49. Arthur S. Miller, *The Supreme Court and American Capitalism* (New York: Free Press, 1970), p. 100. For a complete account of the case, see Maeva Marcus, *Truman and the Steel Seizure Case: The Limits of Presidential Power* (New York: Columbia University Press, 1977). The Court's two basic approaches to the president's use of executive orders, both present in opinions in the Steel Seizure case, are discussed by Cooper, "By Order of the President," 244.

50. *Holtzman v. Schlesinger*, 414 U.S. 1304 and 414 U.S. 1316; *Schlesinger v. Holtzman*, 414 U.S. 1321 (1973). The appellate court then held that Congress' extending the fund cut-off date for funding of the bombing was approved by Congress, 484 F.2d 1307 (2nd Cir. 1973), and other courts held there was no need for judicial decision because the August 15 date indicated an absence of interbranch conflict. See *Drinan v. Nixon*, 364 F.Supp. 854 (D. Mass. 1973).

51. See also *Wright v. United States*, 302 U.S. 583 (1938) (President's return of bill to Senate during three-day recess but with Senate official designated to receive messages).

52. *Kennedy v. Sampson*, 364 F.Supp. 1075 (D.D.C. 1973), 511 F.2d 430 (D.C.Cir. 1974).

53. *Burke v. Barnes*, 107 S.Ct. 734 (1987), vacating *Barnes v. Kline*, 759 F.2d 21 (D.C.Cir. 1985).

54. Glendon Schubert, *Judicial Policy-Making* (Glenview, Ill.: Scott, Foresman, 1965), pp. 59–60.

55. *Williams v. Phillips*, 360 F.Supp. 1363 (D.D.C. 1973), aff'd, 482 F.2d 669 (D.C.Cir. 1973); *Minnesota Chippewa Tribe v. Carlucci*, 358 F.Supp. 973 (D.D.C. 1973); *Local 2677, American Federation of Government Employees v. Phillips*, 358 F.Supp. 60 (D.D.C. 1973).

56. *United States v. Chavez*, 416 U.S. 562 at 580 (1974); see also *United States v. Giordano*, 416 U.S. 505 (1974).

57. *Nader v. Bork*, 366 F.Supp. 104 (D.D.C. 1973).

58. *Mitchell v. Forsyth*, 105 S.Ct. 2806 (1985).

59. *Murphy v. Ford*, 390 F.Supp. 1372 (W.D.Mich. 1975).

60. Quoted in Merle Fainsod, Lincoln Gordon, and Joseph Palamountain, Jr., *Government and the American Economy*, 3d ed. (New York: W.W. Norton, 1959), p. 260.

61. Daniel J. Fiorino, "Judicial-Administrative Interaction in Regulatory Policy-Making: The Case of the Federal Power Commission," paper presented to American Political Science Association, 1975.

62. R. Shep Melnick, *Regulation and the Courts: The Case of the Clean Air Act* (Washington, D.C.: Brookings Institution, 1983), pp. 87, 114, 185–86, 152.

63. *Charles D. Bonanno Linen Service v. N.L.R.B.*, 454 U.S. 404 at 413 (1982).

64. *Federal Election Commission v. Democratic Senatorial Campaign Committee*, 454 U.S. 27 at 37, 39 (1981).

65. *Renegotiation Board v. Grumman Aircraft*, 421 U.S. 168 (1975); *N.L.R.B. v. Sears, Roebuck*, 421 U.S. 132 (1975); *Department of the Air Force v. Rose*, 425 U.S. 352 (1976); *Chrysler Corp. v. Brown*, 441 U.S. 281 (1979).

66. *Kissinger v. Reporters Committee for Freedom of the Press*, 445 U.S. 136 (1980).

67. *Industrial Union Department v. American Petroleum Institute*, 448 U.S. 607 (1980).

68. Albert R. Matheny and Bruce A. Williams, "Regulation, Risk Assessment, and the Supreme Court: The Case of OSHA's Cancer Policy," *Law & Policy* 6 (October 1984):441–42.

69. *Motor Vehicle Manufacturers Association of the United States v. State Farm Mutual Automobile Insurance Co.*, 463 U.S. 29 (1983).

70. *United States v. Midwest Video Corp.*, 406 U.S. 649 at 676 (1972).

71. *Weinberger v. Hynson, Westcott & Dunning*, 412 U.S. 609 (1973) (drug application); *Citizens to Preserve Overton Park v. Volpe*, 401 U.S. 420 (1971) (interstate highway); *Vermont Yankee Nuclear Power Corp. v. Natural Resources Defense Council*, 435 U.S. 519 (1978) (procedural requirements).

72. Cooper, "Due Process, the Burger Court, and Public Administration," p. 85.

73. Phillip J. Cooper, "Conflict or Constructive Tension: The Changing Relationship of Judges and Administrators," *Public Administration Review* 45 (Special 1985): 643.

74. *American Textile Manufacturers Institute v. Donovan*, 452 U.S. 490 at 523 (1981).

75. *Federal Communications Commission v. WNCN Listeners Guild*, 450 U.S. 582 at 593, 595 (1981).

76. On patent law, see Martin Shapiro, *The Courts and the Administrative Agencies* (New York: Free Press, 1968), pp. 143–226; Lawrence Baum, "The Federal Courts and Patent Validity: An Analysis of the Record," *Journal of the Patent Office Society* 56 (December 1974): 758–87.

77. Joseph Tanenhaus, "Supreme Court Attitudes Toward Federal Administrative Agencies," *Vanderbilt Law Review* 14 (1960–1961): 473–502; Bradley C. Canon and Micheal Giles, "Recurring Litigants: Federal Agencies Before the Supreme Court," *Western Political Quarterly* 25 (June 1972): 183–91; Glendon Schubert, *The Constitutional Polity* (Boston, Mass.: Boston University Press, 1970), pp. 37–38.

78. Jerry L. Mashaw, *Bureaucratic Justice: Managing Social Security Disability Claims* (New Haven, Conn.: Yale University Press, 1983), p. 19.

79. Harold J. Spaeth and Stuart H. Teger, "Activism and Restraint: A Cloak for the Justices' Policy Preferences," in *Supreme Court Activism and Restraint*, eds. Halpern and Lamb, pp. 299, 278–80. See also Harold J. Spaeth and Michael F. Altfeld, "Felix Frankfurter, Judicial Activism, and Voting Conflict on the Warren Court," *Judicial Conflict and Consensus*, eds. Goldman and Lamb, pp. 86–114.

80. Tanenhaus, "Supreme Court Attitudes"; Canon and Giles, "Recurring Litigants," pp. 189–90.

81. Spaeth and Altfeld, "Felix Frankfurter," pp. 98, 104.

82. Spaeth and Teger, "Activism and Restraint," p. 282.

10 The Supreme Court's Impact

THE EXPECTATION OF IMMEDIATE, unbegrudging, and total obedience to the Supreme Court's rulings is widely held, particularly by those who fail to recognize that the Court is an actor in a political system. Compliance receives little attention and noncompliance is newsworthy—a further indication of the expectation that compliance should be the norm and the belief that it is. Recognition of the Court's political role should carry with it an understanding of the inevitability of negative reaction to its rulings, including noncompliance with them, particularly when important constitutional questions are at stake or controversial issues are being decided. Yet abundant hostile rhetoric aimed at the Court's rulings interpreting, sustaining, or overturning federal and state statutes is not always consonant with broader response, and those rulings do produce results. For example, one gets two very different estimates of reaction to the abortion rulings by looking at (a) the hate mail received by Justice Blackmun after he wrote the opinion, demonstrations at the Court against the rulings, and efforts to amend the Constitution to prohibit abortions and (b) public opinion polls, which show increasing support for a woman's right to obtain an abortion, not to mention (c) the increase in the number of abortions performed—even if only part of that increase is attributed to the Court's rulings.[1]

Individually or cumulatively, Supreme Court decisions have had definite impact (effects). Some rulings have produced support and compliance; others have resulted in opposition. Search warrants are now obtained where police would not have bothered to do so earlier; police now give the "*Miranda* warnings.*" Despite such clear effects, because the Court's rulings are often only one of multiple causes of events, it is often difficult to tell whether the Court has produced social change, increased its pace, merely served as a catalyst, or had no effect. Southern schools are desegregated, but it is hard to tell how much as a result of *Brown v. Board of Education* and how much as a result of the statute providing for the cutting off of federal funds to government units that discriminate. Except in the Deep South, changing public opinion, itself a result of World War II, might have led to some change without court rulings, but changed national opinion certainly made it easier for the Court to rule as it did. Before Congress acted, *Brown* itself had not produced much activity except resistance in the Deep South, making it largely a symbolic ruling. However, it served to stimulate the civil rights movement, in part because the movement's "street activists" rejected litigation when the "great victory" of *Brown* produced few tangible results, and parts of the 1964 Civil Rights Act and the subsequent desegregation guidelines issued by the Department of Health, Education and Welfare (HEW) might not have occurred without *Brown*.

Decisions on desegregation and the perhaps even more widely disobeyed school prayer rulings were highly visible and affected many people, average citizens as well as officials. Other rulings, such as those on reapportionment or criminal procedure, have their basic direct effect on government officials, through structural or organizational changes, although changes in policy may ultimately affect citizens. Some effects can be relatively diffuse, as when the Court affects the nation's political agenda by helping focus attention on a subject like abortion. At other times, effects are specific. They may even be limited to a particular industry or individual company, for example, when the Court's 1987 ruling upholding the requirement that Texaco post a bond before it could appeal an adverse multimillion dollar state court ruling against it pushed Texaco closer to seeking bankruptcy protection. That a decision can have both specific and diffuse effects is seen in the increase in the number of abortions obtained and the wide variety of "Right-to-Life" activities following *Roe v. Wade*.

Most decisions have an economic effect. The visibility of that effect may differ. Sometimes it may come through costs imposed, for example, by increasing the number of people eligible for welfare. At other times, the effect may be costs removed, as in the 1976 invalidation of the federal minimum wage for state and local employees. In other situations, economic activity may be limited, as observers suggested would be the effect of the Court's 1987 ruling (*CTS Corp. v. Dynamics Corp. of America*) sustaining state laws limiting takeovers of corporations: "Ebb in Takeovers Foreseen" was a headline at the time.

The imposition of costs tends to attract more attention. This was true recently when Supreme Court rulings allowing antitrust actions against cities led to large damage awards—and to countervailing action (see page 311). It was also true when the Court struck down so-called shared-time provisions under which school districts, with federal funding, had provided parochial schools with some services; concern about parochial schools' ability to fund the remedial programs led to efforts—by and large successful—to delay implementation of the Court's ruling.

The Supreme Court's rulings can have an effect on federalism; some have been said to alter our federal system of government. As Charles Warren stated years ago, "To untrammeled intercourse between its parts, the American union owes its preservation and strength. Two factors have made such intercourse possible—the railroad, physically; the Supreme Court, legally."[2] At times the Court's rulings have affected the bargaining relations between federal and state levels of government. Thus when the Supreme Court ruled that the national government, in setting aside a particular national forest, had not reserved certain uses of river waters, the ruling, which "had the effect of maintaining in state hands title to a potentially valuable and arguably federal resource," "created a potential instrument for state influence upon national forest management."[3]

Because the Fair Labor Standards Act covers all the states, 3,000 counties, 19,000 townships, 15,000 school districts, and 29,000 other special districts, with 7,000,000 full-time employees, the Court's rulings on whether FLSA could be applied to those governmental units had significant effects, perhaps greater at the local than state level, with local governments more financially hurt than state governments, the latter likely to have to assist in resolving the problem.[4] Rulings that local government activities authorized by the state would be exempt from antitrust laws might have led to increased workloads for state legislative and executive agencies engaged in supervision of local governments but that burden was lowered when the Court ruled that active supervision by the states is not required for local governments to be exempt from antitrust attack.[5]

Despite this variety of impacts stemming from the Court's decisions, we must be careful not to attribute to it more power than it may actually have when put to the test, as we do at times in our tendency to make the Court a scapegoat for phenomena like increased crime rates that we cannot easily explain. Measuring impact can be quite difficult. We don't even know whether certain laws or other government actions struck down by the Supreme Court "would have soon fallen at the hands of the political process even without judicial intervention." Separating the effects of Supreme Court rulings from other events, difficult to begin with, becomes more difficult over time, as "the repercussions of all government actions ramify indefinitely and interrelate with other phenomena, both public and private, many of which simply cannot be quantified and indeed often cannot even be identified."[6] Actions we tend to attribute to the Supreme Court may result from other, less visible or less immediate, matters. Thus a decrease in civil liberties is less likely to result from Supreme Court rulings than from war and economic depression or from an event like the mid-1980s panic over cocaine and AIDS. The difficulty of determining impact is perhaps shown well when the Court's rulings are said to have produced opposite or competing effects. For example, the Court's decisions have been said to have produced segregation—or retarded it; to have increased crime—or protected people's rights; to have expanded free speech—or allowed our morals to sink by facilitating the sale of indecent literature. Likewise, the Court helped force a president from office, while increasing the president's power by recognizing executive privilege.

It needs to be recognized that the Court cannot act solely by itself to produce impacts, because it cannot always effectively control the consequences of the policies enunciated in its opinions and must rely on others to implement them, that is, to put them into effect. Put another way, the Supreme Court may make law, or the law may be what the Supreme Court says it is, but *only after all others have had their say.* Whether much will happen even if the rulings are fully communicated to those who should know about them and a serious effort is made to implement them is problematic. While most political controversies do arrive at the Supreme Court, the Court's decision of cases will not end those controversies, which often are far too deep-seated to be ended by a single pronouncement from nine justices.

We begin this chapter with a brief look at some historical instances of impact. This is followed by an examination of the Supreme Court's place in public opinion, both historically and especially in recent years. Then we turn to a discussion of terms like "impact " and "compliance," followed by a detailed look at channels through which decisions might be communicated to those expected to know about and follow them, and at some of the factors that help to explain both communication and impact across different policy areas. We conclude with a more detailed discussion of the Supreme Court's impact concerning church-state relations and criminal procedure. [7]

Impact in History

Supreme Court decisions have produced controversy (one type of impact) and other substantial effects throughout the nation's history, perhaps starting with the Eleventh Amendment, a direct and immediate result of *Chisholm v. Georgia* (1793), allowing a suit against a state. The growth of a national economy was aided by Chief Justice Marshall's broad interpretation of national government power, for example, in sustaining the National Bank against state efforts to tax it (*McCulloch v. Maryland,* 1819) and of commerce when striking down a state steamboat monopoly in *Gibbons v. Ogden* (1824). The economy was also affected by the *Dartmouth College* case (1819) on the sanctity of contracts, which states could not abridge, and the *Charles River Bridge* case (1837), allowing establishment of competing transportation companies.

The Court has also had long-term effects on American federalism, particularly when the states as states resisted national supremacy. In the controversy over the fugitive slave laws, the Court ruled that Congress' jurisdiction over fugitive slaves was exclusive, with a federal statute on the subject preempting conflicting state law, and the Court also denied a state court the authority to order federal officials to commit an act in conflict with a federal court decision.[8] Indeed, conflict has been quite likely whenever the Court has ruled that federal activity prevents the states from taking action.

Another important ruling on federalism that stirred the anger of those supporting "states' rights" was the 1920 decision in *Missouri v. Holland* that a federal treaty (with Canada) concerning migratory waterfowl supplanted Missouri's hunting regulations. The Court's statement that in implementing a treaty the national government could go beyond the constitutional powers it would have in the treaty's absence led to later attempts to amend the Constitution to limit the president's treaty-making power.

One of the most important instances of impact was *Dred Scott*. By saying that Congress could not limit slavery in the states, the Court destroyed congressional compromise. The decision had a number of other impacts, one of which is said to have been that the Court badly damaged itself. However, the extent to which the ruling "undermined the Court as an institution has in fact been greatly exaggerated." Those opposed to the decision wanted to change the Court's membership (and decisions) but "not its structure and functions"; moreover, "hostility to the Supreme Court as a whole . . . was confined to a small though at times highly vocal minority."[9] As is often the case, "the response to the decision proved to be much more important than its direct legal effect." Because of the Civil War itself, the expansion of slavery permitted by the decision did not occur; the owner of the slave whose freedom the Court had denied manumitted him (set him free). However, by legitimating the South's proslavery argument, thus increasing its confidence and making it more inflexible, and by increasing Northern hostility to the *South* (instead of to slavery as such), "as a public event, the decision aggravated an already bitter sectional conflict and to some degree determined the shape of the final crisis."[10]

As these few historical instances indicate, the Court not infrequently has created adverse reaction on questions bearing on the structure of the federal system, "particularly when it has validated exertions of national power against the plaint of states' rights," perhaps thus helping create enemies willing to join those "who oppose judicial activism in defense of personal liberties"[11]—the area in which most recent noncompliance has occurred.

The Supreme Court and Public Opinion

One effect of the Supreme Court's decisions is opinions about them, whether held by newspaper publishers, political elites, members of the "attentive public," and "average citizens." Public opinion about the Court itself, for example, the confidence that people express in it, is both another impact of the Court's decisions and a more general reflection of the impact of the Court's individual rulings. A large part of the opinion about the Court reported in the media is criticism of the Court; one only infrequently hears general support for the Court, although some of its decisions may be defended. Political campaigns for more than 20 years have included criticism of the Supreme Court, most notably starting with George Wallace's and then Richard Nixon's "law and order" campaigns with their attacks on the Warren Court's criminal procedure rulings (indeed, Republican candidates since Goldwater in 1964 have run against Earl Warren). Ronald Reagan openly criticized particular decisions. Most recently, potential Republican candidate Pat Robertson took a broad swing at the Court's very position in our system, saying that its rulings were "not the law of the land." If such attacks attract attention—and themselves potentially affect public opinion about the Court—what do we know about public opinion with respect to the justices and their Court?

In this section, we examine a number of aspects of that subject. After treatment of editorial reaction to some of the Court's major rulings, we turn to extended treatment of public opinion polls—both those of the general public and more specialized and focused surveys. Through such polls, we examine the Court's overall rating in the eyes of the public, the public's confidence in the Court, and public reaction to specific decisions. We also can learn the extent to which people have information about the Court on which their opinions might be based; their belief (or disbelief) in the "myth" that the Court finds rather than makes the law; and elements—apart from information—that underlie the extent of their general and specific support of the Court.

Early History and Editorial Reaction

The Supreme Court's decisions produced effects on public opinion long before the days of public opinion polls. Public reaction to the decisions was often mixed. When the Court invalidated state fugitive slave statutes, "the decision was equally unsatisfactory to both pro-slavery and anti-slavery men" because the former were upset at the blow to states' rights and the latter, who disliked the federal fugitive slave law, thought the Court was backing the South. [12] The Court also suffered in the public eye when, shortly after being enlarged and only a year after it had held in the first Legal Tender Case that the Union government could not require that debts made before the passage of the Legal Tender Act be paid in paper money, it reversed itself. Although the legal community felt that the Legal Tender Act was constitutional, the reopening of the case was "a mistake which for many years impaired the people's confidence, not in the honesty, but in the impartiality and good sense of the Court." [13]

In the New Deal period, divided reaction was again evident. When the Court invalidated the National Industrial Recovery Act, "the more conservative sections of the press welcomed it as putting an end to unsound experiments in government regulation of industry," labor opposed the decision, and the business community was divided. [14] However, more and more elements of the public were alienated by the Court's continued striking down of New Deal legislation, and "each new adverse decision in the winter and spring of 1936 brought new bursts of hostility." [15] The farmers were upset about invalidation of the Agricultural

Adjustment Act, the voiding of the Bituminous Coal Act irritated workers, and the minimum wage rulings "alienated nearly everybody"—including supporters of earlier decisions. Only 10 of 344 editorials approved the decision on the minimum wage, with some 60 papers, including a number of conservative ones, calling for a constitutional amendment on the subject.

Editorial reaction to decisions is one measure, although an indirect one, of public opinion, and it has thus received some attention. Twenty-four large-circulation newspapers generally favored separation of church and state after three of four major Supreme Court church-state decisions; the exception was the *Zorach* ruling upholding New York's released time program, which the papers favored. The *McCollum* ruling striking down religious classes on school property was the most favorably received (eight papers favoring and two opposing), with editorials on the school prayer case closely divided (13 favoring, nine opposing). Support for the released time ruling may have resulted from that program's milder link between church and state, more conservative public attitudes toward civil liberties in 1952, liberal Justice Douglas' authorship of the Court's opinion, and the general tendency of newspapers to support the Court. Newspapers' editorial positions on church-state matters were affected by a city's political climate (the more Democrats, the more likely a paper to favor church-state separation), the publisher's politics (same relationship, but stronger), and the publisher's religion (higher support for the Court if Catholic or Episcopalian).[16] Later the Court showed it could still obtain general support from editorial writers for leading daily newspapers. Although majorities of the editorial writers opposed the school prayer ruling and one of the major aid-to-parochial school cases (*Wolman v. Walter*, 1977), otherwise either a plurality or majority of them approved of most of 11 leading church-state cases.[17]

Despite public outcry in some circles about the Court's rulings on race relations, in 17 cases a majority of the editorial writers for the major daily newspapers approved of the decisions, and a plurality approved of all the others but one. Indeed, their only disagreement came when the Supreme Court avoided a decision—by declaring moot the first affirmative action case it accepted for review (*DeFunis v. Odegaard*, 1974). For subsequent affirmative action cases, a plurality approved of each, with editorial confusion evident in the responses to the *Bakke* ruling, in which the Court was severely divided.[18] Editorials on race relations cases could not be explained in terms of partisan affiliation of the papers, but such partisanship did serve to explain reactions on defendants' rights, where "responses . . . are much more 'bipolar' than responses to race cases."[19]

More in line with general public opinion was the editorial and cartoon reaction of 63 papers of a wider range of circulation. Opposition to the school prayer ruling was stronger in those papers in the upper Midwest, with more Southern papers neutral or favorable. Editorial reaction among these same papers to the Court's first reapportionment decision was generally favorable, and the papers' editorial position affected news coverage: those supporting the Court presented a more restrained account of the Court's rulings in both headlines and reportage of critical reaction to the decision than did papers opposing the decision.[20]

Public Opinion Polls

Despite the frequency with which public opinion polls on a wide variety of topics appear, no unified statement about public opinion about the Supreme Court has yet been developed. We can, however, provide a basic picture from scattered items in the Gallup and Harris surveys and from more intensive studies conducted by political scientists.

In the 1960s, national polling organizations began to ask how people rated the Supreme Court. Overall ratings remained fairly constant in the mid-1960s. A November 1966 Harris Poll showed the public giving the Court an overall negative rating (46%–54%). Younger people, the better educated, and blacks backed the Court, while southerners, older people, and the less well educated were the Court's severest critics. Similar results appear in a 1967 Gallup Poll. The Court's work was rated excellent by 15 percent, good by 30 percent, fair by 29 percent, and poor by 17 percent, resulting in an almost even balance between favorable and unfavorable reactions. The June 1968 Gallup Poll rating showed how quickly opinion can change. Evaluations had shifted to 36 percent favorable, 53 percent unfavorable, with only 8 percent rating the Court's work as excellent. Republicans were most critical of the Court, and those with less than a college education were also negative; Democrats and those with a college education were evenly divided.

Although the Burger Court's criminal procedure rulings were more in tune with public opinion, they did not produce an improvement in the Court's overall rating. The Court received only a slightly higher Gallup Poll rating in 1973 than it had received in 1969—a rating much lower than the Court's mid-1960s ratings. In 1973, 37 percent rated the Court's work good or excellent, but only 6 percent rated it excellent. Thirty-five percent thought the Court too *liberal*, while 26 percent thought it too conservative. Who liked the Court had also changed. Decreased approval of the Court was shown by the college educated, those 21 to 29 years old (who showed the greatest drop), westerners and easterners, and Democrats, but ratings were up among those age 50 and over, southerners, and Republicans (up 12%).[21] A 1986 *New York Times*/CBS News poll found 46 percent rating the Court's work as either excellent (7%) or good (39%), considerably higher than the 37 percent Gallup Poll figure of 13 years earlier and even marginally higher than the 43 percent Gallup figure of 25 years before; nonetheless, more rated the Court fair or poor than rated it good or excellent. More of those who said in 1986 that the Court was conservative approved the Court's work than did those who said it was too liberal.

Polls also show shifts in the public's confidence in the Court as an institution. A 1966 Harris Poll majority (51%) expressed a great deal of confidence in the Court—almost 10 percent more than did so for either Congress or the executive branch but less than for medicine, colleges, or the military. A related finding came in a 1967 Gallup Poll, which indicated that almost half the public thought the Court had been impartial, but 30 percent—particularly older citizens, Republicans, and southerners—believed the judges showed favoritism toward some groups.

An indication of the extent of variation in the public's confidence in the Court can be seen from 1972 poll results showing only 21 percent of Harris Poll respondents expressing a great deal of confidence in the Court. Although confidence in the Court rose from 1972 through 1974 (to 40% expressing a great deal of confidence), it dropped substantially—back to 22 percent in 1976. It then rebounded to 31 percent in early 1978. By 1984, the figure was roughly the same. In general, the proportion of the public expressing confidence in the Court was higher than the proportion expressing confidence in other government institutions, and when confidence began to increase from its low point, the Supreme Court registered larger gains than did Congress or the president, an indication that the Court's place in public opinion, although partly a function of confidence in all government institutions, is to some extent independent of the public's view of those institutions. Yet confidence in the Court was responsive "to the happenstances of political events" such as Watergate and President Nixon's resignation and to inflation (although bad economic times had little effect). Of particular interest, given public attention to the Court's criminal procedure rulings, is that increases in the FBI's crime index had no effect on the public's view of the Court. However, the Court's decisions favoring criminal defendants did cause the public to lose confidence in the Court.[22]

Another indication of the Court's position in public opinion is the 1975 Harris survey finding that 38 percent of the respondents felt that those in charge of the Supreme Court "really know what most people they represent or serve think and want," somewhat better than Congress, the White House, or the executive branch. However, more—43 percent—said the Court was out of touch with those it served, and 19 percent did not know, higher than for any other institution. By 1977, the percent saying the Supreme Court was "mostly out of touch" had risen to 47 percent. In 1981, only 17 percent of those polled said the Supreme Court had too much power, with more than twice that proportion (39%) saying the Court was carrying out proper responsibilities.

In addition to their general evaluation of the Court, the public expressed reaction to specific decisions. Thus the 1966 Harris survey showed the public, despite its overall negative rating of the Court, favoring rulings on reapportionment (76%–24%) and desegregation of schools and public accommodations (both 64%–36%). Only reapportionment received approval in the South, where only 44 percent of the public supported school desegregation. Opinion was evenly divided on the Court's having forbidden the State Department to deny passports to Communists, but the school prayer and *Miranda* rulings were disliked (30%–70% and 35%–65%). A 1973 Gallup Poll revealed that 58 percent favored the Burger Court's conservative ruling on obscenity, but roughly the same percentage disapproved of the Court's 1972 invalidation of the death penalty. (President Nixon's appointees, who had dissented, were closer to public opinion.) The rulings denying news reporters a First Amendment right to protect confidential sources and invalidating aid to parochial schools were also opposed by majorities of those questioned. Recent polls reveal potentially conflicting findings. In early 1981, 74 percent of the public opposed busing their children to another part of town for desegregation, but a year later, a majority opposed a federal law prohibiting the Department of Justice and federal courts from ordering school busing to achieve racial balance.

When we look at instances where the public was asked about a particular issue before and after a relevant Supreme Court ruling, we find no clear pattern of Supreme Court effects: in some instances, the shift was positive, in some instances negative, but the "shifts very nearly balanced out," leaving as an average "very nearly a zero shift." When the Court decided a case with full opinion, the public was more likely to move toward the Court's position, as it was when it overturned the law or policy challenged in the Court, and when noneconomic issues were before the justices; if all three factors occurred in the same case, the shift in public opinion in the direction of the Court's position would be roughly 15 percent.[23]

The opinions of those in the legal community might be thought to be particularly important because of the possibility that lawyers might be able to affect the opinions of average citizens. Although at the present time, the American Bar Association, the lawyers' principal national organization (although containing far fewer than half the nation's attorneys), generally supports the Court, that has not always been the case. Indeed, the ABA's unwillingness to back the Court against its critics during the early Warren Court—the period of liberal internal security rulings and of desegregation—and reports by ABA committees criticizing the Court's controversial decisions led Chief Justice Warren to resign his ABA membership.[24] An intensive survey that showed lawyers in a specific community more dissatisfied with the Court than was the Gallup Poll's national sample of the same time was a 1970 poll of Providence, Rhode Island, lawyers. They were also more undecided than the national sample's college-educated and business and professional groups, with their indecision coming from indifference rather than ambivalence. The criminal procedure decisions seemed most important for the lawyers who criticized the Court; they tended to hold a "traditional" attitude toward the Court—including the idea that the Court only finds law—and wanted "strict constructionist" judges. Those favoring the Warren Court were more likely to approve of judges engaging in lawmaking.[25]

In 1967, four-fifths of the police officers in four medium-sized Wisconsin cities disapproved of *Miranda*. There was no relationship between attitude and amount of formal education, but those with least police experience approved of the decision the least.[26] Five years later, Illinois and Massachusetts small-town police chiefs did not show this same resistance to *Miranda*, as most officers had learned to live with the ruling. However, although Massachusetts officers generally favored the (*Mapp*) rule excluding illegally seized evidence from trials, it was hard to find an Illinois officer who could say anything good about that doctrine. The chiefs' views were not related to their formal education, but those who had had law enforcement training before becoming officers were somewhat more likely to view the rule positively. A study of officers in 29 St. Louis area police departments carried out at the same time, however, showed weak relationships between training and attitudes.[27]

More than three of four federal judges, state supreme court judges, and lawyers responding in early 1977 to a *U.S. News & World Report* survey preferred the Burger Court to the Warren Court. Although two-fifths thought the Court was still taking questions the respondents felt better left to the legislative or executive branches of government, 84.2 percent thought the Burger Court less likely to do so than the Warren Court, and only 2.4 percent thought the Burger Court *more* likely to do so. Over half of those in the poll approved of the Court's making it more difficult for citizens to use the federal courts to obtain redress of grievances and just under half (48.4%) said that the Court *was* making it more difficult. A majority of those surveyed approved of the Burger Court's decisions and direction in all areas except obscenity and pornography.

More Extensive Surveys

These polls do not provide information about the public's knowledge of the Court or reveal deeper orientations toward it. Detailed local, state, and national surveys indicate low levels of knowledge, broad general support, and low specific support.

Information. The public generally lacks knowledge about the legal system; lack of specific knowledge about the Supreme Court is part of that pattern. One small instance is that in July 1986, when the nominations of Justice Rehnquist to be Chief Justice and of Judge Scalia to be an associate justice were pending, only 26 percent of those questioned could identify Rehnquist as a Supreme Court justice and only 16 percent could identify Scalia as a Supreme Court nominee.[28] For all the attention given to cases in the media, "only a few cases are sufficiently dramatic to rise above the public's threshold of attention."[30] This is clear from a 1965 survey of Seattle residents and from respondents' inability in 1964 and 1966 University of Michigan Survey Research Center (SRC) national postelection surveys to name good or bad things the Court had done and their attribution to the Court of cases it had *not* decided. It is also clear from the fact that one-fourth of a 1968 Missouri sample declined to comment on the Court or pleaded ignorance. In a 1966 Wisconsin survey test of knowledge about decisions, only 2 percent of respondents had all items correct and only 15 percent had more than half correct; 12 percent had every answer wrong. This lack of awareness extended even to criminal procedure decisions about which there had been open controversy and to reapportionment despite redistricting in the state, indicating that people have difficulty relating decisions to their personal lives.[30] Less than half (45.2%) of those in the 1964/1966 national SRC survey could name any Supreme Court decision they liked or disliked, although by 1975 over 60 percent of those in the same sample who had been located indicated specific knowledge of Supreme Court decisons. Despite this improvement, in both years less than half could answer open-ended questions about specific likes and dislikes.[31]

By comparison, more than three-fourths of the attentive public (those generally better informed about public events) could indicate specific likes and dislikes among Supreme Court rulings. Elite groups—congressional administrative assistants and Princeton students—had still higher recall levels: 86 percent could name a recent Supreme Court policy they liked or disliked; not surprisingly, 99 percent of lawyers could do so.[32] Similar differences between the general population and those politically active were evident in a 1976 Wisconsin survey. Overall, only one-third could identify a Supreme Court decision; over half of those politically active had such knowledge, while only one-fourth of the inactives did. Yet only slightly more than one-fifth of the activists identified more than one subject on which the Court had ruled, support for the proposition that likes and dislikes about the Court are based on limited aspects of the Court's work.[33]

School prayer rulings have been among the most salient of the Court's decisions and, along with civil rights rulings, account for more than two-thirds of the 1964 likes and dislikes about the Court; by 1966 most likes and dislikes were accounted for by criminal procedure decisions, indicating volatility in the public's views. In the 1975 reinterviews, references to schoool prayer had decreased but other issue-areas salient in 1966 (civil rights, school prayer, criminal defendants' rights) were still salient; specific references to capital punishment (on which the Court had begun to rule in 1972) had increased. The school prayer decisions were "unknown only to the same seemingly irreducible number of persons who have managed to remain unaware of the segregation decisions."[34] However, because some in the Missouri survey who did not read newspapers knew of at least one Court decision, it appears that "issues which gain the court renown (or notoriety) are so salient that they come through even to people virtually isolated from the printed word."[35]

Support. What about support for the Court's actions? A recent summary suggests, "There is . . . little evidence of widespread public support for the justices' specific decisions; and the Court does not appear to command sweeping generalized approval."[36] In the earlier national surveys, those giving the Court diffuse (general) support outnumbered four-to-one those giving it specific support (that based on particular decisions). Only about 20 percent were negative as to diffuse support, but one-third were negative on specific support; moreover, almost three times as many people named only decisions they *dis*liked as named only those they liked.

Putting together the data on general support and that on specific support shows that some of those opposing particular decisions provided general support, as did some of those least knowledgeable about the Court—who also seemed most trusting of government. Among 1966 SRC respondents reinterviewed in 1975, support for the Court decreased, on almost every measure, although by modest amounts, so that support levels, overall, were not substantially different from 1966 levels: "In the aggregate, diffuse support for the Supreme Court, despite tremors that shook the entire political system, proved comfortingly resilient."[37] This is further evidence for the view that "public orientations toward courts apparently change slowly over time if at all, as decisions and popular policy preferences (and other factors) interact."[38] Such interaction is evident in the responses to civil rights matters, particularly busing, where from 1966 to 1975 we find the proportion of negative mentions had increased, with the proportion of positive references decreasing by an even greater amount (from 46.5% to 25.8%); far higher proportions of whites than blacks oppose busing, but not all blacks support it.

Explaining Support. What explains support for the Court? Higher knowledge about the Court has regularly seemed to correlate with greater *dis*approval of the Court, although the relationship might be complex. For example, a person's support for procedural rights might affect what that person heard and read about the Court, which in turn would affect support for the Court. Level of knowledge of the Court and race are related, affecting blacks' support for the Court. The 1966 SRC survey showed a majority of blacks to be among those unaware of even the desegregation decisions. Waterloo, Iowa, surveys in 1970 produced similar results: for 49 percent of blacks but only 32 percent of whites, the Supreme Court "as a regime institution is not salient."[39] A 1975 survey of students at Kentucky universities showed that blacks attributed more legitimacy to the Supreme Court than did whites but were more likely to be found in the midrange of support for the Court than were whites, a result of blacks' having less knowledge about the Court's decisions. Whites, aware of more decisions, favored and disfavored them about equally.[40]

What about partisanship and ideology? Degree of political activity seems to correlate with support. Wisconsin activists indicated opposition to most major Supreme Court decisions but nonetheless provided higher levels of specific support than those politically inactive.[41] Political party identification affected attitudes toward the Court in some but not all surveys; in some situations, the relationship was indirect, for example, being a Democrat influenced what one heard, affecting current attitudes. In the 1966 Wisconsin survey, approval of the president and approval of the Court were positively related regardless of one's party, but part of Republicans' unhappiness with the Court seemed to stem from

Democratic control of the White House.[42] However, 1975 SRC reinterviews produced no evidence that the public evaluated the Court in terms of who was president, and, more important, showed party identification "useless in explaining change in diffuse support."[43] Among those surveyed in Wisconsin in 1976, among the politically inactive the level of hostility exceeded 80 percent for both Republicans and Democrats, with Republicans somewhat more hostile. Differences between Democrat and Republican activists were much greater, with the Democrats far more favorable to the Court's decisions (59.3%–39.5%).[44]

Respondents' attitudes (liberal/conservative) best explained support for the Court in the SRC national surveys. Congruence between liberals' political positions and the Warren Court's decisions meant that liberals gave the Court more support at that time. Strong effects of ideology also appeared in the 1976 Wisconsin survey. Although activists supported the Court much more strongly than inactives, it was the combination of liberalism *and* activism, not activism alone, that operated to provide strong commitment to the Court.[45]

Related to diffuse and specific support is public belief in the myth that the Court is a legal rather than a political body. Less than 10 percent of the Missouri sample associated the Court directly with the Constitution, although respondents' references to constitutionality increased the proportion to one-sixth. Just under one-third referred to law and a similar proportion to courtlike functions. Although 60 percent saw the Court in terms of symbols and beliefs, less than half the comments (46.7%) contained positive symbols regarded as legitimators of the Court's authority. In less than one-fourth of all responses was the Court seen primarily as a political institution. This led to the conclusion that "the Court's myth enjoys widespread diffusion," although members of the public were not fully dependent on external symbols to legitimate their belief in the Court. Particularly important is that education *increased* rather than reduced belief in the myth: those who did not believe in the myth were not more politically sophisticated but actually were less well socialized into prevailing norms.[46] Similarly, in the 1975 survey in Kentucky universities, whites, who "exhibited a greater mythical belief" than did blacks, and those from higher status families "seem to accept conventional political values and attribute fine qualities to the Court" more than blacks and lower-status whites.[47] The continuing strong hold of myth is also shown in the 1976 Wisconsin survey: although one-half the respondents held a "realist" perspective, one-third were classified as myth holders, with a higher proportion among the more politically active. What the picture would be today is not known, but a book like *The Brethren*, revealing as it did—to a large audience—the inner workings of the Court and the bargaining and compromise that takes place there, might well lead to a decreased belief in the myth of lawmaking, particularly among those of higher education, who would have been more likely to have read at least parts of the book.[48]

A question following from people's myth-holding, related to functions thought appropriate for the Court to perform, is whether people can think it proper for the Court to produce changes in governmental structure or process, such as those required by the reapportionment decisions, that is, whether the Court could "legitimate regime change." A Supreme Court ruling can perform such a function only for those who satisfy three conditions: they must perceive, that is, be aware of, the Court, recognize that it may properly interpret and apply the Constitution, and feel that the Court was acting competently and impartially. According to the 1964/1966 surveys, 40 percent satisfied neither of the first two conditions, while roughly one-fourth satisfied both; only about one-eighth satisfied all three. Ten years later, asked to indicate their preference as to whether Congress or the Supreme Court should resolve disagreements over national policy, more Wisconsinites chose Congress (40.4%–35.3% overall), although the politically active chose the Court by a 6-5 ratio. Perhaps a reflection of Watergate, far more respondents picked the Court over the president (54.2%—19.4%); activists were even more likely to choose the Court.[49]

Action from Opposition? If we wish to know more fully about the Court's place in public opinion, we need to know whether those opposed to the Court will act on their beliefs. Those who think the Court's performance is poor are "most likely to act to change a decision" but "they are neither numerous nor particularly rebelliously inclined."[50] In Wisconsin only a few of those who said they would do something to change a Supreme Court decision they disliked would try to develop further opposition to those decisions among the public. Half would work through members of Congress, and another one-fourth would "act within the established legal processes." Virtually no Illinois or Massachusetts small-town police chiefs said they would refuse to go along with a court ruling. Over half the Illinois officers said, however, that they would do something about a decision they disliked, but for most, this was only to talk about the disliked decisions, complain, and "gripe." In Massachusetts, most spoke of writing to the authorities, including their commanding officers or other chiefs, in order to express their opinions, while a couple would have acted through the legal system.

These responses lead to the remark made about the Wisconsin sample: "This is quiescence indeed" and to the conclusion that "the decisions of the Supreme Court have had more effect on the reputation of the Court than the activities of its antagonists."[51] Yet we have seen repeated attacks on the Court, from the conservative end of the political spectrum, in the 1970s and 1980s. More specifically, the Court's abortion ruling produced clear, even violent, opposition; the ruling aroused Right-to-Life groups and propelled them into politics. (In somewhat the same way, the Court's school prayer rulings helped to arouse religious fundamentalists and to stimulate their entrance into political activity.) There were annual demonstrations, on the anniversary of *Roe v. Wade*, aimed at the decision; interference with those seeking to enter abortion clinics; and even bombings of clinics where abortions took place. Continued legislative efforts to overturn the abortion rulings also demonstrated that those opposing a ruling could indeed become active. (In response, those supporting a "pro-choice" position realized that they had to demonstrate in support of the ruling—and to get those who had had abortions to come forward to speak out in favor of the Court's action.)

What protects the Court if such active opposition—generally restricted to a few rulings—does occur? A distinct possibility is "the complex interaction between ideological activists, ideological elites, the nation's institutional and structural arrangements, and the character of dominant political majorities in the United States."[52] Liberal activists provide support for the Court. That support reinforces liberal officeholders' will to resist attacks and to use the complexity of the policymaking process (such as the number of points that a proposed statute or constitutional amendment must "clear") to delay and defuse opposition attacks. The requirement of extraordinary legislative majorities and strong executive support to enact anti-Court policy works to liberals' advantage as they seek to protect the Court, evident in the 1982 filibusters by liberal senators against school prayer and abortion measures.

Impact and Compliance

The terms *impact* and *compliance* are both used to refer to effects of Supreme Court rulings, but they do not have the same meaning.[53] *Compliance* may mean several things. One can distinguish between impact and compliance by saying that impact stands for the consequences of a policy—including but not limited to compliance—while compliance refers to the process, which occurs prior to impact, by which individuals accept decisions, although the process by which decisions are enforced can also be referred to as *implementation*. Or one can define compliance differently, saying that a person cannot comply with a law unless that person knows of its existence. In this definiton, compliance is obedience to a ruling *because* of that ruling, particularly when a person through either opposition or neutrality did not previously intend to take the action required by the decision. One *can* say that a person is compliant when the person's behavior is parallel to, or in *conformity* with, the requirements of the Court's ruling— when the person would, in any event, have done what the Court requires—but that weakens the meaning of compliance; at best one can say the person is *not noncompliant*. One can further distinguish between "acceptance decisions," involving changes (or nonchanges) in attitude, and "behavioral responses," involving changes (or maintenance of) policies.[54]

Compliance is relevant when decisions *demand* or *require* certain actions; other *permissive* decisions *allow* governments or private actors to take certain actions, called *adopting* behavior. With the latter, because no one is required to do anything, there can be no noncompliance. Thus, after the Court, in *Ginsberg v. New York* (1968), upheld New York's statute prohibiting the sale to children of materials "harmful" (a standard less strict than "obscene") to them, several states adopted that type of statute. Cases on jury size and unanimity are other examples of permissive decisions: when the Court ruled that state noncapital criminal juries could be smaller than 12 people (*Williams v. Florida*, 1970) and nonunanimous (*Johnson v. Louisiana*, 1972), the Court was saying only that nonunanimous juries and juries of less than 12 were acceptable, not that they were required, so a state retaining unanimous, 12-person juries was *not* disobedient.

Even when part of a ruling is mandatory, some implications may be permissive, leaving certain actions optional. For example, *Roe v. Wade* told states to stop criminalizing abortions, at least during the first trimester of pregnancy if the woman and her doctor thought an abortion appropriate, and placed strict limits on regulation of abortions during the second trimester. Because the Court did not order doctors or hospitals to participate in abortions, on this score the ruling was permissive for hospitals. Nonetheless, the decision "appears to have had a substantial impact on hospital abortion policies," with almost half changing their policy. Most expanded abortion services to include elective as well as therapeutic abortions, with a smaller number changing from no abortion services to providing elective abortions. [55]

Determining what is compliant is difficult, but there is little question that noncompliance exists. By any standard, some resistance is obvious, for example, Virginia's plan of Massive Resistance to school desegregation and its closing of schools in Prince Edward County. Other types of resistance, such as attempts to override the Court by constitutional amendment, may be accompanied by some limited compliant behavior. This mix of compliant and defiant behavior, which when combined appears to fall between outright defiance and full acceptance, is one type of *evasion*. Evasion also occurs when the Court's ruling is accepted, but only literally and narrowly while other ways are sought to achieve goals with which the ruling has interfered. For example, after the Court said in 1917 that whites could not enact laws to prevent blacks from residing in particular neighborhoods (*Buchanan v. Warley*), they developed private racially restrictive covenants and enforced those covenants in state courts. Another type of evasion is the misapplication of Supreme Court standards or the substitution of other standards for the Court's, particularly when those doing so (for example, state supreme court judges in establishment of religion cases) do "not admit their noncompliance but rather attempt to portray their decisions as consistent with previous Court decisions and the standards enumerated in them."[56] When those affected move only a small distance from invalidated statutes, evasion is close to disobedience. Many statutes enacted after the 1973 abortion ruling, particularly those that outlawed the use of saline solution for abortions and thus interfered with medical decisions, fell in this category.

Impact includes all effects resulting from a decision regardless of whether people knew about the decision. There may, of course, be situations of "nonimpact" in which nothing happens. For example, after the Court ruled that states may block construction of nuclear power plants, there was no apparent effect on construction. And, five years after the *Bakke* affirmative action ruling, there appeared to be little effect one way or the other in the proportion of minority students in college or professional school—although effects of the ruling could have been offset by other phenomena. In another instance, after the Court upheld Illinois' "group libel" statute prohibiting unfavorable references to minority racial or religious groups (*Beauharnais v. Illinois,* 1952), no other states adopted a similar statute. More recently, when the Court in *Cox Broadcasting Co. v. Cohn* (1975) allowed the use of the name of a rape victim by the media if that name was in public court records, newspapers for the greatest part continued to adhere to the older ethic of not reporting the name: nothing much changed as a result of the decision.

Impact may well begin *before* the Court hands down a decision, perhaps even before litigation commences, as a controversy produces a series of effects on those involved. Impacts may also be unintended, such as extra work for federal district judges as a result of new standards for deciding habeas corpus petitions; "white flight" after desegregation rulings; or a complete stop in the building of public housing in Chicago after the Court in *Hills v. Gautreaux* (1976) ordered desegregation of public housing in the Chicago area.

Impact includes a wide variety of behaviors. When a statute from one state is struck down, officials elsewhere may reexamine their own laws to determine whether they remain valid. This is part of the Court's ability to affect others' *agendas*: a Supreme Court ruling may well force legislative, or executive, attention to issues that had been ignored or neglected. *Brown v. Board of Education* certainly placed school desegregation on the agenda of school boards and state legislatures, and *Reynolds v. Sims* forced legislatures to deal with reapportionment, just as the recent *Davis v. Bandemer* (1986) ruling on partisan gerrymandering will prompt greater attention to districting.

If, after a Court ruling, it is not clear whether statutes or regulations differ in significant particulars from those on which the justices have ruled, uncertainty will result, as it does when the Court's ruling is not comprehensive and thus does not encompass laws elsewhere. For example, when the Court ruled in the 1982 *Rowley* case that a school district did not have to provide a sign language interpreter for a deaf fourth-grade child, school administrators were unsure what services school districts would have to provide to handicapped children. An important element of uncertainty is fear of litigation.

Fears of a Court ruling's effects, which are often highest immediately after the decision, may be shown to have been exaggerated and to have resulted from claims made in defending the challenged action. For example, fears that the Court's ruling requiring Texas school districts to provide tuition-free education for children of illegal aliens (*Plyler v. Doe,* 1982) would result in substantial enrollment increases were not borne out at the beginning of the 1982–83 school year. Similarly, when the Court ruled in *Baxstrom v. Herold* (1966) that prisoners could not be retained in an institution for the criminally insane beyond the end of their maximum prison sentence unless they were provided a hearing to determine their dangerousness, the state feared that dangerous individuals would create violence in mental hospitals outside the prison system or would be assaultive if released into the community. Again, none of these fears was borne out: levels of violence in civilian mental hospitals were less than expected, and there was less assaultive behavior, both there and "outside," than expected.[57]

There are both first-order and second-order impacts, which parallel the distinction between impact and outcomes. For example, the *impact* of a judicial ruling ordering desegregation would include not only immediate resistance to or acceptance of the decision but also the actual desegregation of schools. Second-order impact or *outcomes* would include desegregation's effect on children's education, including increased disciplinary action against black children; removal of black teachers and administrators; and population movement, such as "white flight" to the suburbs. If the impact of reapportionment is redrawn legislative districts and increased numbers of minority legislators, outcomes would include public policy changes enacted by the newly constituted legislature, such as increased welfare benefits or general state expenditures that were not as substantial as some anticipated.[58] If the impact of the Court's 1973 abortion ruling was invalidation of most criminal abortion statutes and changes in hospital policy, outcomes included a substantial increase in abortions: the Court's ruling did not command but only facilitated abortions for women desiring them.

This range of impacts involves several relevant "populations": an "interpreting population," usually a lower court, that refines—makes clearer—the higher court's policy; an "implementing population" that applies the Court's basic policy directive; a "consumer population" for whom the directive was intended and to whom it is applied; and a "secondary population." This last group includes the general population not included in the consumer population—for example, for school desegregation, perhaps those without children in school, as well as both governmental and nongovernmental "attentive publics"—those interested in but not directly involved in the particular policy and its implementation.[59]

Not only are several populations involved, but to get a full picture of impact one must look at both short-term and long-term effects of cases and at the effects of *sets* (or a "line" of) decisions in a policy area. Thus to determine impact in the criminal justice area, we would not look only at *Mapp* or *Miranda* but at the whole set of rulings "nationalizing" defendants' rights, which as one effect led state court judges to master federal law. Looked at this way, impact involves not only one-way effects of Court on relevant populations but also feedback, the transmission of reactions back to the Court, in short, reciprocal interaction over time between the Supreme Court, lower courts, legislatures, and executive branch agencies. An important part of feedback is *anticipatory compliance*, in which lower courts, in an example of interlevel interaction, see the direction in which the Supreme Court is heading and hand down rulings that take the law beyond the last Supreme Court decision, with the Court then adopting this forward movement as its own. Evidence of this behavior is quite clear in libel law where the Supreme Court itself invited lower courts to extend the test it had developed in *New York Times v. Sullivan* (1964), limiting public officials' ability to obtain libel judgments.[60]

Communication of Decisions

Communication and response or impact are intimately related. In some instances, people may not know much about the actual outcomes that result from the Court's rulings but may respond to the Court because of effects the media have attributed to a decision. Those expected to respond to a decision cannot do so if they do not learn of the ruling. If they receive an incomplete or otherwise distorted version of the ruling, their response may diverge from what the Court anticipated. Because compliance or impact will vary even if justices' opinions come through "loud and clear," communication and compliance are related but communication does not control compliance. The means by which decisions—or information about them—are communicated are quite important, particularly because few among those who might be affected by rulings—whether police affected by criminal procedure decisions or booksellers by decisions on the meaning of "obscenity"—seek out that information. Thus it must be brought to them if they are to obtain it.

Only a "small minority" of booksellers questioned in one multistate survey knew about the Supreme Court's obscenity decisions, and only 3 percent of those responding sought legal advice on more than "isolated occasions" about sexually explicit books they sold. In a study of 18 communities that had experienced censorship campaigns, newsdealers did know the Supreme Court had handed down rulings on obscenity and that those rulings "restricted 'obscenity' to a very narrow class of publications," but they were nonetheless "generally unclear about specifics."[61] These studies also indicate the complexities of the relationship between information about the Court's rulings and other factors. For example, in the former study, those who did know and who allowed their activities to be regulated were the most restrictive in their attitudes toward what they would sell, that is, they engaged in "self-censorship." In the 18-community study, however, "attitudes of the wholesalers and retailers toward sexual speech yield[ed] very limited insight into merchandising practices." One reason was that some retailers did not have to self-censor because their wholesalers did so; another, pointing in the opposite direction, was that customer demand for sexually explicit material made it difficult for retailers to limit the items they made available for sale; moreover, publishers exerted pressure on sellers to stock disputed items. Quite relevant to wholesalers' and retailers' actions was their view of "whether their rights . . . could be defended without great cost or anguish" and their recognition that if they cooperated with censorship groups, the demands of those groups often became excessive—requiring resistance by those in an economically marginal situation.[62]

What *are* the ways in which the Court's decisions are communicated?[63] Figure 10.1 depicts the basic channels through which information about the

Figure 10.1

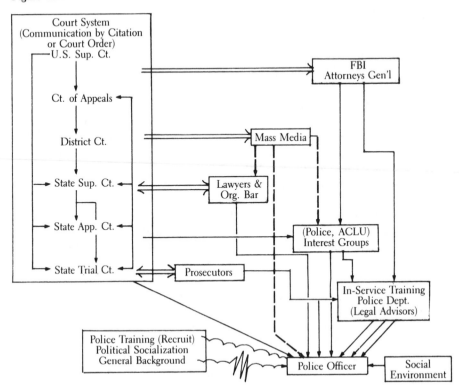

Source: Stephen L. Wasby. *Small Town Police and the Supreme Court* (Lexington, Mass.: Lexington Books, 1976). p. 43.

decisions might flow. One obvious means would be the Court's own opinions, available in several forms, including the "slip opinions" handed out on Decision Day, the advance sheets published by private companies soon thereafter, and, in due course, bound volumes. These circulate among at least some attorneys and others interested in the Court's work. The actual availability of the decisions at the local level where people might want to use them is generally unsatisfactory, particularly in the more rural states, where a set of the *United States Reports* may be found only in the few larger cities. In many counties in the United States, a set is simply not available, and the reported decisions of the courts of appeals and district courts are even less likely to be accessible. However, even in larger cities, only a few of the larger law offices—and the county law library—may have copies.

Lower Courts

The court system itself can serve as a means of communication. The decision in a case is generally sent to a lower court for "proceedings not inconsistent with this opinion." As a result, "the formal judicial structure . . . provides an important channel through which a ruling is transmitted to those directly under obligation to act."[64] But Supreme Court decisions often are not communicated directly to others, instead slowly working their way down to implementing populations through intervening layers of federal and state courts. At times not even the trend in the high court's decisions gets adequately communicated, at least as measured in lower court rulings. The relationship of the highest court and the courts below it, despite the court system's official structure, is not hierarchical and bureaucratic. Indeed, "communication channels may be so poor that subordinates do not become aware that a superior has issued a directive," particularly the further away they are from the Supreme Court.[65]

Notwithstanding these difficulties, major changes in law, particularly if they are clear, can be heard and understood by the lower courts. Thus when the Supreme Court gave a liberal reading to private causes of action under the securities law, "it is hardly surprising that the lower courts did encourage private litigation and the statutes were read very flexibly indeed."[66] When the rulings are not clear—true of Burger Court rulings weakening *Miranda*—there will be less effect; as a result, those rulings "did not result in as much erosion of the *Miranda* principles by state supreme courts as observers seemed to expect."[67] When the Supreme Court ruled that pretrial proceedings could be closed to the public, judges closed their courtrooms much more frequently, an indication—although not proof—that they were well aware of the ruling, one to which they were likely to pay more attention because it directly affected their control of their courtrooms.

Appellate judges also obviously hear the Court's rulings. For example, the U.S. courts of appeals and state supreme courts, despite the major change in libel law the Supreme Court directed in *New York Times v. Sullivan*, complied in 86 *percent* of their relevant cases, with federal courts complying somewhat more than the state courts. This compliance by the appellate courts was particularly important, because, although the present evidence is mixed, in those libel cases that went to trial, the press was likely to lose there, with the juries, despite Supreme Court statements disfavoring punitive damages, often adding punitive damages to the general damages award. Libel lawyers, and lawyers for the media, are also said to have paid closer heed to stories to check them for accuracy before they were printed or aired, and lawyers in libel suits have made greater use of the discovery process ever since the *Herbert v. Lando* decision that journalists' "state of mind" was relevant to the "actual malice" test.[68]

Lower courts' acceptance of Supreme Court rulings can also be seen in their response when the Supreme Court remands a case after reversing the lower courts. Somewhat more than a majority of those who have won in the Supreme Court in civil as well as criminal cases were able to preserve that victory on remand. Civil liberties and criminal procedure cases received less support than economic regulation decisions, partly because the Supreme Court gave the lower courts considerable discretion in criminal procedure cases. There were no differences in outcomes on remand between federal and state courts, but courts two levels away from the Supreme Court were less supportive than were those only one level away, such as the U.S. courts of appeals. In addition, the longer the time after the Supreme Court's ruling, the less likely was the Supreme Court victor to prevail on remand.[69]

If the high state courts often follow the Supreme Court's rulings, state judges have nonetheless engaged in sarcasm or injected "organizational contumacy" into communication channels by criticizing the rulings, by stating concern for the effect of those decisions on the public's safety, and by challenging the factual premises underlying the rulings. At times they have gone beyond criticism to urge lower state courts not to extend disliked Supreme Court rulings beyond absolute necessity so as not to unsettle the state judiciary. When enforcement is thus based less on "genuine enthusiasm" than on "a sense of hierarchical duty," with courts indicating they are acting because they have to do so, they are not likely to kindle much enforcement activity by implementing populations.[70]

Trial court judges are crucial in the transmission of the Supreme Court's rulings to particular recipients, such as the police. "To the average officer 'the law' concerning arrest, search, and other police practices is in large measure represented by his direct and indirect knowledge of the attitudes of the local judiciary."[71] Yet trial judges seldom explain their decisions, most trial court decisions are either unwritten (announced from the bench) or unpublished, and few local government units have established methods for systematically gathering and transmitting information from the courts.

Most trial court judges are not likely to obtain information about Supreme Court rulings through vertical channels. They are more likely to learn about them "horizontally" or laterally from other judges at the same jurisdictional level, who thus can be crucial in the transmission of the rulings. However, even when they correctly apply the Supreme Court's rulings, they may do so narrowly. For example, lower courts' reaction to *Firefighters v. Stotts* (1984), invalidating an affirmative action consent decree involving layoffs, was to say that the quotas in their cases were either voluntarily agreed upon in negotiations or that actual racial discrimination had been shown, making quotas an appropriate remedy.[72] In interpreting some Supreme Court rulings narrowly, lower courts may take their lead from higher state courts to which they are likely to pay more attention. Lower court judges who did not like the *Escobedo* ruling—that a suspect being interrogated had to be allowed access to his lawyer—refused to apply *Escobedo* to anyone who did not already have a lawyer. Similarly, judges who did not like the *Miranda* ruling did not require warnings to be given to those not in custody, and then defined "in custody" as narrowly as possible. They were thus much like state supreme court justices in their interpretation of *Escobedo*. Only four state supreme courts followed the letter and spirit of *Escobedo*, while 37 followed the letter but violated the spirit by refusing to extend the ruling beyond its specific facts; five openly criticized the decision. On the other hand, all but two of the courts interpreting *Miranda* complied, with 14 classified as "liberal" in their interpretations.[73]

In evaluating state judges' performance, we should not assume that all lower courts—even those at the same jurisdictional level—are the same. They may vary in general orientation to legal matters, to their local community, and to important "relevant others" with whom the judges interact. For example, in the area of juvenile justice, courts differ in the extent to which proceedings are adversary in character and emphasize treatment. Some local criminal courts are characterized more by "community mediation" than by imposition of formal penalties. One would expect Supreme Court rulings requiring increased due process requirements to be more readily accepted and implemented in those courts with a more formal orientation—although the judge's ideology about defendants' rights would also have an effect.

At times the pressures from their local "constituency" under which lower courts operate—whether or not the judges are elected—can be severe, as it was on southern judges, both state and federal, asked to enforce desegregation in the decade and more after *Brown v. Board of Education*. Some were aggressive, active enforcers of individual rights; others, more gradualist, although probably having personal attitudes not congruent with the rights required by the Constitution and statutes, would enforce the law if they were given enough evidence. Similarly, although some state supreme court judges (States' Righters) have emphasized local needs and problems and stressed the primacy of state law and state judicial processes, others (Federals) have been willing to take their cues from higher federal courts and from the Supreme Court's interpretation of the national Constitution.[74] If some local judges were to do what the Supreme Court wanted and to resist pressures from the communities to which they had ties, they needed a "hierarchy of scapegoats" as well as more specific guidance about how to achieve desegregation.[75] It was also easier for state judges to sustain civil rights when they could avoid mentioning the U.S. Constitution and could emphasize state legal symbols (the state constitution and state cases). If constituency pressure can work against acceptance of Supreme Court rulings, it can also support it. Liberal lower court judges, particularly if elected, may be hesitant to diverge from Burger Court criminal procedure rulings for fear of being labeled "soft on crime."

Lower courts' resistance to a controversial set of Supreme Court civil liberties decisions undoubtedly overstates the degree to which the judges react negatively to the Court's rulings overall. Lower court judges' preferences and interests do run in opposite directions from Supreme Court rulings from time to time, particularly in new areas of the law. Also, some trial judges may not pay much heed to the Supreme Court—particularly if they have adopted a position on an issue before the Court has spoken or if their attitudes are "unfavorable to the intrusion of 'law' into court proceedings which are highly routinized."[76] Yet in the broad range of cases, resistance occurs relatively seldom. Most policies enunciated by the Supreme Court fall within lower court judges' "zone of indifference," the area in which their feelings are not strong; because the judges have been socialized to accept the authority of higher courts—coupled with the potential sanction of reversal—they usually do what is expected of them, led to do so because "the judge's sense of professionalism and obligation will overcome any personal reaction he or she might have to the higher court's policy."[77]

Lawyers

Lawyers play an important role in communicating Supreme Court rulings, both to clients seeking advice about the legality of past or proposed behavior, and to judges as well. With few judges monitoring higher court decisions, a Supreme Court ruling may come to a judge's attention only when a lawyer presenting a case cites it. Indeed, many judges, partly because of work pressures that limit their reading, intentionally wait until attorneys bring new legal doctrine to their attention. Yet if attorneys are unaware of cases and thus do not cite them, the judges may never be apprised of new rules, and defense lawyers' negative feelings about their clients do serve to limit their learning about the rulings. Where a substantial number of attorneys practice a particular specialty, they may have an informal organization for circulating information about relevant cases, and lawyers arguing appellate cases are particularly likely to know about relevant higher court decisions. (Nonlawyers generally must rely on the interest groups to which they belong to provide such information, but most interest groups do this only sporadically.[78])

Attorneys general and prosecuting attorneys are among the lawyers playing a most important role in the process of communication and impact. We can see this from another study of the disposition of cases on remand after the Supreme Court has ruled. Of the over 1,100 criminal cases in fiscal years 1975–79 that resulted in reprosecution, a majority led to results different from the original trial; however, the changes resulted largely from actions of prosecutors, not the judges, with motions filed by U.S. Attorneys producing most of the changed results. In those instances where there was a retrial to final verdict, however, only one-fourth resulted in acquittals.[79]

The advisory opinions of state attorneys general, which may incorporate Supreme Court rulings, do not have the force of law but are often given great weight by officials contemplating the legal ramifications of proposed actions. However, the advisory opinions usually are issued only on a public official's request and are not widely circulated, thus limiting their use as a means of communication. More important are informational meetings on new developments in the law and bulletins published for law enforcement officials, in which Supreme Court decisions are related to state statutes and judicial rulings and thus made more relevant to local officials' immediate concerns. Within organizations, lawyers—in an agency's legal division—can play an important role not only in communicating the requirements of a court ruling to agency employees but also in developing alternatives to the court's ruling or rationales for retaining previous agency policy.[80]

Local prosecutors, although they could play a large role in the communications process, may not be knowledgeable even on the subjects of cases they have tried. For example, Wisconsin district attorneys involved in obscenity cases felt some books and magazines "cleared" by the Supreme Court were obscene and other prosecutors gave many wrong answers to factual questions about Supreme Court obscenity cases. Only 20 percent of the prosecutors were rated as having high perception of Court policy (medium perception: 42%; low: 20%).[81]

Regardless of their knowledge, however, even where the police would like them to do so, prosecutors rarely undertake the task of telling the police about Supreme Court decisions or about how police practices might be altered to comply with those decisions. Similarly, a regular link with local police departments through which the information could be transmitted is likely to be lacking, so officials who obtain legal information from the prosecutor usually must do so informally. This lack of legal information from the prosecutor has led an increasing number of large police departments to hire police legal advisers—lawyers whose task includes interpretation of Supreme Court decisions, the development of teaching materials, and training within the department.[82] Small departments, which cannot afford to hire these advisers, are thus left without systematic means of acquiring appropriate legal information.

Media

Although sources of legal information inside the legal community are important, there are sources outside the judicial system and legal community. There is no radio or television coverage of the Supreme Court's oral arguments or its announcement of decisions, although the media have made repeated efforts to obtain access to the Court for that purpose, especially for oral argument in such important cases as the challenge to the Gramm-Rudman-Hollings budget law. Chief Justice Burger said television coverage would not occur "until after my funeral" and argued it would be a distracting influence—an argument more appropriate to television of trial court proceedings—and his colleagues apparently agreed, as did the membership of the Judicial Conference. There is, however, speculation that Chief Justice Rehnquist, a more open person, will bring about a change in that policy.

In any event, the mass media serve as an important initial source of information about cases. Television is the principal source for most members of the general public, as well as the source given most credibility; newspapers, on the other hand, provide more detail, although most papers rely on the wire services for coverage of the Court rather than using their own reporters or even their own Washington, D.C., bureaus. Despite many Americans' reliance on English-language media, media in other languages may be quite important, particularly where there are concentrations of people speaking or reading only those other languages. Thus many refugees from Central America did not learn about the Supreme Court's 1987 ruling on the standards for obtaining political asylum (*I.N.S. v. Cardoza-Fonseca*) for some time after it was handed down, when Spanish-language newspapers (many of them weeklies) began to publish information about it.

In the 1960s, reporters covering the Supreme Court were frequently criticized for not being well trained, and for being passive and uncritical in their reporting of the Court.[83] Since then, however, the accuracy of reporting has increased; most reporters covering the Supreme Court for major newspapers, the wire services, and the television networks either have law degrees or have spent some time studying law. This results in greater legal sophistication in coverage of the Court, and one now seldom finds such errors as reporting a denial of review as a full decision of the Court, although this does still occur.

Nonetheless, reporters covering the Court operate in a situation where the public seems not to have an expectation of accurate reporting about the Supreme Court, or perhaps the public's low level of knowledge about the legal system makes it difficult for the newspaper reader or television viewer to know whether information presented is accurate. Nor does there appear to be an expectation of complete reporting about the justices' activities, unlike expectations that the media will report the work of Congress and the president and the president's activities fully and *accurately*. For example, reporters covering the Court did not mention a speech problem (stammering, slurred words) exhibited by Justice Rehnquist in 1982 until after he was hospitalized. Only from George Washington University Hospital's spokesman were other doctors able to identify the drug (for a back problem) that had probably caused the difficulty. Nor did reporters seem to complain when the Court's Information Officer was typically uncommunicative on the matter, and the Court did not issue a clear or full statement of the sort the reporters would *demand* of the president's press secretary. Some commentators actually defended the silence, saying the Court was sufficiently close-knit to take care of the problem. However, such statements ring false, given the Court's difficulty in getting a disabled Justice Douglas (like other disabled justices before him) to leave even when the Court's work was being affected.

The media do not transmit Supreme Court decisions intact; few newspapers even print portions of the most important cases. Nor could they, not only for reasons of space but because the Court's opinions are too complex in their original form to be understood by most people. One can see this in a humorous vein in the accompanying "Supreme Court Roundup," a parody of typical wire-service summaries of the Court's decisions.

SUPREME COURT ROUNDUP
by *Veronica Geng*

Washington, May 8—*The Supreme Court took the following actions today:*

First Amendment

In a landmark decision, the Court ruled unanimously in favor of a twelve-year-old plaintiff who sought damages on account of being denied the chance to audition for the Clint Eastwood role in the motion picture "Maddened Rustlers." The Court's opinion, written by Chief Justice Happ, argued that exclusion of the little girl was "rotten, beastly, a crying shame—really makes the Court sick." The case was not decided, as had been expected, on the ground of sex discrimination; rather, the Justices invoked the First Amendment's guarantee of freedom of expression. The Court thus affirmed for the first time the constitutional right to a screen test.

Search and Seizure

Overturning the "dog's breakfast" doctrine of search and seizure, the Court held unconstitutional the Drug Enforcment Administration's system of obtaining search warrants, under which a judge who issues a warrant receives the rest of the afternoon off, while a judge who refuses a warrant is reclassified as a Controlled Substance. Justice Happsberger, writing for the majority, said that such procedures "lean upon the delicately coiffed maiden of the Fourth Amendment with the great ugly brutish heavily muscled shoulder of procedural error," and cited Judge Cheerful Hand's famous dictum "I shall keep at it with these metaphors until I'm very old and it's unbecoming."

Taxes

Without hearing arguments on the issue, the Court ordered the Internal Revenue Service to desist at once from collecting personal income taxes—a practice that Justice Hapenny defined in his opinion as "inconsiderate" and "the product of diseased minds." He pointed out that the government could easily collect the same amount of money by manufacturing and selling wall plaques that say "UNCLE SAM LOVES YOUR FIRST NAME HERE."

Controversy

In one of their occasional "piggy-back" decisions, the Justices resolved some of the long-standing issues that clog the Court calendar. They ruled that nurture is more influential than nature, that men make history, that Iago is driven by motiveless malignancy, that one isn't too many and a thousand is enough, that there is an earthly paradise, and that Don Bucknell's nephew Ed doesn't look anything like John Travolta. Justice Hapworth dissented but was too polite to say so.

Moral Blight

Citing "want of attractiveness" as a reason, the Court declined, 7-2, to hear an appeal by the publisher of two so-called men's magazines, *Rude Practices* and *Men's Magazine*. In the majority opinion, Chief Justice Happ explained that appellant's arguments were "unprepossessing and—let's be frank about it—just incredibly disingenuous." Dissenting, Justices Happer and Happner said they wanted to pretend to hear the case and then rule against appellant for "putting out such a clumsily edited and typographically unappetizing publication."

In a related decision, the Justices unanimously refused to hear a song written by a Kleagle of the Ku Klux Klan.

Criminal

By a 9-0 vote, the Court held unconstitutional a New York City statute that would have mandated criminal convictions for suspects who fail to take policemen aside and "read them their duties." The statute had required that suspects deliver these "Caliban warnings" to policemen in order to remind them of their power of life and death, their obligation to attend to personal hygiene, etc. The Court, in an opinion by Justice Happell, contended, "Who can doubt that this would be the first step toward compelling suspects to serve their arresting officers creamed chicken on toast points?"

Greed

Splitting 8-1, the Court upheld the constitutionality of a federal program for the redistribution of wealth. Under the program, which is known as "horizontal divestiture," rich people are asked to lie down, and poor people then divest them of their money. Justice Happold, dissenting, said that the program would diminish the impact of a standing Court order requiring that income in excess of $8,000 a year be bused across state lines to achieve bank-account balances.

Gibberish

The Court voted unanimously not to review a case in which a court of appeals struck down a lower federal court's decision to vacate an even lower court's refusal to uphold a ruling that it is not unconstitutoinal to practice "reverse discrimination." Chief Justice Happ, who wrote the opinion, said that the Court "is not, nor will it consent to be, a body of foolosophers easily drawn into jive baloney-shooting." A brief was filed by the Modern Language Association as *amicus curiae* ("curiosity about Don Ameche").

●

As is their custom, the Justices closed the session with an informal musicale, playing a Corelli *gigg*. Justices Hapgood, Hapworth, Happner, and Happer performed on violin, Justice Happell on bassoon, Justice Happsberger on harpsichord, Justice Happold on oboe, Justice Hapenny on flute, and Chief Justice Happ on viola d'amore.

Source: Abridgement and adaptation of "Supreme Court Roundup" (Originally reprinted in *The New Yorker*, May 15, 1978) from *Partners* by Veronica Geng. Copyright © 1978 by Veronica Geng. Reprinted by permission of Harper & Row, Publishers, Inc.

The wire services have been and continue to be the principal source of information about the Court for newspapers and to some extent for television as well. A study of *Baker v. Carr* and the School Prayer Cases in the early 1960s showed that 23 of 25 papers carried reports of the reapportionment ruling on Decision Day, with 14 stories coming from AP, five from UPI, one from the *Herald Tribune* News Service, and only two from the papers' staff writers. The picture was roughly the same for the school prayer rulings. However, starting with the second day after the opinion, although wire service domination continued, more stories were written by staff writers.[84]

In addition to not communicating decisions intact, the media's reporting filters the Supreme Court's rulings in other ways. This is particularly likely when the Court's decisions affect the media themselves. Justice Brennan has suggested that the media's attacks are unreasonable, unintelligent, and inaccurate.[85] The media's views even affect the way opinions are condensed and summarized generally. As Justice O'Connor has observed, "The summaries of the opinions of this Court carried in the media . . . frequently provide a perspective, not only on the work of the Court but also on the perceptions and judgment of the reporters and their editors."[86]

The media deal with some decisions more carefully or more sympathetically than with others. Some rulings are not treated at all, being lost in the deluge of rulings, particularly toward the end of each term of Court. Because the rulings are not directly reproduced, much of the "richness"—including the rationale or reasoning—of the Court's opinions is lost during transmission. The media are thus part of a translation process in which changes are introduced and different elements of a decision and its context are emphasized. Each medium differs in what it emphasizes about what happens at the Court. The wire services, which cover the Court on more days than the newspapers (relatively close behind) or the television networks, appear to have the greatest capacity to handle "raw word flow." Although individual newspapers vary considerably, wire-service and newspaper coverage is closely related to the Court's output, but television coverage is not. When output increases, changes in the pattern of coverage occur, with more attention paid to impact and somewhat less to legal principles; television is more affected by increase in output than are the other media. However, when output reaches a certain level, the ability of the media to expand coverage to match that output ceases and coverage loses most of its "depth," tending to summaries of individual cases.[87]

Each medium also seems to have a different "profile" in relation to "Court time": wire services and television give relatively greater emphasis to predecision coverage; newspapers, more to postdecision coverage. Television seems to add more "contextual information" than do the other media, and to report "informational content" about the decisions least; the newspapers, on the other hand, seem to be most balanced in coverage of various elements—including not only predecision material and the decision itself, but also material on the Court as an institution and trends in the Court's decisions. The inclusion of all this other material makes it difficult for people to find out what the Court has said: they may be able to read about the decision's impact without knowing what it is that is having the impact. Yet if a decision is to be applied to a variety of circumstances, its rationale—not merely the facts and the holding—must be communicated.

For specialized audiences, television is clearly inadequate as a source of needed operational information, and even newspapers are likely to have insufficient material about the Court's decisions. Because of these inadequacies, specialized magazines must perform an information-communication function about judicial decisions. However, while most occupational groups' trade journals can carry such information and some do, it usually is not well developed and is available only sporadically. Another, related source of information about legal decisions is the specialized material prepared for use in training. An advantage of such material is that the law is related to problem situations that those who must implement the rulings will face. Such details, although quite necessary, are not likely to have been provided by the courts. Such material must be written so that it can be understood; for example, materials for police officers must be written without a "dumb cop" image but so that those with a high school education or at most a couple of years of college can understand it.

As this suggests, training serves as a major means of communicating the law (statutory materials as well as court cases) to specific occupational groups like police officers, who tend to rank training as the most effective means of learning about the law. Training takes a variety of forms, including degree programs at two-year and four-year colleges and much shorter two-day or three-day or one-week in-service programs. These education and training programs must cover many subjects, so that coverage of legal matters is likely to constitute only a very small percentage of a total program unless, as is rarely the case, it is devoted solely to the law.

Factors Affecting Communication and Impact

Communication of the Supreme Court's rulings and the impact of those rulings are affected by a variety of factors that alter messages before they reach their intended audience and by the ways in which those audiences respond to the rulings. At times such factors are strong enough to "wash out" most of a decision's intended effect. There is, however, no clearly developed "theory of impact" to tell us exact effects or relative importance of these factors.

Attitudes

Attitudes of those affected by decisions appear to play a particularly important role in the decisions' impact. Relevant attitudes include views of the Court's legitimacy, with distaste for the Court leading people to pay less attention to its decisions. Similarly, a feeling that the Court is not ruling fairly on a subject or is not ruling on the basis of adequate knowledge can interfere with the reception given its decisions. For example, the Court's competence and hence its legitimacy was questioned in the police area when the Court in *Miranda* seemed, at least to law enforcement officers, to be acting without reference to the actualities of police work. This perceived action of the Court made it increasingly likely that the personal and organizational goals of the police would differ from the goals embodied in the Court's ruling. On the other hand, when the Court showed recognition of the dangerous situations in which police find themselves, as in the

Terry "stop and frisk" case, there was less hostility to the decision in the law enforcement community.

Another attitudinal element is an individual's general commitment to "obeying the law." However, "obeying the law," including the dictates of the Supreme Court, plays a limited role when other factors enter the picture. Some people alter their attitudes to bring them more in line with the Supreme Court's position, but many others develop a variety of techniques that allows them to retain their policy preferences without adhering to the Supreme Court's doctrine. Among these techniques are attacks on those who are seeking to enforce the decisions (condemning the condemners); appeals to a "higher morality" (an authority higher than the Supreme Court); denial of responsibility for the present situation, perhaps coupled with a claim that others are preventing compliance from coming about; and beliefs that those the decision is intended to protect (whether blacks or criminal defendants) have not really been injured or are instead the *real* menace to society.

Prior attitudes about policy affect people's reaction to the Court's rulings, as can be seen in responses to the abortion rulings, which also illustrate that there are multiple responses to some rulings rather than a single unitary response. After the abortion rulings, support for abortion when health considerations were involved increased among those who had heard of *Roe v. Wade*; however, among nonwhites and Catholics opposition to "discretionary" abortions increased, and women moved from greater support of abortion than men to slightly greater opposition. In general, "the structure of preferences for discretionary abortions changed in the direction of greater group differences and conflict."[88] That such changes did not occur among those who had not heard of the ruling indicates that the changes were likely the result of the Court's ruling rather than of some other factor. The effect of *Roe v. Wade* was also influenced by attitudes of community leaders, at least as perceived by those implementing the ruling. Community leaders' attitudes were related to post-*Roe v. Wade* changes in hospitals' abortion policies and played a larger role in such changes than did demands for abortions or the activities of interest groups. Similarly the attitudes of hospital governing boards and of doctors and nurses working in the hospitals heavily determined hospital abortion policies.[89]

Basic attitudes help explain parental resistance to desegregation, and the attitudes of decision makers can somewhat moderate local opposition to desegregation. However, sometimes attitudes are superceded by judgments of whether "the utility of noncompliance is greater than the utility of compliance, that is, of engaging in the available alternative activity expected to yield the greatest net gratification." Indeed, desegregation of Georgia school districts provided strong evidence to support a cost-benefit explanation: "In communities in which the costs of compliance were perceived to be high and rewards low, the most severe coercion was required."[90]

Clarity

Characteristics of the Court's ruling itself and the place of the ruling in a pattern of decisions are also important. If those who are expected to implement decisions are to hear about them, the decisions must be highly visible. Because at times people become aware of rulings only after they have been cited by lower courts or commented on in an attorney general's bulletin, that is, only after they have traveled through lengthy communication channels, the initial signal must be strong to overcome interference and delays. Otherwise the message becomes garbled, as in the game of "Gossip." A unanimous opinion is thought easier to transmit than are several opinions from a single case, and thus increases impact. However, if unanimity is achieved at the cost of a murky, unclear compromise, communication will be more difficult and impact may be lessened. Concurring and dissenting opinions not only increase the information to be transmitted but also make it easier for potential opponents of the majority's view to resist compliance. A plurality opinion makes it particularly difficult for others to determine the Court's intent.

As this discussion indicates, the relative clarity or ambiguity of even a single opinion also affects its communicability. There are few decisions that, like *Miranda*, can be reduced to four or five warnings to be put on a "Miranda card." Even when a decision is clear initially, it may become less clear as the Court later explicates or limits it. Thus, the initial clarity of *Miranda* was blurred by rulings on use of confessions obtained without warnings or resumption of questioning after it had been stopped. Greater clarity is generally thought to produce greater compliance; ambiguity, more noncompliance. However, state supreme court reaction to establishment of religion cases did *not* show a relationship between Supreme Court clarity and lower court compliance.[91]

The addition of more and more cases will by itself increase the amount of "noise" in the communication system, particularly if they are decided on the basis of the "totality of circumstances" in the case—the Burger Court's initial preference in the field of criminal procedure—rather than a broad rule such as the Warren Court tended to use. Just as a large number of cases increases distortion, gaps in doctrine may also create ambiguity. Such gaps are inevitable because the number of cases decided by the Supreme Court is very small in relation to the total number of issues on which it is asked to rule. Thus courts can develop a "clear policy line" on only a few issues at any one time, if they can do so at all.

The Court may set off far more of a furor when it first approaches an area of policy, even if its first case in that area has limited scope, than it does later with more far-reaching cases, because its initial action may be unexpected. Thus *Engel v. Vitale*, although invalidating only state-written prayers in schools, drew far more heated reaction than *Abington School District v. Schempp*, which outlawed school prayer and Bible reading, which were far more prevalent. Affecting reaction to these cases was the Court's greater care in delineating its second holding—in saying that not all teaching about religion had to be excluded from the school—than it had been in its first opinion, where important qualifications appeared only in a footnote. Similarly, less negative state court reaction to *Miranda* than to *Escobedo* may have come both from a realization that *Miranda* was likely to follow and from the *Miranda* opinion's greater clarity.

Situation

The ongoing situation into which a Supreme Court decision is injected is another factor affecting the receipt of communications and the decision's impact. A decision handed down in the midst of a crisis is likely to receive less coverage than one announced in "normal" times, unless the decision is perceived as contributing to the crisis or producing one. Compliance with an appellate court decision is assisted because such a ruling "often comes well after the deep feelings in the community [provoked by the litigation] have subsided."[92] However, if a substantial change in the law has taken place immediately prior to the Court's ruling, obtaining further change soon is difficult. Similarly, judges are less likely to go along with the Supreme Court when invalidating local practices is thought likely to be disruptive. Getting people to pay attention to the courts is also difficult when the law is well settled, making it less likely that further substantial change will occur in the short run.

Both a community's long-term history and events of the immediate past may attune potential recipients to what the Court has said; a community with few major crimes is less likely to be "up" on criminal law than one in which a murder has recently occurred or in which the police want to make a major drug bust. A community's general belief system also affects communication of decisions and receptivity to them. Officials in communities that pride themselves on being "up-to-date" or "professional" might be more likely than other communities to seek out information about court decisions and to work to bring local government action into accord with those rulings.

In large measure because "most judicial policies are implemented through organizations,"[93] factors related to organizations play a part in the communication of and compliance with court decisions. Among those factors are "the cost of the policy or program changes to the agency, . . . whether the policy conflicts with an agency's goals or mission, whether the policy conflicts with preferences of key personnel, and whether the agency can effectively resist judicial pressure to implement a policy,"[94] with availability of agency resources for that purpose particularly important. Organizational structure and location are other relevant factors. An organization may be so large that what specialists or others at the "top" of the orgnization learn about judicial rulings cannot be effectively transmitted to the "bottom." Where units are small, division of labor and specialization may be insufficient to have a person assigned to monitor judicial rulings. A small unit located near other units may acquire information from those units "horizontally"; however, when the small unit—like a rural police department—is geographically isolated, it may have few contacts through which to acquire information. Political isolation may be as important as geographical isolation in determining communications received, with community influence in the form of daily pressure affecting how an agency responds to a judicial ruling. Community pressures vary with the size and homogeneity of the community and are particularly severe in small, homogeneous communities where role expectations reinforce each other. And an agency operating in a supportive environment may be more resistant to outside rules that demand change than an agency that is politically vulnerable and may comply to protect its position.[95]

"Follow-up"

Another important part of the postdecision situation is the "follow-up" to a ruling—*who* responds and how they respond. Average citizens and government employees may pay greater attention to subsequent communications about a ruling if elites support it. Even the absence of criticism—when relevant officials merely maintain a neutral posture—may be important. However, communities with homogeneous populations may prove immune to officials' support of a disliked Supreme Court ruling such as school prayer. And if prominent officials immediately oppose a ruling, further communication about it may well fall on plugged if not deaf ears. Agency officials' reactions to the Court's rulings are likely to be a function of the distance between the organization's policy and what the Court suggests, as well as of the agency's commitment to its own program; the greater the change the agency thinks the Court requires, the greater the likelihood the agency will search for alternative policies. Here organizational norms can come into play forcefully; the norm that the organization should make decisions independently, not subject to an external "superior," would encourage noncompliance.[96]

Because the Court's rulings are usually not self-enforcing, the degree to which government officials enforce or attempt to enforce those rulings, part of "follow-up," is critical. (Even where the decisions are self-enforcing, such as decisions allowing sale of material of greater sexual explicitness, officials' actions in responding to or rejecting demands from community groups opposed to the rulings or abstaining from taking action themselves are important in that situation as well.[97]) Executive branch officials do not often directly attack Supreme Court decisons (see pages 314-15), but they may severely damage the possibilities for compliance by refusing to take firm action to implement them. This was true with respect to school desegregation in the Eisenhower, Nixon, and Ford administrations. Eisenhower "declined to state publicly his personal view of the *Brown* decision, thus giving rise to speculation that he disapproved of compulsory desegregation." Although his attorneys general supported desegregation in the courts, "the President's ambiguity and the administration's general inactivity. . .

encouraged white Southern leadership to believe that the federal executive branch would take no forceful action to enforce the courts' orders." The role of southern governors was also vital; the increase in the number of militant segregationist governors after *Brown* certainly did not facilitate compliance.[98]

At the local level, prosecutors' inaction concerning police violations of search and seizure rules does little to encourage compliance. Prosecutors may even approach the Court's rulings negatively, talking to police (in what is called "negative advocacy") about how to "get around" a ruling. People are not encouraged to learn about or to follow the rules if there are no sanctions or only limited ones for not knowing the law, with little if any reward for following Court-established rules. Thus, if new rules are to be carried out, there must be active supervision, not just executive passivity.

Follow-up is also affected by the community pressures that are an important part of an official's "work situation."[99] That work situation also includes the people from whom the official takes cues about how to behave—his "reference group"—that is particularly important when community expectations are contradictory, thus allowing the individual more discretion as to how to act. Some government employees ("locals") take their cues primarily from their own communities, while others ("cosmopolitans," particularly professionals), such as lawyers and doctors, look to those in the same occupation. If, like police officers, individuals spend much time in the company of colleagues and feel the Supreme Court is hurting their work, they may wish to avoid becoming "sore thumbs" or deviants by attempting to follow rules not adhered to by their fellow workers. Such social pressure is increased when the work subculture becomes organized into unions or comparable interest groups.

Impact in Particular Policy Areas

Church-State Relations

The Court's rulings on released time programs (in which children are re leased from public school classes to receive religious education) and those on prayer in the public schools attracted much attention and produced much controversy, which has continued to the present concerning school prayer. Resistance to the Court's school prayer ruling, not typical of reaction to decisions on other church-state issues, has come close to matching resistance to school desegregation in both intensity and openness. For example, when the Supreme Court in 1981 invalidated a Kentucky law that required the posting of the Ten Commandments in public school classrooms *(Stone v. Graham)*, many school districts left them posted despite a state attorney general's opinion that this was improper even if the Commandments were donated by a private group.

Released Time. When the Supreme Court in the 1948 *McCollum* case invalidated a program of religious instruction operated on school property by religious pesonnel, those operating other programs attempted to differentiate theirs, and some were modified. Programs most likely to continue where those with long-standing enabling legislation. Some on-premises programs continued, with state attorneys general doing little to stop them; opponents of the programs tended to be religious minorities who lacked the political weight necessary to produce change.[100]

After the 1952 *Zorach* decision sustained religious programs held *off* school grounds during school hours, attendance at such denominational activities returned to pre-*McCollum* levels, but subsequent growth was small. Some people interpreted *Zorach* to require, rather than merely to permit, released time programs, but states did not enact new programs, a fact that raises further questions about the force of the Court's power to legitimate a policy. Nor was much done to eliminate continuing noncompliance with *McCollum*, even though off-premises programs could have been adopted with relative ease to produce compliance.[101] (Another impact of *Zorach* stemmed from Justice Douglas' dictum, "We are a religious people whose institutions presuppose a Supreme Being": it was often quoted subsequently by those favoring a variety of programs supporting religion.)

School Prayer. The school prayer decisions of 1962 and 1963—*Engel v. Vitale*, invalidating a state-composed prayer, and the *Schempp* case, striking down recitation of the Lord's Prayer and readings from the Bible—produced far more outcry than the released time rulings. Local and state officials played a key role in deflecting the requirements of the school prayer rulings. Where a superintendent opposed the practices, he was able to use the Supreme Court's ruling to change local practices but needed the decisions to do so. However, far more numerous were officials who wanted to avoid conflict with small-town local power structures, often because the officials had other, more important goals to achieve. The large number of local districts provided necessary *opportunities* for noncompliance that must accompany depth of feeling before noncompliance can actually occur. Local officials' claims that their districts were in compliance when the truth was otherwise also made it difficult to constrain disobedience. The officials either presumed that compliance was taking place and did not check for violations or turned their heads after making a perfunctory statement that prayer and Bible reading were to be stopped, thus allowing teachers to continue the practices. Lawsuits were the only practical way of challenging the practices, but little litigation occurred because it was extremely expensive and often had few supporters and because, as in the post-*McCollum* period, those in the minority on this emotional issue were unwilling to subject themselves to the pressure they would have felt had they attacked local practices.[102] Where policy was made primarily at the state level, compliance was more likely both because there were fewer actors to be constrained and because the education "establishment" actively enforced compliance.[103]

There were major regional differences in compliance. Where the practices had been most widespread, in the East and particularly the South, they were least likely to be given up, but school prayer was far more likely to be discontinued in the Midwest and West. Some areas had had long-standing prohibitions against such devotional activities; areas that had adopted the practices without explicit requirements found it easy to give them up. Those areas that retained school prayer were likely to have had constitutional or statutory requirements underlying the practices. In the East, formal requirements were eliminated, leading to compliance. But in the South, requirements were not removed and were at times supplemented, making it unlikely that the practices would be changed.[104]

After the Court's ruling, the national incidence of classroom prayers as reported by teachers decreased from 60 percent to 28 percent in 1964–65; Bible reading decreased from 48 percent to 22 percent. It could thus be said that "the average teacher did feel the impact of the Supreme Court decision."[105] The largest number of teachers said there was no school policy on prayer or that matters were left up to them. School policies did have an effect: compared to an incidence of 40 percent in schools with no policy, only 4 percent of teachers in schools that opposed the prayers said them, but of teachers in schools favoring the prayers, 43 percent led prayers. For Bible reading, the figures were much the same. Yet teachers' own religious practices affected compliance: those who attended church more frequently were more likely to lead prayers in the classroom—both before and after the Court ruled. Conservative Protestants were most likely to have said prayers before the ruling and were least likely to comply with the Court's ruling. Jews and Catholics, who, along with liberal Protestants, were less likely to have led classroom prayer before 1963, were most likely to comply. A teacher's seniority also had an effect on compliance: the greater the seniority, the less the change in practice.

Among those who did not change their views about religious practices, there were several types of responses.[106] The "backlashers," committed to defiance of the Court's ruling, tried to bring religious activities into the schools whenever they could and took a negative stance toward the Court itself. On the other hand, the "vindicateds" were critical of "schoolhouse religion" both before the decision and afterward. Others who did not change their personal views complied with the decisions because they generally believed or led themselves to believe that they had no choice but to comply; these were the "nulists." There were also many who changed their views toward religion in the school, but not all did so in the same way. The "converts" came to believe in the Supreme Court ruling and were committed to enforcing it, while the "liberateds" softened their views about religion in the school and moved toward convergence between their own views and what the Court required. The "reverse liberateds," however, became more rather than less favorable to schoolhouse religion; they moved away from the Court's position, not toward it.

The school prayer issue is also one that illustrates continuing effects, not one in which there is great short-term controversy and then compliance and quiet. As a March 11, 1984, New York Times headline indicated, "Prayer in Many Schoolrooms Continues Despite '62 Ruling." The Bible is read, prayers are recited, and hymns sung in some schools; in many more, there is a moment of silence—also struck down by the Court, at least where the legislature enacting the provision intended it as prayer (*Wallace v. Jaffree*). Efforts aimed at amending the Constitution to provide for "voluntary" prayer or for silent meditation have been made regularly, with such efforts defeated in Congress as recently as 1984. Statutory efforts also continued; a bill sponsored by Senator Jesse Helms (R-N.C.) to prevent federal court challenges to organized prayer in public school was defeated in September 1985. However, Congress did pass a bill to allow student-sponsored religious groups to meet in public high schools as long as nonreligious groups were permitted to use school facilities for meetings—but only after protection for political groups' use of the facilities was provided.

Criminal Procedure

Most of our knowledge about communication of Supreme Court decisions comes from the field of criminal justice. In the least professionalized of four police departments in medium-sized Wisconsin cities (Green Bay), the greatest proportion (more than one-third) of the officers found out initially about the *Miranda* decision from a newspaper. About 75 percent cited the newspaper as either an initial or later source, and the same proportion heard about the ruling from a superior officer. Only slightly fewer officers were exposed to the case by television, and somewhat over 60 percent heard of it in training sessions. Although a full 40 percent of the department's officers ultimately read the opinion itself, the evidence confirms that "people who have no formal connection with the judiciary may be a more important source of information than any judicial authority."[107] The newspaper was also the most common initial source in the most professional of the four departments (Madison), but more than 90 percent of the officers there were exposed to the decision in conference-and-training; roughly three-fourths heard about it from each of three sources—newspapers, a superior officer, and the attorney general. In Racine, where there was a captain of detectives on whom others relied for legal information, a high proportion of the officers received their first information about *Miranda* from superior officers—who were also the predominant overall source of information.

The greater the professionalism of the department, the larger the number of sources of information and the greater the percentage of officers who received information from training sessions. Formal law enforcement sources were stressed more in the more professionalized departments. However, none of the departments had much contact with "outside" information that might have proved helpful in understanding the decision. Professionalization did not bring increased contact with nonpolice groups, but instead tended to bring about well-developed lines of intradepartmental communication. Outside groups were listened to more frequently in the more professionalized departments, but that was because the groups furnished information that reinforced professional ideology. In all four departments, conference-and-training was rated the best source of information by the most people, with opinions as to the next best source varying. Those approving and those disapproving of the decision did not differ much in selecting the best source of information. However, those approving of the decisions were more likely to have received information at training sessions than were those who disapproved. Although professionalization affected the way *Miranda* was communicated and received, after the decision as before, "there was no real hierarchy through which binding directives regarding the implementation of the *Miranda* decision could flow." Thus *Miranda* "did not basically change the decentralized and often unsystematic communications processes used to inform police departments about innovation."[108]

In small (two- and three-officer) Wisconsin departments, the primary initial source of information about criminal justice rulings was also the newspaper—also the predominant general source of information and the one thought best. Other sources were police magazines and the attorney general's office—despite the lack of personal contact with the latter. Conferences and training sessions, attendance at which gave the officers prestige, were mentioned in connection with *Miranda* and received high ratings.[109]

Small-town police chiefs in southern Illinois and western Massachusetts interviewed in 1972 were most likely to have found out about Supreme Court decisions from other sources—bulletins and other specialized or professional literature. However, of the few chiefs who considered training programs a primary source of information about the Supreme Court, most felt they had not learned enough about the Supreme Court from such programs. In large city departments throughout the country, three types of sources of information about Court decisions predominated: the decisions themselves, specialized police publications, and the district attorney. The media were cited as a source by only about 10 percent of the departments.[110]

Small-town chiefs saw the Court's decisions—which they believed nonlawyers could understand—as the most effective means of communication, with state and local prosecutors a close second; mass media and personal friends were thought highly *ineffective* means of communication. Written communications were seen by most as more effective than oral communications, although some thought a combination (training materials discussed at a conference) better still. The officers seemed to want something like a regular (monthly) bulletin or newsletter that digested cases and provided updated information for the individual officer, not just the department. They also saw the local prosecutor—in Massachusetts, along with the attorney general—as having responsibility for providing legal advice to the police. However, many officers said they were not provided sufficient material or access to it. However, differences between states can be seen in the fact that, although most Illinois chiefs did not know where the Supreme Court's decisions were available, those in Massachusetts often had copies of the decisions in their offices—and read them.

Right to Counsel. The Massachusetts and Illinois police chiefs certainly felt that the Supreme Court had affected police work, although these chiefs thought the effect had occurred primarily in large cities, not in their small towns. The Court's decisions (mainly Warren Court rulings) were thought to have improved the quality of police work. Although "old-timers" had been reluctant to "get involved" with cases, newer officers were more accustomed to the new rules and not scared by them.

Another long-term impact of the Court's rulings was on the environment in which law enforcement personnel operated. *Gideon v. Wainwright*, requiring representation of indigents at trial, played a major role in shaping this environment. It led to creation or expansion of public defender programs and, coupled with other Warren Court broad rulings on confessions and searches, to attorneys' greater persistence in pursuing criminal cases, particularly at the appeals stage. Courts interpreting *Gideon* had usually adopted a narrow view of its requirements and imposed a "variety of different lines . . . as to where the cut-off point" came for providing counsel.[111] However, a year after *Argersinger v. Hamlin* (1972), which extended the right to counsel at trial for any situations in which a jail term was imposed, most jurisdictions except for rural southern counties were complying with the Court's directive. Most locations appointed counsel even in traffic cases where imprisonment was a reasonable possibility, although they did not do so for nonserious traffic cases, which usually involve only a fine. A somewhat later study did suggest, however, that compliance with *Argersinger* had been only "token," with judges encouraging waiver of counsel and with "no coherent development of defense systems to meet the need for quality representation" that the spirit of the ruling demanded. Appointed counsel—often assigned immediately before a trial—were frequently inexperienced and not well prepared to represent their clients.[112] In the early 1980s, state funding cutbacks seriously affected both public defender agencies and reimbursement of appointed counsel. Appointed counsel resisted working without pay, and in at least one state (Missouri) judges had to impose compulsory service without compensation on attorneys so that defendants would be represented.

Even when there was an increase in appointment of counsel under *Argersinger*, staffs of public defender offices increased in only a small proportion of all counties, primarily the larger ones. This increased staffing did *not*, however, produce the expected great increase in nonguilty pleas in misdemeanor cases. Rates of guilty pleas were somewhat—but not much—lower than when counsel were not frequently present, and presence of defense counsel did not result in a greater frequency of trials. However, provision of counsel may have delayed the guilty pleas that most misdemeanor defendants intended to enter when they came to court. (More frequent case dismissals and charge-and-sentence concessions may have, however, benefited defendants.) Cases did seem more "stretched out" when defense counsel were present than when they were not. Apparently courts' administrative burdens were not affected by lawyers' actions, for misdemeanor judges did not perceive their ability to handle their caseload was being hindered by greater use of defense counsel.[113] Defense counsel—whether assigned counsel (used primarily in small counties) or public defenders (used in larger jurisdictions)—now had to help process guilty pleas. Thus the rationale of *Argersinger*—that the trial proces should become more adversary in nature—was not carried out.

Exclusionary Rule. The two most crucial Supreme Court criminal procedure decisions were *Mapp v. Ohio* (1961), imposing the exclusionary rule on the states, and *Miranda v. Arizona* (1966), on the admissibility of confessions. Questionnaire responses from police chiefs, prosecutors, defense attorneys, judges, and American Civil Liberties Union (ACLU) officials indicated that as a result of *Mapp*, search and seizure questions were raised more frequently at trial but that there had not been overall change in police effectiveness. Attitudes were reported to have altered as a result of the ruling, with a general movement toward agreement with statements that the same rules should exist for federal and state police, that the legality of searches should be broadened, that more flexible search warrants were needed, and that safety should be emphasized more and liberty less.[114] Increased police adherence to legality in searches between 1960 and 1963 was reported, with a high positive correlation between increased police education on search and seizure and adherence to legality.

Mapp also produced a substantial increase in police education, including development of courses at police academies, adult education programs, colleges, and universities. In fact, it was among the "key factors in increasing the attempts at centralization and formalization of police training procedures."[115] In New York, retraining sessions "had to be held from the very top administrator down to each of the thousands of foot patrolmen and detectives engaged in the daily basic enforcement function," with "hundreds of thousands of manhours" devoted to the task.[116] Training improved in previously nonexclusionary rule states, and the FBI increased its training of state and local officers, but the exclusionary rule did not guarantee that good police training on arrest and search would take place, with pre-*Mapp* exclusionary rule states among those doing the least. Four years after *Mapp*, training remained "very spotty in both quantity and quality."[117]

States that had a pre-*Mapp* exclusionary rule appeared to differ from those without the rule prior to 1961. Courts in the former states seem to have been *less* likely to adopt federal search and seizure precedents after *Mapp*, particularly if they had already begun to develop their own lines of precedents. Thus "where a state judiciary *anticipates* a federal rule, but with variations of its own, those variations are going to prove very hard to kill."[118] Making this conclusion problematic is that states previously adopting an exclusionary rule had seldom invoked it or had interpreted it narrowly when they did. We are thus left with "virtually no relationship between adoption and implementation of *Mapp*."[119] Nor was there a great deal of post-*Mapp* judicial action to implement the ruling. Supreme courts in 18 states did not deal with more than two of 16 basic search and seizure questions, and thus did not provide the law enforcement community with statements on much of what constituted an unreasonable seizure. For only three questions did two-thirds or more of the state courts rule evidence inadmissible; five of the questions were settled in a manner limiting *Mapp's* application, in line with not uncommon explicit resistance to *Mapp* by judges, who often indicated that they had little use for it. Overall, nine states responded positively to *Mapp*, 14 were in an intermediate category, and nine were rated negative.[120]

The most important potential effect of *Mapp* was on police actions—arrest and search warrants—where changes could have resulted from increases in particular types of crimes (guns, gambling, drugs) as well as from the decision itself. Disagreement abounds about the decision's effects, with different studies cited on either side of the argument that the costs of the rule are too high to retain it. It has also been suggested that "in the vast majority of criminal cases," those costs and benefits are not involved because seizure of evidence does not occur.[121] In the study cited most by opponents of *Mapp*, Dallin Oaks, relying primarily on data from Chicago and Cincinnati, concluded that "the data contains little support for the proposition that the exclusionary rule discourages illegal searches and seizures, but it falls short of establishing that it does not." However, in a stronger statement, he argued, "As a device for directing or deterring illegal searches and seizures by the police, the exclusionary rule is a failure." He went on to say that police conduct not leading to prosecutions was unlikely to be affected by the rule, with little deterrent effect on prosecution-oriented activity.[122]

Analysis of arrest, warrant, and disposition data for the immediate post-*Mapp* period and for later years (to allow the decison's long-term effects to be ascertained) raises doubts about these conclusions.[123] In 14 cities without a pre-*Mapp* exclusionary rule, few search warrants had been used, but the proportion of constitutional searches, although varying from city to city, increased after the Court's decisions. Officials in large-city police departments attributed the increase in search warrants primarily to the increase in narcotics traffic, with less of the change accounted for by increased numbers of police, better training, and other judicial rulings. In roughly one-third of the cities, court decisions were not thought to have had much effect on recent increases in the numbers of search warrants, but in approximately one-fourth of the cities, judical action was thought to be a major if not the total cause. The data did suggest an interplay between increased narcotics use and judicial rulings as causes of increased warrants. Police decisions to use rather than not use search warrants turned on the existence of the exclusionary rule, but the increased use of narcotics largely explained substantial increases in use of search warrants from the late 1960s through the early 1970s. Charges dropped by police departments and prosecutors because evidence was improperly seized did not show evidence of widespread police violation of the exclusionary rule, but there was also little evidence that the rule was having a very substantial effect. It was also the case that many officers saw the exclusionary rule as creating problems, including frustration and irritation at the granting of motions to suppress evidence.

Debate about effectiveness and costs of the exclusionary rule has continued in the 1980s but still has failed to resolve the central issue. One cannot yet determine which of several possible effects of the exclusionary rule has been predominant. The rule "might have induced police officers to observe Fourth Amendment requirements" or it might have led them to lie about improper searches without defense attorneys being able to penetrate the perjury. On the other hand, the defense attorneys may not have worked hard to overturn improper searches. Still another possibility "is that evidence has been rarely suppressed because judges and prosecutors have winked at Fourth Amendment violation."[124] A 1980 National Center for State Courts study in several locations suggests that all of these effects may have occurred. Because police found the warrant process "burdensome, time-consuming, intimidating, and confusing," search warrants were sought only infrequently, and police often found alternative ways to conduct searches; there were also few challenges to warrants (to suppress evidence).[125] Such a picture would suggest that the Supreme Court's shift to a "good faith" exception to the exclusionary rule might make relatively little difference, but many observers feel it would encourage even looser police practices.

The debate about the exclusionary rule has been fueled by exchanges between law professors and judges,[126] continuing suggestions by Chief Justice Burger and (now) Chief Justice Rehnquist that the rule be replaced, and additional studies of the rule's effects. The General Accounting Office (GAO) reported that motions to suppress evidence under the Fourth Amendment led to exclusion of evidence in only 1.3 percent of the federal prosecutions examined; the motions, filed in less than one-fifth of the cases, were denied most of the time when they led to formal hearings; and prosecutors dropped less than 1 percent of cases because of search and seizure problems. A subsequent study conducted for the Senate Judiciary Committee, focusing on 13 state juridictions, where the greatest effect of the rule had been alleged, also revealed a low proportion of cases dropped at the prosecution screening stage because of due process problems, with the rule having little overall impact on prosecutions. Another study, of reasons why felonies were rejected by prosecutors when they screened cases in six jurisdictions, revealed that the rule "and other due process related issues . . . appear to have little impact on the overall flow of criminal cases after arrest," accounting "for only a small portion of rejections at screening—from 1 to 9 percent."[127] Such findings may mean that the rule's opponents have exaggerated the extent to which the rule has resulted in "criminals running loose on the street because of technicalities," or that cases come to prosecutors in better shape, with fewer due process problems than earlier because police have "cleaned up their act"—an indication of the rule's effectiveness. However, there are other possibilities—and other arguments. A 1983 study by the National Institute of Justice, based on California data for the late 1970s, concluded that the rule did affect felony case processing in important ways, accounting for up to 5 percent of prosecutors' rejections of felony charges across the state, and more in large cities like Los

Angeles and San Diego; effects were greatest in drug cases (where seizure issues are most likely to occur and to be raised).[128] That study, however, has been severely criticized for being misleading—in particular for relying on statistics showing what proportion of the *reasons for rejection* were search related rather than focusing on the proportion of *arrests rejected* because of improper searches. Attention to the latter measure, a critic suggests, indicates rejection of less than 1 percent of all felony arrests—and only 2.4 percent of drug arrests—because of improper searches.[129]

Confessions. If we turn our attention to *Miranda,* in the period shortly after the decision, we find that in New Haven and Washington, D.C., not all four warnings required by the decision were given in all situations at the stationhouse and in some instances none were. An even lower rate of warning-giving occurred "on the street."[130] Warnings given at the stationhouse did not silence all defendants for several reasons: detectives effectively used a variety of elements of psychological interrogation, those informed of their rights did not understand the warnings, or they could not take advantage of them because they did not know how to contact an attorney. Yet even when stationhouse counsel was promptly available, many suspects talked before an attorney could arrive to assist them. Nor was this simply a result of lack of formal education. Yale University graduate students interrogated by the FBI in connection with draft-card violations were generally unaware of their *Miranda* rights until law professors called the warnings to their attention; even then, many continued to participate in the interrogations.[131]

In four Wisconsin cities (see above), police knowledge of *Miranda's* requirements was relatively high, but the decision appeared to produce little change in the conduct of interrogations. Police department statements of rules and procedures for interrogators to give warnings to suspects before interrogation were undermined by the interrogators' discretion and by their habit of giving the warnings but not following through on department policies of allowing counsel to be present at interrogations. In short, compliance was "formal, perfunctory or rhetorical" without behavioral changes. Detectives said that *Miranda* had changed the way they had to obtain evidence, particularly by forcing them to obtain it prior to beginning interrogation, but observations suggested instead that "all the departments continued to rely first on interrogations. If that failed, either because of lack of relevant information or because of a lawyer's refusal to allow questioning, only then were alternative methods relied upon."[132]

These effects were from the relatively short term. What about the longer term? For one thing, generational effects exist, with newly trained officers accustomed to the warnings from the beginning of their police service. In addition, the Burger Court's cutting back on *Miranda* might have affected the degree to which law enforcement officials applied it. Yet in 1979 prosecutors in counties with 100,000 or more population strongly supported *Miranda,* with younger prosecutors more strongly supportive than older ones. The prosecutors also supported the

Burger Court's changes in requirements for compliance with *Miranda*, of which they were well aware. However, they did not think the changes significant, nor did they believe the Burger Court rulings had had "a significant, or even a moderate, effect on their decisions to prosecute." Over half reported that the Burger Court's *Miranda*-related rulings had had limited or nonexistent effects, and less than 10 percent said that their prosecutorial decisions had been significantly affected.

The greatest change came where the Supreme Court's change had been clearest—in allowing use of improperly obtained statements to impeach a defendant's credibility. Yet even on this point, less than half the prosecutors were more likely to use confessions this way. Other differences in the types of confession-related cases prosecutors were likely to pursue closely paralleled the relative clarity of the Court's rulings: the less the clarity in Burger Court rulings, the less likely the prosecutors to use a confession obtained under the circumstances covered in the Court's opinion. A factor more important than the Supreme Court's clarity affecting prosecutors' actions was local judicial standards. Because local judges either had not relaxed *their* application of *Miranda* or had become more strict since the first Burger Court ruling (1971), "the Burger Court's weakening of *Miranda* has not been duplicated at the local level."[133]

Concluding Comments

Despite all the obstacles both to communication of the Supreme Court's rulings and to compliance with those rulings that have been enumerated and discussed in this chapter, compliance with the Court's decisions does occur and those decisions have substantial impact. If that were not the case, we would hear far less objection to them. More important, without them, racial and sexual equality, freedom of speech and religion, and defendants' rights, as well as economic regulation, would not take the form in which they now exist. The resistance to implementation of those decisions serves all the more to remind us that the Supreme Court is not merely a "finder" of the law but an active policymaker.

Despite the views that many people have of the Court, which do not cast it in such a role, and despite the public's general lack of awareness of what the Court has done—even how it operates—the justices maintain a commanding presence. Other officials must at least take them into account before they act; nor has the Court, even when publicly adopting a general posture of "self-restraint," been hesitant to strike down the actions of both of its coordinate branches at the national level of government and of the state governments as well. In perhaps the most important test, attacks on the Court's major rulings have only very infrequently been successful, although the Court has at times backed off from some of its strongest positions. It is doubtful that we have "judicial supremacy" as the Supreme Court's harshest critics have argued from time to time, but we do have in the Supreme Court of the United States a body of individuals who, operating within the constraints of the nation's legal system, through both the full-dress treatment given some cases and the variety of other, less visible actions they take, regularly make policy for that system and the larger political and social system.

Notes

1. For an examination of the impact of the abortion ruling, see Charles A. Johnson and Bradley C. Canon, *Judicial Policies: Implementation and Impact* (Washington, D.C.: Congressional Quarterly Press, 1984), pp. 4–14.

2. Charles Warren, *The Supreme Court in United States History* (Boston: Little, Brown, 1922), vol. 1, p. viii.

3. Jeff Romm and Sally K. Fairfax, "The Backwaters of Federalism: Receding Reserved Water Rights and the Management of National Forests," *Policy Studies Review* 5 (November 1985): 423–24. The case was *United States v. New Mexico*, 438 U.S. 696 (1978), involving the Rio Mimbres and the Gila National Forest.

4. See S. Kenneth Howard, "A Message from *Garcia*," *Public Administration Review* 45 (Special 1985): 738–41.

5. *Town of Hallie v. City of Eau Claire*, 105 S.Ct. 1713 (1985). See Stephen Chapple, "*Community Communications v. City of Boulder*: An Intergovernmental Paradox," *Public Administration Review* 45 (Special 1985): 732–37.

6. Jesse Choper, "Consequences of Supreme Court Decisions Upholding Individual Constitutional Rights," *Michigan Law Review* 83 (October 1984): 7.

7. Some of the material presented here, revised and updated, was first presented in Stephen L. Wasby, *The Impact of the United States Supreme Court* (Homewood, Ill.: The Dorsey Press, 1970).

8. *Ableman v. Booth*, 21 How. 506 (1859); *Prigg v. Pennsylvania*, 16 Peters 539 (1842).

9. Don Fehrenbacher, *The Dred Scott Case*, pp. 454, 576.

10. Ibid., pp. 3, 449, 493.

11. Jesse Choper, *Judicial Review and the National Political Process*, pp. 231–33.

12. Warren, *The Supreme Court*, vol. 2, p. 358.

13. Ibid., vol 3, p. 244. That Justices Strong and Bradley, who helped produce the second decision, were named to the Court on the day of the first decision did not help matters.

14. Merle Fainsod, Lincoln Gordon, and Joseph Palamountain, *Government and the American Economy*, pp. 540, 541.

15. Arthur M. Schlesinger, Jr., *The Politics of Upheaval* (Boston: Houghton Mifflin, 1960), p. 489.

16. Stuart Nagel and Robert Erickson, "Editorial Reaction to Supreme Court Decisions on Church and State," *Public Opinion Quarterly* 30 (Winter 1966–67); 647–55; also in Nagel, *The Legal Process from a Behavioral Perspective*, pp. 285–93.

17. William Haltom, "Editorialists and the High Court: Race, Crime, and Religion," paper presented to New York State Political Science Association, 1986, p. 5.

18. See William Haltom, "Virtues Passive and Active: Supreme Court Opinions and the Attentive Public," paper presented to American Political Science Association, 1985, p. 12.

19. Haltom, "Editoralists," pp. 4, 9.

20. Chester Newland, "Press Coverage of the United States Supreme Court," *Western Political Quarterly* 17 (March 1964): 15–36.

21. See Richard Claude, "The Supreme Court Nine: Judicial Responsibility and Responsiveness," in *People vs. Government: The Responsiveness of American Institutions*, ed. Leroy N. Rieselbach (Bloomington, Ind.: Indiana University Press, 1975), particularly Table 1, p. 123.

22. Gregory A. Caldeira, "Neither the Purse Nor the Sword: Dynamics of Public Confidence in the Supreme Court," *American Political Science Review* 80 (December 1980): 1219–23.

23. Thomas R. Marshall, "Legitimation, Public Opinion, and the Supreme Court: Old Polls, New Evidence," paper presented to Midwest Political Science Association, 1986.

24. See account in Bernard Schwartz, *Super Chief*, pp. 282–86.

25. Edward N. Beiser, "Lawyers Judge the Warren Court," *Law & Society Review* 7 (Fall 1972): 139–49.

26. Neal Milner, *The Supreme Court and Local Law Enforcement: The Impact of Miranda* (Beverly Hills, Calif.: Sage Publications, 1971).

27. Stephen L. Wasby, *Small Town Police and the Supreme Court: Hearing the Word* (Lexington, Mass: Lexington Books, 1976), p. 82; Dennis C. Smith and Elinor Ostrom, "The Effects of Training and Education on Police Attitudes and Performance: A Preliminary Analysis," unpublished ms., 1973, p. 11.

28. "What America Really Thinks About Lawyers," *National Law Journal*, August 18, 1986, p. S–6.

29. John H. Kessel, "Public Perceptions of the Supreme Court," *Midwest Journal of Political Science* 10 (May 1966): 175.

30. See Kessel (Seattle); Walter Murphy and Joseph Tanenhaus, "Public Opinion and the United States Supreme Court: Mapping of Some Prerequisites for Court Legitimation of Regime Change," in *Frontiers of Judicial Research*, eds. Joel B. Grossman and Joseph Tanenhaus (New York: John Wiley, 1969), pp. 273–303; also Walter F. Murphy, Joseph Tanenhaus, and Daniel L. Kastner, "Public Evaluation of Constitutional Courts: Alternative Explanations," Sage Professional Papers #01-045 (Beverly Hills, Calif.: Sage Publications, 1973) (1964 and 1966 SRC); Gregory Casey, "The Supreme Court and Myth: An Empirical Investigation," *Law & Society Review* 8 (Spring 1974): 385–420 (Missouri); Kenneth Dolbeare, "The Public Views the Supreme Court," in *Law, Politics and the Federal Courts*, ed. Herbert Jacob (Boston: Little, Brown, 1967), pp. 194–202 (Wisconsin).

31. See Joseph Tanenhaus and Walter F. Murphy, "Patterns of Public Support for the Supreme Court: A Panel Study," *Journal of Politics* 43 (February 1981): 24–39.

32. Walter F. Murphy and Joseph Tanenhaus, "The U.S. Supreme Court and Its Elite Publics," paper presented to International Political Science Association, 1970, p. 22.

33. The 1976 Wisconsin survey is reported in David Adamany, "Public and Activists' Attitudes Toward the United States Supreme Court," paper presented to Ameican Political Science Association, 1977, and David Adamany and Joel B. Grossman, "Support for the Supreme Court as a National Policy Maker," *Law & Policy Quarterly* 5 (October 1983): 405–37.

34. Dolbeare, "The Public Views the Supreme Court," p. 199.

35. Casey, "An Empirical Investigation," p. 397.

36. Adamany and Grossman, "Support for the Supreme Court," p. 409.

37. Tanenhaus and Murphy, "Patterns of Public Support," p. 29.

38. Kenneth Dolbeare, "The Supreme Court and the States: From Abstract Doctrine to Local Behavioral Conformity," in *The Impact of Supreme Court Decisions: Empirical Studies*, eds. Theodore H. Becker and Malcolm Feeley, 2d ed. (New York: Oxford University Press, 1973), p. 203.

39. Edward N. Muller, "A Test of a Partial Theory of Potential for Political Violence," *American Political Science Review* 66 (September 1972): 940.

40. Dean Jaros and Robert Roper, "The U.S. Supreme Court: Myth, Diffuse Support, Specific Support, and Legitimacy," *American Politics Quarterly* 8 (January 1980): 100.

41. Adamany and Grossman, "Support for the Supreme Court," p. 412.

42. Kenneth M. Dolbeare and Phillip E. Hammond, "The Political Party Basis of Attitudes Toward the Supreme Court," *Public Opinion Quarterly* 31 (Spring 1967): 23–24.

43. Tanenhaus and Murphy, "Patterns of Public Support," p. 36.

44. Adamany and Grossman, "Support for the Supreme Court," p. 428.

45. Ibid., pp. 415, 418.

46. Casey, "An Empirical Investigation" pp. 398, 402.

47. Jaros and Roper, "Specfic Support and Legitimacy," p. 95.

48. See Ronald J. Fiscus, "Studying *The Brethren*: The Legal-Realist Bias of Investigative Journalism," *American Bar Foundation Research Journal* 1984 (Spring): 487–503.

49. Murphy and Tanenhaus, "Public Opinion and the United States Supreme Court," p. 282; Adamany, "Public and Activists' Attitudes," p. 26.

50. Dolbeare, "The Public Views the Supreme Court," p. 208.

51. Kessel, "Public Perceptions," p. 191.

52. Adamany and Grossman, "Support for the Supreme Court," p. 426.

53. Discussion of terminology can be found in Wasby, *The Impact of the United States Supreme Court*, pp. 27–42; in several of the articles in *Compliance and the Law*, eds. Samuel Krislov et al. (Beverly Hills, Calif.: Sage Publications, 1972); and in Robert V. Stover and Don W Brown, "Understanding Compliance and Non-compliance with Law: The Contributions of Utility Theory," *Social Science Quarterly* 56 (December 1975): 363–75.

54. See Johnson and Canon, *Judicial Policies*, pp. 14–15.

55. Jon R. Bond and Charles A. Johnson, "Implementing a Permissive Policy: Hospital Abortion Services after *Roe v. Wade*," *American Journal of Political Science* 26 (February 1982): 4.

56. G. Alan Tarr, *Judicial Impact and State Supreme Courts* (Lexington, Mass.: Lexington Books, 1977), pp. 54–55.

57. See Henry Steadman and Joseph J. Cocozza, *Careers of the Criminally Insane* (Lexington, Mass.: Lexington Books, 1974), and Steadman and G. Keveles, "The Community Adjustment and Criminal Activity of the Baxstrom Patients: 1966–1970," *American Journal of Psychiatry* 129 (1972): 304–10.

58. See Roger A. Hanson and Robert E. Crew, Jr., "The Policy Impact of Reapportionment," *Law & Society Review* 8 (Fall 1973): 70–93.

59. Charles A. Johnson, "The Implementation and Impact of Judicial Policies: A Heuristic Model," in *Public Law and Public Policy*, ed. John A. Gardiner (New York: Praeger, 1977), pp. 107–26. See also Johnson and Canon, *Judicial Policies*, pp. 15–20.

60. John Gruhl, "Anticipatory Compliance with Supreme Court Rulings," *Polity* 14 (Winter 1981): 308–9.

61. James P. Levine, "Constitutional Law and Obscene Literature: An Investigation of Bookseller Censorship Practices," in *The Impact of Supreme Court Decisions: Empirical Studies*, ed. Theodore L. Becker (New York: Oxford University Press, 1969), pp. 129–48; Harrell R. Rodgers, Jr., "Censorship Campaigns in Eighteen Cities: An Impact Analysis," *American Politics Quarterly* 2 (October 1974): 376.

62. Rodgers, "Censorship Campaigns," pp. 376, 378.

63. An earlier version of this section, which has been updated, appeared in Wasby, *Small Town Police and the Supreme Court*, chapter 2, pp. 25–55.

64. Richard Johnson, *The Dynamics of Compliance* (Evanston, Ill.: Northwestern University Press, 1967), p. 61.

65. Walter F. Murphy, "Lower Court Checks on Supreme Court Power," *American Political Science Review* 53 (December 1959): 1017–31; Lawrence Baum, "Implementation of Judicial Decisions: An Organizational Analysis," *American Politics Quarterly* 4 (January 1976):94.

66. Barbara Ann Banoff and Benjamin S. DuVal, Jr., "The Class Action as a Mechanism for Enforcing the Federal Securities Laws: An Empirical Study of the Burdens Imposed," *Wayne Law Review* 31 (1984): 21.

67. John Gruhl, "State Supreme Courts and the U.S. Supreme Court's Post-Miranda Rulings," *Journal of Criminal Law & Criminology* 72 (Fall 1981): 911.

68. John Gruhl, "Patterns of Compliance with U.S. Supreme Court Rulings: The Case of Libel in Federal Courts of Appeals and State Supreme Courts," *Publius* 12 (Summer 1982): 109–26; Gruhl, "The Supreme Court's Impact on the Law of Libel: Compliance by Lower Federal Courts," *Western Political Quarterly* 33 (December 1980): 502–19; Michael Massing, "The libel chill: How cold *is* it out there?" *Columbia Journalism Review* 24 (#1, May/June 1985): 31–43.

69. Richard Pacelle and Lawrence Baum, "Supreme Court Authority and the Judicial Hierarchy: A Study of Remands," paper presented to Midwest Political Science Association, 1982.

70. Bradley C. Canon, "Organizational Contumacy in the Transmission of Judicial Policies: The *Mapp, Escobedo, Miranda,* and *Gault* Cases," *Villanova Law Review* 20 (November 1974):69.

71. Wayne LaFave and Frank Remington, "Controlling the Police: The Judge's Role in Making and Reviewing Law Enforcement Decisions," *Michigan Law Review* 63 (April 1965):1005.

72. Robert Pear, "Judges Continuing to Uphold Quotas," *New York Times,* February 10, 1985, pp. 1, 28.

73. Neil T. Romans, "The Role of State Supreme Courts in Judicial Policy-Making: *Escobedo, Miranda* and the Use of Judicial Impact Analysis," *Western Political Quarterly* 27 (March 1974):38–59.

74. Charles Hamilton, *The Bench and the Ballot: Southern Fedeal Judges and Black Voters* (New York: Oxford University Press, 1973); Kenneth N. Vines, "Southern State Supreme Courts and Race Relations," *Western Political Quarterly* 18 (March 1965):5–18.

75. J.W. Peltason, *Fifty-Eight Lonely Men: Southern Federal Judges and School Desegregation* (Urbana: University of Illinois Press, 1971 [1961]), pp. 245–46. See also Kenneth Vines, "Federal District Judges and Race Relations Cases in the South," *Journal of Politics* 26 (May 1964):337–57; Micheal W. Giles and Thomas G. Walker, "Judicial Policy-Making and Southern School Segregation," *Journal of Politics* 37 (November 1975):917–36.

76. Baum, "Implementation of Judicial Decisions," p. 95.

77. Lawrence Baum, "Lower-Court Response to Supreme Court Policies: Reconsidering a Negative Picture," *Justice System Journal* 3 (Spring 1978):208–19. See Johnson and Canon, *Judicial Policies,* p. 38.

78. Alan Schechter, "Impact of Open Housing Laws on Suburban Realtors," *Urban Affairs Quarterly* 8 (June 1973):439–65.

79. Robert T. Roper and Albert P. Melone, "Does Procedural Due Process Make a Difference? A Study of Second Trials," *Judicature* 65 (September 1981):136-41.

80. See Johnson and Canon, *Judicial Policies,* p. 100.

81. Thomas E. Barth, "Perception and Acceptance of Supreme Court Decisions at the State and Local Level," *Journal of Public Law* 17 (1968):308–50.

82. See Gerald Caplan, "The Police Legal Advisor," *Journal of Criminal Law, Criminology, and Police Science* 58 (September 1967):303–9, and Frank Carrington, "Speaking for the Police," ibid., 61 (June 1970):244–79.

83. See David L. Grey, *The Supreme Court and the Mass Media* (Evanston, Ill.: Northwestern University Press, 1968).

84. Chester Newland, "Press Coverage of the United States Supreme Court," *Western Political Quarterly* 17 (March 1964):15–36.

85. William Brennan, Address at Rutgers–Newark School of Law, October 17, 1979, *Rutgers Law Review* 32 (July 1979):173–83.

86. *F.B.I. v. Abramson,* 456 U.S. 615 at 641 n. 12 (1982).

87. See David W. Leslie, "The Supreme Court in the Media: A Content Analysis," paper presented to International Communication Association, 1976, and Leslie and D. Brock Hornby, *The Supreme Court in the Media: A Theoretical and Empirical Analysis* (Final Technical Report to National Science Foundation, 1976, Grant GS 38113).

88. Charles H. Franklin and Liane C. Kosaki, "The Supreme Court and Public Opinion: The Abortion Issue," paper presented to Law & Society Association, 1986, p. 10.

89. Bond and Johnson, "Implementing a Permissive Policy," pp. 13–19.

90. Stover and Brown, "Understanding Compliance," pp. 369–70; Harrell R. Rodgers Jr., and Charles S. Bullock III, *Coercion to Compliance* (Lexington, Mass.: Lexington Books, 1976), p. 65.

91. Tarr, *Judicial Impact,* p. 199.

92. Frank Sorauf, *The Wall of Separation,* p. 287.

93. Johnson and Canon, *Judicial Policies*, p. 210.

94. Ibid., p. 94.

95. Michael Ban, "The Impact of *Mapp v. Ohio* on Police Behavior," paper presented to Midwest Political Science Association, 1973, p. 33 (study based on Boston and Cincinnati).

96. Charles A. Johnson, "Judicial Decisions and Organizational Change: Some Theoretical and Empirical Notes on State Court Decisions and State Administrative Agencies," *Law & Society Review* 14 (Fall 1979):27–56.

97. Bond and Johnson, "Implementing a Permissive Policy," pp. 13, 15.

98. Harold C. Fleming, "Brown and the Three R's, Race, Residence, and Resegregation," *Journal of Law & Education* 4 (January 1975):10; Earl Black, *Southern Governors and Civil Rights: Racial Segregation as a Campaign Issue in the Second Reconstruction* (Cambridge, Mass.: Harvard University Press, 1976).

99. For a discussion of the police work situation, see Neal A. Milner, "Supreme Court Effectiveness and Police Organization," *Law and Contemporary Problems* 36 (Autumn 1971):467–87.

100. Gordon Patric, "The Impact of a Court Decision: Aftermath of the McCollum Case," *Journal of Public Law* 6 (Fall 1967):455–65.

101. Frank J. Sorauf, "Zorach v. Clauson: The Impact of a Supreme Court Decision," *American Political Science Review* 53 (September 1959):777–91.

102. See Johnson, *The Dyanmics of Compliance*. Among the other important studies are those by Donald Reich, "The Impact of Judicial Decision-Making: The School Prayer Cases," in *The Supreme Court as Policy-Maker: Three Studies on the Impact of Judicial Decisions*, ed. David Everson (Carbondale, Ill.: Public Affairs Research Bureau, Southern Illinois University, 1968), pp. 44–81; and Robert Birkby, "The Supreme Court and the Bible Belt: Tennessee Reaction to the Schempp Decision," *Midwest Journal of Political Science* 10 (August 1966); 304–19.

103. Sorauf, *The Wall of Separation*, p. 304.

104. Kenneth Dolbeare and Philip Hammond, *The School Prayer Decisions: From Court Policy to Local Practice* (Chicago: University of Chicago Press, 1971).

105. H. Frank Way, Jr., "Survey Research on Judicial Decisions: The Prayer and Bible Reading Cases," *Western Political Quarterly* 21 (June 1968):191.

106. See William K. Muir, *Prayer in the Public Schools: Law and Attitude Change* (Chicago: University of Chicago Press, 1967).

107. Milner, *The Court and Local Law Enforcement*, p. 47.

108. Ibid., pp. 52, 226.

109. Larry Berkson, "The United States Supreme Court and Small-Town Police Officers: A Study in Communication," unpublished manuscript, 1970.

110. Data from Illinois and Massachusetts in this and the following paragraph from Stephen L. Wasby, *Small Town Police and the Supreme Court*; large-city data from a study by Bradley C. Canon, also reported in ibid.: see p. 96, and chs. 5 and 6, pp. 119–98, passim.

111. Barton L. Ingraham, "The Impact of Argersinger—One Year Later," *Law & Society Review* 8 (Summer 1975):616.

112. Sheldon Krantz et al., "The Right to Counsel in Criminal Cases: The Mandate of *Argersinger v. Hamlin*," Summary Report (Washington, D.C: National Institute of Law Enforcement and Criminal Justice, Law Enforcement Assistance Administration, Department of Justice, 1976), pp. 2–3.

113. Ingraham, "The Impact of Argersinger"; James J. Alfini and Patricia M. Passuth, "Case Processing in State Misdemeanor Courts: The Effect of Defense Attorney Presence," *Justice System Journal* 6 (Spring 1981):114.

114. Stuart Nagel, "Testing the Effects of Excluding Illegally Seized Evidence," *Wisconsin Law Review* 1965 (Spring):283–310; also in Nagel, *The Legal Process from a Behavioral Perspective*, pp. 294–320.

115. Milner, *The Court and Local Law Enforcement*, p. 52.

116. Michael J. Murphy, "The Problem of Compliance by Police Departments," *Texas Law Review* 44 (1966):941.

117. Wayne R. LaFave, "Improving Police Performance through the Exclusionary Rule: Part II: Defining the Norms and Training the Police," *Missouri Law Review* 30 (Fall 1965): 594–95.

118. David Manwaring, "The Impact of *Mapp v. Ohio*," in *The Supreme Court as Policy-Maker*, ed. Everson, p. 26.

119. Bradley C. Canon, "Reactions of State Supreme Courts to a U.S. Supreme Court Civil Liberties Decision," *Law & Society Review* 8 (Fall 1973):126–27.

120. Ibid.; and Canon, "Organizational Contumacy."

121. Albert W. Alschuler,"'Close Enough for Government Work': The Exclusionary Rule After Leon," *The Supreme Court Review 1984*, eds. Kurland, Casper, and Hutchinson, p. 368.

122. Dallin H. Oaks, "Studying the Exclusionary Rule in Search and Seizure," *University of Chicago Law Review* 37 (Summer 1970):655, 667.

123. Bradley C. Canon, "Is the Exclusionary Rule in Failing Health? Some New Data and a Plea Against a Precipitious Conclusion," *Kentucky Law Journal* 62 (1973–1974):708–9. See also Canon, "Testing the Effectiveness of Civil Liberties Policies at the State and Federal Levels: The Case of the Exclusionary Rule," *American Politics Quarterly* 5 (1977):57–82.

124. Alschuler, "Close Enough," p. 349.

125. Richard Van Duizend, L. Paul Sutton, and Charlotte A. Carter, *The Search Warrant Process: Preconceptions, Perceptions, Practices* (Williamsburg, Va: National Center for State Courts, 1984).

126. See Yale Kamisar, "Is the Exclusionary Rule an 'Illogical' or 'Unnatural' Interpretation of the Fourth Amendment?" *Judicature* 62 (August 1978):66–84; Malcolm Richard Wilkey, "The Exclusionary Rule: Why Suppress Valid Evidence?" *Judicature* 62 (November 1978):214–32; Kamisar, "The Exclusionary Rule in Historical Perspective: The Struggle to Make the Fourth Amendment More Than An Empty Blessing," *Judicature* 62 (February 1979):336–50; Wilkey, "A Call for Alternatives to the Exclusionary Rule: Let Congress and the Trial Courts Speak," *Judicature* 62 (February 1979):351–56. For an exchange on empirical evidence with respect to the rule, see Canon, "The Exclusionary Rule: Have Critics Proven That It Doesn't Deter Police?" *Judicature* 62 (March 1979):398–403, and Steven R. Schlesinger, "The Exclusionary Rule: Have Proponents Proven That It Is A Deterrent to Police?", *Judicature* 62 (March 1979):404–9.

127. Kathleen B. Brosi, *A Cross-City Comparison of Felony Case Processing* (Washington, D.C.: Law Enforcement Assistance Administration, 1979), pp. 18–19.

128. National Institute of Justice, *Criminal Justice Research Report—The Effects of the Exclusionary Rule: A Study in California* (Washington, D.C.: Department of Justice, 1982).

129. See Thomas Y. Davies, "A Hard Look at What We Know (and Still Need to Learn) About the 'Costs' of the Exclusionary Rule: the NIJ Study and Other Studies of 'Lost Arrests'," *American Bar Foundation Research Journal* 1983 (Summer): 611–90.

130. Michael Wald et al., "Interrogations in New Haven: The Impact of Miranda," *Yale Law Journal* 76 (July 1967):1519–1648; Richard J. Medalie et al., "Custodial Police Interrogation in Our Nation's Capital: The Attempt to Implement Miranda," *Michigan Law Review* 66 (May 1968):1347–1422; Albert J. Reiss, Jr., and Donald J. Black, "Interrogation and the Criminal Process," *The Annals* 374 (November 1967):47–57.

131. John Griffiths and Richard E. Ayres, "A Postscript to the *Miranda* Project: Interrogation of Draft Protestors," *Yale Law Journal* 76 (December 1967):300–319.

132. Milner, *The Court and Local Law Enforcement*, pp. 229, 217.

133. John Gruhl and Cassia Spohn, "The Supreme Court's Post-Miranda Rulings: Impact on Local Prosecutors," *Law & Policy Quarterly* 3 (January 1981):29–54.

Table of Cases*

*All cases the names of which appear in the text are included here, as are other important cases appearing in the notes. When the case name is not mentioned in the text, the reference is to the notes at the end of each chapter, from which the reader can refer to the appropriate place in the text.

Index

abortion, 3, 16, 18, 20-22, 33, 35, 97, 105, 123, 146, 170, 176-77, 195, 268, 306, 308-9, 315-16, 339, 352-54, 356, 359
abstention, 183-85. *See also* federalism
access, 162-78, 286; Burger Court, 165-66; judges' values, 166. *See also* causes of action; courts; Supreme Court
Access to Justice Act, 154
accountability, 6-8
activism, 3-4, 8, 11, 143, 163, 178, 183-87; Burger Court, 286; off-Court, 287. *See also* Supreme Court
administrative agency: *see* regulatory agencies
Administrative Office of the U.S. Courts, 49, 64-65, 70-71, 300; and Congress, 53, 69; director, 70-71; and Judicial Conference, 70-71
Administrative Procedure Act, 327-28, 330
admiralty, 192, 200
adversary legal system, 138, 165
advisory opinions, 80, 165, 174-75, 322
affirmative action, 16, 21, 27, 143, 146, 177, 275, 315, 344, 354, 360; in judge selection, 97, 102-3
age: of justices, 118, 247; and public opinion, 345-46. *See also* senior judges
agenda: of justices, 120, 199; of solicitor general, 146-47; of Supreme Court, 199, 203
Agricultural Adjustment Act, 344
aliens, 328, 355
Allen, Florence, 115

amendment: *see* Constitution
American Bar Association, 26, 63, 95, 293, 309; Committee on Federal Judiciary, 107, 109; criticism of, 110; criticism of Court, 347; ethics code, 122, 221; guidelines, 108-9; in judicial selection, 99, 101, 103, 123-24; ratings, 97, 103, 107-10, 124; and Senate, 105; and women, 108-9
American Civil Liberties Union (ACLU), 110, 123, 152, 155-56, 159, 221-22, 370
American Law Institute, 293
American Liberty League, 150
Americans for Effective Law Enforcement, 150
amicus curiae, 150-52, 155, 290; by solicitor general, 144-46
antitrust, 200-201, 266, 312, 339-40
appeals, 73-74, 202; dismissal, 202, 204; factors affecting, 148-49; jurisdictional statement, 202; lawyers' role, 138, 148-49; scope, 74; and solicitor general, 144, 146; types of, 58. *See also* Supreme Court
appellate courts: *see* courts of appeals; Supreme Court
Article I: *see* courts
Article III, 30-31, 42, 164, 167-68. *See also* courts; judges; jurisdiction
Articles of Confederation, 10, 76-77
Asian-Americans: as judges, 115
attitudes: and impact, 368-69, 375, 379
attorneys: *see* lawyers
attorney's fees, 154

Stephen L . Wasby

The Supreme Court in the Federal Judicial System
Third Edition

0-8304-1175-5